Mental Health Practice

A Guide to Compassionate Care

For Elsevier:
Commissioning Editor: **Steven Black/Mairi McCubbin**
Development Editor: **Ailsa Laing**
Project Manager: **Emma Riley**
Designer: **Sarah Russell**
Illustrations: **Kirsteen Wright, Gillian Richards**

Mental Health
Practice

A Guide to Compassionate Care

Peter N. Watkins MEd RMN RNT DipN DipHumPsych
Cert Systemic Family Practice

Mental Health Nurse with the Ipswich Outreach Service,
Suffolk Mental Health Partnerships NHS Trust,
Formerly Senior Lecturer in Mental Health at Suffolk College,
Ipswich, UK

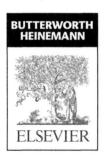

BUTTERWORTH HEINEMANN

ELSEVIER

Edinburgh   London   New York   Oxford   Philadelphia   St Louis   Sydney   Toronto   2009

BUTTERWORTH
HEINEMANN
ELSEVIER

First edition 2001
Transferred to Digital Printing, 2011

ISBN 978-0-7506-8881-9

British Library Cataloguing in Publication Data
A catalogue record for this book is available from the British Library

Library of Congress Cataloging in Publication Data
A catalog record for this book is available from the Library of Congress

Note
Neither the Publisher nor the Author assumes any responsibility for any loss or injury and/or damage to persons or property arising out of or related to any use of the material contained in this book. It is the responsibility of the treating practitioner, relying on independent expertise and knowledge of the patient, to determine the best treatment and method of application for the patient.

The Publisher

ELSEVIER your source for books,
journals and multimedia
in the health sciences
www.elsevierhealth.com

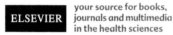
Working together to grow
libraries in developing countries
www.elsevier.com | www.bookaid.org | www.sabre.org
ELSEVIER   BOOK AID International   Sabre Foundation

Printed and bound in the United Kingdom

Transferred to Digital Print 2011

The Publisher's policy is to use paper manufactured from sustainable forests

Dedication

To the memory of my mother Ruby Miriam Watkins, who taught me about caring, and my father Albert Henry Watkins, who taught me about courage.

Dedication

Contents

Contents

viii

Preface to the first edition

This book is a reflection on mental health care. At its core is an exploration of the helping relationship and the caring process. During the 40 years that I have been a psychiatric nurse I have come to believe strongly in compassionate care as the mainspring of recovery. Unfortunately, over the last few decades the compassionate care of deeply troubled people has come to be valued less than the 'psycho-technologies'. These days everyone wants to be a therapist! You will find very little 'therapy' in this book; what you will find is an exploration of the nature of restorative care in the context of the mental health services.

Most of my experience over the years has been with people who have struggled not only with their own disabling distress but also with the oppression and stigma that comes with enduring mental health problems. Many of them have been inspiring examples of the indomitable nature of the human spirit when faced with continuing anguish and adversity. I often ask myself how I would cope with the afflictions and deprivation that many users of the mental health services survive and recover from. What sustains the human spirit through such troubled states of mind, when distress is so enveloping that everyday living becomes difficult, if not impossible, is the empathic and compassionate presence of another who can be a caretaker of hope. You cannot work in an enabling way with people unless you believe in the potential of everyone to grow and change in the direction of becoming a fully functioning person. A person who is able to manage the challenges and opportunities of living more effectively, discover a personal identity that is not circumscribed by vulnerability and disability and recover an ordinary life that offers a measure of the joys and satisfactions we all seek. In making this point, I am not suggesting that the recovery pathway is one that is easily found or taken. Many people get stuck in a psychiatric system that so often sees people as prisoners of a neurologically based psychopathology, a perspective from which the best one can hope for is some degree of symptom relief mediated by drugs.

Throughout the book I have tried to avoid the conventional language of psychiatry, which can be mystifying and excluding. Biomedical psychiatry has, over the years, erroneously acquired the status of a scientific truth, a status that confers enormous power on those who hold this knowledge. To claim an empirical understanding of human vulnerability to disabling distress simply from the biomedical perspective is arrogant nonsense. As individuals we have a uniqueness and complexity that defies such a structuralist approach. A similar charge can be levelled against psychological models, which locate the cause of distress in the inner world, largely ignoring the social context in which people live their lives. As mental health professionals we need to take a more holistic, person-centred view of human distress, seeing the client as the only true expert, the only person who has knowledge of the lived experience that has influenced their way of being in the world. We have the privileged role of standing alongside people in the landscape of their lives. If we can listen empathetically enough, we can witness the journey that has brought them to their present place and offer companionship, guidance and encouragement to continue their journey along a more sustaining path.

The first part of the book is an exploration of the experience of severe and disabling distress, the recovery process and the values that underpin a person-centred approach to therapeutic care. Part two examines the nature of the working alliance between people who use the mental health services and mental health professionals. The third part of the book goes beyond the working alliance to consider the various forms the intentional use of self can take in aiding the process of recovery. In the final section, the focus is on the interface between the professional and personal. It argues that the art of compassionate care depends on a commitment to personal development as an integral part of our growth as mental health professionals. If we are to give of our best, we have a responsibility to sustain our capacity to care compassionately through recognising and respecting our own needs and vulnerabilities.

Significant learning is a process not just of engagement and assimilation but of integration. Making new learning a part of ourselves, part of the way we think, feel and act involves an interaction with the material not just cognitively, but affectively and behaviourally. The self-enquiry exercises that form part of the text are offered as a structured invitation to interact with the key themes. The personal narratives that appear in the book are largely authentic though of course altered to protect anonymity. It has been the experience of disabling distress of the people I have worked with over the years that has taught me most and it is the glow of their testimonies that I hope illuminates the text.

The book has been written as a foundation for good practice in mental health care. I have intentionally used the generic term mental health practitioner extensively in the text as the book will have a direct relevance to the core skills of nurses, social workers, occupational therapists, psychologists, arts therapists, psychotherapists, psychiatrists and to mental health support workers who have come to play an increasingly important role within the voluntary sector. It is my hope that the book will also be read by people using mental health services and by carers and that they will find in the text something insightful, uplifting and encouraging.

The key theoretical influences on my thinking will be readily apparent, even from a cursory glance at the text. The ideas of Carl Rogers, John Heron and Gerard Egan have been sustaining for me, both philosophically and practically, throughout much of my career. What links them is their humanistic orientation and it is in the fertile soil of humanistic psychology that the contents of this book have their deepest roots. But it is not just the work of these innovative thinkers that has informed this text. It has been my good fortune to work with many gifted educationalists and clinicians whose teaching and practice has exemplified compassionate care and I am conscious that something of their work has been distilled into the pages of this book.

My heartfelt thanks to those close to me for their patience, encouragement and support throughout the book's long 'gestation'. I owe a special debt of gratitude to my partner Ann Baeppler, who has spent long hours helping me refine the text. It might have remained simply a good idea without the enthusiasm and belief of the former commissioning editors at Butterworth Heinemann, Mary Seager and Susan Devlin, who conjured up a 'fresh breeze' during periods when both I and the book have been in the doldrums.

Preface to the second edition

In the seven years since the first edition of *Mental Health Practice* was published, the evolution of mental health services in the UK has continued apace with a more defined community service emerging, embodying many of the aspirations of the National Service Framework (Department of Health 1999a) and able to respond to a broad spectrum of mental suffering. I would like to be able to say that a more human service was emerging but I do not detect any fallback from the conception of states of psychological overwhelm as an illness caused by aberrant neurones, nor from drug-oriented treatment, despite the call to re-vision psychiatry from the critical psychiatry movement (Thomas & Bracken 2004) and from the increasingly confident, questioning voice of the consumer/survivor movement. I despair at the increasing number of young people who are being prescribed powerful antipsychotic drugs for prolonged periods of time – despite having shown no clear signs of symptom relief or relapse prevention, with all the unknown long-term implications for health this has. Where are the alternative recovery programmes for those who do not respond to medication? Where is the vision of humanity that recognises the seeds of madness in us all; a vision that also recognises our potential for creative, harmonious living, a potential realised through sustained relational experience in which a person feels accepted, valued and understood.

What is still so often missing is the human face of psychiatry, a recognition of the importance of the quality of the interpersonal contact between mental health practitioners and the people using services. The increase in workloads, the escalating demands for data demonstrating that targets are being met, the reduction in professional development opportunities, and a management style based on masculine values all conspire to create a workforce that struggles to find the emotional energy to sustain recovery relationships. Despite this, some amazing work continues to be done within the statutory services, within the voluntary sector and through user-led resources. There are many guardians of good practice; practitioners who do not feel compelled to try and find prescriptive solutions to people's suffering, who know that the essence of therapeutic care is to be with people in their overwhelmed troubled states of mind in a way that is compassionate and healing.

More than ever we need to get back to the heart and soul of mental health care: the healing relationship. No significant relationship is ever neutral – it is either enhancing and growthful or restrictive and damaging. We must be committed to our own personal growth and to our own healing if we are to be compassionate and enabling companions to clients on their own journeys of growth and recovery. We must all be more insistent on having an organisational culture that sustains our practice, that recognises its workforce as its most valuable resource, a resource committed to the mental health of the community. I see around me many colleagues who come to mental health care out of a strong sense of vocation – although many might be uncomfortable with the term, who are altruistically motivated to help those that suffer. Yes of course there are other, more personal, motives involved and that is why an organisation that exists to provide mental health care must, above all, maintain a learning/healing culture in which staff are sustained emotionally and can grow personally and professionally. To ensure that a learning/healing ethos runs through an organisation in these target-driven times of economic stringency, requires a creative management team whose values are deeply rooted in feminine principles, able to resist the drift of psychiatry back into the paternalism and masculine values that dominated past eras.

It seems to me that a vision of psychiatric practice which is more cognisant of the potential of an individual to *live well* than of the dysfunctional facets of their state of being offers a profoundly worthwhile opportunity to all mental health practitioners to become compassionate allies to people on a journey of growth and healing. Being that compassionate ally is what this book is about.

The first edition appeared as a nursing title, though it was never my intention to write purely for nursing colleagues and the text was and remains strongly multidisciplinary. Compassionate caring is at the heart of the work of all practitioners whatever their professional discipline and I hope the loss of the word 'nursing' from the title will give the book a more inclusive feel. I have been gratified to receive generous feedback from service users and carers in response to the first edition, many of whom have found the text insightful, uplifting and encouraging and in revising the book I have been particularly mindful that caring is rooted in the heart of communities and is not an exclusively professionalised commodity, though there is a danger of it becoming just that.

In this second edition, several chapters have been substantially rewritten and updated and the book has been restructured to make it more accessible and readable. Some chapters have been discarded as they now seem to clutter rather than enrich the book. I have perhaps gone further in my use of nontechnical language, believing as I do that diagnostic labels and the mystifying jargon of psychiatry serve no useful purpose, are more damaging than helpful and must, at some point, be consigned to the dustbin of history, one that is already quite full of psychiatric follies.

The book remains deeply rooted in humanistic psychology which I believe has had a considerable, though largely unacknowledged, influence on interpersonal practice and the therapeutic use of self. I have included in this edition a guide to humanistic psychology, as I recognise that many colleagues will not be familiar with the width and depth of this field of study of human potential.

Some themes have become more visible in the second edition. Action research seems to offer a particularly exciting methodological approach to personal and professional growth (McNiff & Whitehead 2006). I have included a personal perspective on action research and its value to the relational aspects of mental health work. More attention has also been given to the organisational culture of mental health services which have such an influence on the delivery of compassionate, therapeutic care (Hawkins & Shohet 2000). Organisations are living systems that can enhance the growth and wellbeing of its workforce or be limiting and sick making. It is difficult to sustain care that has at its heart the intentional and therapeutic use of self in a work culture in which the growth and wellbeing of that self is not nurtured. This edition has, I hope, a more holistic feel in that I have become increasingly aware over the past decade that eco-psychology or eco-consciousness is missing from much of the discourse on mental health. Undeniably our wellbeing is connected to that of the planet. We have an evolutionary based affiliation with nature – if we damage the ecosystem we damage ourselves.

Revisiting the book again at some depth has for me been a joyful contemplation, reaffirming my belief in the worthwhileness of the work. The book is a quiet celebration of the extraordinary depth and creativity of the healing and growthful relationships I have witnessed over the years between my practitioner colleagues and people who come, or are sent, to mental health services at times of great suffering; times when their lives have become unbearably discordant. There is of course a shadow side to psychiatry and we must not deny that, but the much greater force is found in the capacity of many if not most mental health practitioners for loving kindness and compassion.

Compassion is not a word that sits comfortably in the lexicon of contemporary health care professionals. It has religious connotations which can seem to elevate the practice of caring to a vocational height too lofty for modern practitioners. More than that, allowing oneself to be moved to feeling and action by the suffering of another grates against the dispassionate professional stance, a dubious hallmark of proficiency many practitioners seek to maintain. But I make no apology for making compassion the central theme of this book. For all psychiatry's technical expertise and voluminous knowledge base, the essence of healing the mind is still predicated on this deeply human response. To practise compassionately is to liberate within us all that is good in humankind – love, kindness, empathy, acceptance, forgiveness; and living those values in our work and beyond brings a measure of meaningfulness and happiness to our own lives.

My gratitude and heartfelt thanks goes to Dr Suzanne Thompson whose perceptive review of the first edition provided me with a wealth of ideas for a revision of the text. My thanks also go to my colleagues in the Ipswich Outreach Team who unknowingly have inspired much of the content of the book. Finally I am indebted to my editors at Elsevier, Stephen Black and Susan Young, who have been able to share my vision of all that is best in the practice of psychiatry enough to publish this second edition.

Ipswich, 2008   Peter Watkins

Part 1

Meaning and behaviour

Introduction

Over the latter decades of the 20th century a quiet revolution has taken place in mental health care as humanistic ideas have gradually permeated and embedded themselves in practice, education and management. It is the premise of this part of the book that a humanistic psychology/philosophy provides the most relevant theoretical foundation on which to build the practice of mental health care and understand the nature of human suffering.

Chapter 1 applies the humanistic lens to the experience of disabling distress which, it is argued, can only be understood from the perspective of the individual seeking help. It takes a holistic view, seeing distress behaviour as an outcome of disharmony in the biological, psychosocial, spiritual and ecological dimensions of human experience.

Chapter 2 argues that wellbeing depends, not just on inner harmony, but also on the social context in which we live out our lives. The social context of distress and dysfunction has been a neglected aspect of mental ill-health over the past few decades, decades which have been dominated by psychobiological research. Overcoming the social disadvantage and exclusion that are so often the precursors and/or the consequences of mental suffering is one of the biggest challenges facing people in their recovery.

Chapter 3 considers the transcultural dimension of psychiatry. We live in an increasingly multicultural society in which differences in tradition, beliefs and lifestyle are generally accepted, often celebrated, though perhaps not widely understood. But there is of course a shadow side expressed in the prejudice that continues to exist in the hearts and minds of the majority white British segment of society and by extension mental health practitioners, that to our shame is reflected in the racial bias seen in the treatment and care of ethnic minorities. Compassionate care, if it is authentic, cannot be limited or conditional; it has to transcend cultural differences.

Chapter 4 reflects on gender issues as a cause of distress. It is no accident of fate that anxiety states and depression are one and a half to two times more common in women in the UK than in men. Nor is it without significance that more young men than women are likely to seek to resolve identity and belongingness issues in addictive behaviour, violence and suicide; or that they are likely to experience an earlier onset of psychosis which has a tendency to be more persistent and disabling (Department of Health 2002b). The significant changes in traditional gender roles over the last fifty years have been joyfully emancipating for many women and men but have also created new developmental challenges.

Chapter 5 addresses the theme of working creatively with people in crisis. Distress can at times be so overwhelming that a person's mental and social functioning becomes seriously disturbed. Currently a lot of endeavour is going into developing crisis services in which crisis is perceived, not as a sign of failure on the part of the service user or the practitioners, but as a learning opportunity. A crisis is seen not as another breakdown but as another opportunity for a breakthrough.

Chapter 6 considers working with risk. We cannot eliminate risk from life nor from the process of care and recovery. Positive risk-taking is a necessary element in personal growth and the emergence of socially constructive behaviour; in risk-averse conditions of care, personal development and social adjustment are likely to be impeded by oppressive regimes. The danger exists that increasing litigation consciousness and a fear of the savage publicity which follows tragic cases of homicide and suicide will lead to mental health services adopting more defensive if not oppressive practices.

Chapter 7 outlines a holistic, person-centred, approach to assessment. It steers a course away from the pseudo science of assessment tools and diagnostic interviews that attempt to fit the experience of individuals into pathologised conceptions of distress. It argues instead for an empathic, dialogical enquiry in which the experience of the client is made known and its emergent meaning understood by both client and practitioner.

Chapter 8 focuses on the recovery process. Recovery can be seen as a continuing journey towards higher levels of functioning and wellbeing and in that sense is a journey we all share. Psychiatry is not very good at sowing seeds of hope. A culture of maintenance, rather than recovery, has dominated the psychiatric stage, in which the troubled individual is cast as a prisoner of their aberrant biology and destined to live a life circumscribed by a continuing vulnerability. The missing ingredient here is realistic hopefulness. Hope for a less anguished, problematic way of being in the world. Hope for an ordinary life containing a measure of the joys and satisfactions we all seek. Mental health professionals need to be able to hold that hope for those seeking care and become companions to people on their journeys.

Chapter 9 is an exploration of a philosophy of care based on humanistic values. Compassionate care is the art of being rather than doing. It starts from the position that people are OK, although they might need help recognising it; that people know what they need, although they might need help expressing it; that people can discover their own meaning, although they might need help doing it; that people can take responsibility for themselves, although they might need encouragement to take it. In the context of a sustained relationship embodying these values, a troubled individual is able to move in the direction of becoming a fully functioning person, finding within themselves the resourcefulness to manage the problems and opportunities of living.

The nature of human distress

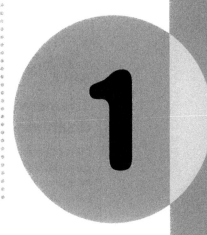

The humanistic approach to understanding and helping people who are deeply troubled is rooted in the phenomenological tradition of Western philosophy. The phenomenological view of man does not try to impose any theoretical construct on that experience but seeks to make sense of distressed and disturbed behaviour principally through an understanding of a person's subjective world. In doing so it unshackles differentness from pathology and as Bentall (2003) argues, takes us to a position where:

> We should abandon psychiatric diagnosis altogether and instead try to explain and understand the actual experiences and behaviours of psychotic people. (p. 141)

Experiencing the world or oneself in unusual ways may be problematic and disturbing for the individual and others but it is not a phenomenon outside the range of 'normal' human experience. The assumption of a discontinuity between ordinary experience and psychotic experience is illusory. Joseph & Worsley (2005) in their exploration of person-centred psychopathology suggest:

> It is probably more accurate to conceptualise the experiences that constitute the so called (psychiatric) disorders as lying along a continuum, ranging from low levels of distress and dysfunction to high levels of distress and dysfunction. (p. 3)

Many people have strongly held unusual beliefs, which have many of the characteristics of beliefs that in a psychiatric context would be considered delusional and symptomatic of psychosis. Such beliefs may be discordant with prevailing norms, divergent from consensual reality, and a potential source of conflict; but however unusual and troubling those beliefs might be they belong in the panoply of ideas that spring from the perceptual world of individuals and are not the product of a malfunctioning brain. Similarly, voice hearing may be a cause of distress and problematic behaviour, but many people who are not considered psychotic experience voices. Romme & Escher (1993, 2000), in their seminal work on voice hearing, make the case that the nature and content of voices always has meaning in the context of the person's life. Morrison et al (2003) highlight how traumatic experience, such as physical or sexual abuse, frequently reveals itself in the themes expressed in delusions and in auditory hallucinations.

Ian's story

Theme: vulnerability to psychosocial overwhelm and disabling distress

I've been seeing psychiatrists for the last 10 years for schizophrenia. I'm not really sure what that means, I just think I'm an outsider. I used to feel drugged up, like my body didn't belong to me. Now I have quite a low dose of my medication and take extra tablets if I feel I need it. What stresses me most is feeling bored and lonely. My life feels empty a lot of the time. It's then that my voices become worse and bother me more. I hear several voices, usually bad mouthing me, calling me 'a loser'. Sometimes I feel depressed about my life and think about ending it; I did stab myself in the stomach once. Often it's difficult to make sense of things. Little things can trouble me for ages. I saw some girls laughing in town the other day, one of them was on her mobile phone and I thought why am I suffering and they're laughing. Then I began to think I was a scapegoat, carrying all the blame for other people. I got the feeling I had been banished and that everyone wanted me gone.

What I need is a girlfriend and a job. But that's difficult. I haven't got much confidence and I worry about how people will react when they know I've been in hospital and I'm on medication. It's hard to get a foothold in the world when you've been ill. I remember when I came out of hospital the second time, I felt utterly helpless; I just couldn't cope and went high. I started thinking I was on TV, a star in a soap and that cameras were filming me. I miss that feeling of being high even though I know I had some crazy ideas. It was a bit like taking a holiday in an exotic place.

It would be easy to become a 'full time patient', mix with other service users, go to the resource centre, but I want an ordinary life. I did 3 months voluntary conservation work three summers ago and I was hoping to do a part-time environmental studies course but I became unwell again just before the term started. Now I'm not sure I could cope with it.

I think my mental illness started when I was a child. My father left when I was seven. I used to see him at weekends, then he got married again and stopped coming. I wasn't important enough to him I suppose. Then my mother's new partner couldn't stand to have me around so I went and lived with my grandma for about a year till my mother left him. I hated school. I was an outsider even then and was bullied from when I was about nine until I was thirteen. The teachers used to say I was 'vacant' and I was. I went a long way away, deep inside and lost myself.

Perhaps, as Rogers (1978a) suggests, there is not one reality but multiple realities experienced at both a cultural and individual level.

> The only reality I can know for certain is the world as I perceive and experience it at this moment. The only reality you can know for certain is the world as you perceive and experience it at this moment. The only certainty is that they are not the same! (p. 424)

Rogers argues that, rather than try to change a person's reality, the task of helping is to respect and understand his view of himself in the world. If we can relate to people in respectful, authentic and empathic ways, the most troubled and alienated person will be literally brought to his senses. That is, he will become more in touch with his true being and become more fully, rather than selectively, aware of the physical and interpersonal world in which he lives. Reality is largely relational with us testing out the validity of our perceptions and experience in the social matrix of our everyday lives, thus creating a consensual reality. Though differing fundamentally from Rogers' approach, cognitive behavioural ways of working with unusual beliefs that are problematic and distressing, are in essence, a strategic way of reality testing and central to this process is establishing that what the client experiences is a belief and not objective reality.

We live in a rationalist culture, but this has not always been so. In many traditional societies, for example, it is still not unusual to have a more animate view of the world, that is, to experience the world as a living entity with which we can interact (Harding 2006). It is not unusual in some societies to seek to live life in a way that harmonises with the spirit world, often experienced as resident in nature. Harding argues that in Western culture we are socialised to think more than we feel, sense or intuit and as a result these attributes remain underdeveloped. This is at some cost to our wellbeing, for, as Jung suggested, the balanced use of these mental functions is necessary for mental health (Fig. 1.1). In our rationalist, left-brain dominated culture we have suppressed our emotional, intuitive and sensory functions, subdued our imagination and become disconnected from the natural world of which we are a part, with disastrous consequences. Could it be that an individual we regard as showing psychotic behaviour is in fact someone who tends to perceive the world more through the other mental functions than through dispassionate rationalism? A kind of awakening that could be overwhelming! I have no wish to romanticise what can be a devastating experience, but often there seems a kernel of truth in the unusual perceptions of people who enter these extraordinary states of consciousness we choose to call psychosis. To shift from a state of being in the world informed primarily by rational thought to a way of being informed primarily by the senses, feeling, intuition and imagination would make it difficult to 'know' any longer what is real.

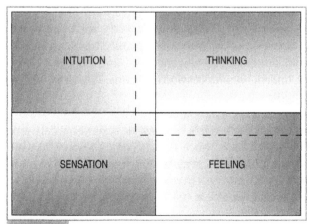

Figure 1.1 ● Jung's four mental functions. In Western culture left brain activity, i.e. logical thought, is more developed than emotional intelligence, sensory awareness and intuitive knowing.

Self-enquiry box

You may find it helpful to consider your own functional style in relation to Jung's categorisation. Most people have one or more mental functions that are underdeveloped, mainly as a consequence of the value that the family, the educational system and the wider culture you have been exposed to places on these respective functions. One way of approaching this self-enquiry is to keep a diary for a month recording your reflections on key moments day to day. At the end of each week highlight, using different coloured markers, those passages that are a reflection on thoughts; those that are a reflection on feelings; those that are a reflection on sensory experience; and those that are a reflection on intuitive awareness. This should give you some insight into the interplay of the four functions in your working and personal life. Relating deeply to the experience of others is enhanced if we are able to bring not only our heads and our hearts but a developed capacity for sensory and intuitive awareness into our work. You may find it useful to explore aspects of your diary work in supervision.

Another useful way of identifying and changing your functional style is to spend time looking at art images either in books or galleries. Be aware of how you approach a piece of art; is your response intellectual, reaching for a cognitive understanding; or is your response an emotional one, using your feelings as a way into the painting; are you primarily transfixed by the sensory experience, what you notice about the work of art; or finally do you allow an intuitive awareness of what the artist was communicating to arise unbidden into your consciousness?

The fully functioning self

The humanistic view of humankind is basically optimistic, holding that, given favourable conditions for development, we move towards becoming fully functioning people who behave in socially constructive ways. Rogers characterised the fully functioning person as someone open to the experience of themselves, others and the world. If we can be sufficiently open to experience and not subject it to defensive distortion, we are able to engage more freely and creatively in the process of living. Rogers argues that the more open to experience we are, the more we are able to trust our emotional intelligence and intuition, in concert with cognitive evaluation, to inform our choices and decisions. This more holistic way of being leads to wise action.

The journey towards becoming more fully ourselves, what Abraham Maslow referred to as self-actualisation, lies at the heart of humanistic and existential thinking about psychological wellbeing and disturbance. If we become alienated from our true selves and live our lives in an inauthentic way, we will find it difficult to know what we truly think or feel and consequently act in unconstructive ways when faced with the challenges of living. We will then be at risk of becoming overwhelmed by accumulating distress.

The quest for selfhood begins in infancy and childhood, during which time our emergent sense of self is particularly vulnerable to approval and validation by the significant caregivers in our lives. In unfavourable circumstances, the care we receive may be conditional on being and behaving in certain ways, which limits the expression of our unfolding self. In these circumstances, our self-concept is created out of the internalised conditions of worth imposed by others, rather than by the prompting of our true self. The internalised beliefs and values of others may be difficult to live up to. We will often fall short of those standards and as a consequence develop a deeply negative sense of self which, once established, will produce behaviour that reflects and confirms our negative self-evaluation. Similarly, traumatic experiences of loss or abuse that deprive us of secure, nurturing relationships can dislocate us from what we have the potential to be. People with deeply negative self-concepts do not have that inner core of self-worth that comes from the experience of having one's emergent self prized and nurtured during early development. Their self-esteem will be low and externally regulated, vulnerable to the rejections, disappointments and failures that are inevitably part of human experience.

Dissenting voices

This way of conceptualising growth as a realisation of the attributes that define us as individuals and human beings is but one view and a view challenged by some who regard the idea of self as highly individualised and autonomous as an ethnocentric Western concept. In many non-Western cultures, the self is constituted much more by the social context, within which integration and harmony are valued. Fernando (2002) argues that integration, balance and harmony within oneself and within the family and community are important aspects of what may be considered mental health in traditional non-Western cultures, while in the West self-sufficiency, autonomy, the enhancement of self and self-esteem are important criteria. Westernised constructs of mental health and psychological distress and disturbance universally applied in a multi-ethnic society are untenable. Knowledge of what is normal and what is divergent is shaped by cultural definitions of personhood, social identities and role expectation (Ahmed & Webb-Johnson 1995). Any psychiatric assessment must take into account a person's culturally determined beliefs about the cause of their distress and what *they* think would be acceptable and helpful interventions in restoring their wellbeing. For some clients, spiritual care from leaders of their faith community, or holistic care from an alternative therapist or traditional healer may be seen as more relevant than a pharmacological or psychotherapeutic intervention.

Another challenge to the concept of separation and individuation has come from feminist writers who argue that this is more a male conceptualisation than female. Women, it is argued, don't set themselves so sharply apart. The boundaried self is more permeable and their way of being in the world more relational than for men. For women, connection and embeddedness within social groups are of vital importance for the emergence of identity. The 'me' is derived from 'we' (Josselson 1987). Unlike males, who grow up in a culture that stresses self-assertion, mastery, individual distinction and separation, women are raised in a culture that emphasises communion, where skill and success in relatedness become the keystones of identity.

Stress, vulnerability and overwhelm

The theory of distress and disorder that has gained most credibility over the past two decades is the vulnerability-stress model (Zubin & Spring 1977). Unfortunately this model has been hijacked by biomedical psychiatry to advance the theory that genetic based dysfunction of neurotransmission is the dominant cause of vulnerability. This narrows down what was originally intended as a broad focus on the aetiology of troubled states of mind. In its original conception the model postulated that the vulnerability to psychological overwhelm could occur as a consequence of exposure to adverse psychosocial events in our developmental history and current experience. Bentall (2003) redraws this broader picture, concluding that there is good evidence that adverse family relationships and interactional patterns contribute to a vulnerability to psychosis in adult life. The more distress is attributed to some internal psychobiological disease process, the more the origins of that distress become obscured. A person's experiential knowledge is thus invalidated in the process of becoming a patient. They begin to distrust their own feelings, thoughts and perceptions, and their volitional urge to find meaning in their suffering and their quest for a way of resolution gradually diminishes. Trapped in a state of confusion, passivity and helplessness, they come to see themselves as victims of some powerful pathological process over which they have little control.

Most of us accumulate some distress as we grow up and grow older (Fig. 1.2). This distress is held in the body and mind and we acquire various strategies to defend ourselves against it surfacing into awareness and overwhelming us. Those who carry high levels of distress are likely to lead a life restricted by defensive behaviour. They live on the edge of their distress and are at risk of being emotionally overwhelmed by everyday problems of living. Accumulated distress is always

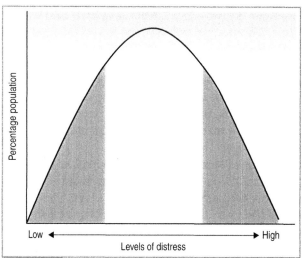

Figure 1.2 ● Levels of distress in the general population. Levels of distress sufficient to cause dysfunctional behaviour occur in 10–25% of the population annually and 2–4% will experience severe and disabling degrees of distress (Bird 1999).

likely to be reactivated by stressful events in the here and now, particularly those that in some way mirror earlier experiences. People who are highly vulnerable to this psychosocial overwhelm may adopt extreme strategies in order to try and cope. They may secrete themselves behind a wall of depression, escape into manic flights, displace their distress into somatic complaints, self-harm, or seek to reduce their emotional pain with alcohol or street drugs. All of these behaviours may be seen as strategies to deal with overwhelming feelings of despair, fear, helplessness, anger, guilt or self-loathing. For some people – those whose attribution style or source monitoring has become skewed in the course of their developmental history, affecting their capacity to make sense of experience – inner distress may manifest itself as voices or unusual beliefs. Such individuals may become so withdrawn and anxious, threatened and hostile, or over-aroused and excitable, that they find it difficult to engage with others and lose their foothold in consensual reality and their place in the community.

So universal is the phenomenon of unconsciously held distress that it is frequently represented in folk tales by the image of the dragon's cave. This is portrayed as a fearful place, which the hero enters, usually after a perilous journey, to defeat the dragon and discover the treasure that the dragon guards. It involves facing what is difficult to face, discovering the treasure within and emerging with a stronger sense of self, a more positive self-evaluation and less reliance on defensive behaviour. This heroic journey can be seen as a metaphor for therapeutic endeavour, often undertaken with help and companionship. I do not mean to suggest by this some 'revelatory, cathartic, couch experience', more a continuing journey of self-discovery that is part of a living–learning experience (Watkins 2007).

The almost exclusive focus on psychobiological research in recent decades has obscured the fact that a high proportion of people who experience severe and disabling levels of distress are individuals who have experienced trauma, family dysfunction or other disadvantageous life circumstances (Morrison et al 2003). We should not be surprised that sexual abuse, violence, parental loss or neglect in childhood, often exacerbated by re-traumatisation in adult life, are significant in the aetiology of psychotic disorders, just as they are in less disabling manifestations of distress. Morrison et al also draw attention to the trauma of incipient psychosis and the experience of becoming a patient. Follow-up studies of people admitted to psychiatric facilities with a diagnosis of psychosis show that around 52% experience post-traumatic stress disorders as a consequence, a phenomenon that is given very little therapeutic focus by mental health professionals (Frame & Morrison 2001, Shaw et al 2002).

It is an undeniable fact that, as with physical disease, psychological dis-ease is more prevalent in poorer communities than affluent ones. As we shall see in the next chapter, substantial evidence exists connecting poverty, ethnicity and gender causally to disabling distress, yet these issues are seldom adequately addressed by medically oriented psychiatry. Read (2004) points to a cycle of oppression that exists when poorer people enter the psychiatric system where they are more likely than their more affluent counterparts to be diagnosed psychotic, a label which serves to impoverish their lives further socially and economically.

If the social causation of distress has been relegated to a position of minimal aetiological significance, then the spiritual dimension of suffering has been virtually ignored by psychiatry. Many of us in the Western world seek a meaningful existence in acquisitive and hedonistic lifestyles, what the psychoanalyst and philosopher Eric Fromm has called the *having mode* of existence (Fromm 1979). Unsurprisingly we remain largely unfulfilled, suffering as a consequence a deep spiritual malaise. This we seek to cure with even more self-indulgence and, if the spiralling prescriptions of psychoactive drugs are anything to go by, mood-altering drugs. In today's secular culture we have largely forgotten what it means to live soulfully, with this absence expressing itself in a profound sense of meaninglessness, emptiness and disillusionment – *a great sadness of the soul* (Inglesby 1998). For some people, recovery from a troubled state of mind is synonymous with a spiritual journey, a journey that gives a greater sense of meaning and wholeness to their lives. This may be through one of the world religions; through Eastern practices and philosophies such as meditation, yoga, tai chi and mindfulness; or through one of the emergent spiritual movements such as Creation Spirituality. Inglesby likens this journey to a pilgrimage to the unknown realms of the psyche to find salvation in our true selves and to reconnect with the joy of being.

Finally, we can no longer ignore the pressing problem of the continuing exploitation and pollution of this biosphere that sustains us. Eco-consciousness is no longer a peripheral issue but is central to our wellbeing and survival. We have an evolutionary based affiliation with the animate world; we are part of the community of life and if we damage our world we damage ourselves. It is the contention of many people that quite apart from the clear and present danger to physical wellbeing of the toxic environment we are creating, the increasing levels of psychological dis-ease are also related to our estrangement from nature and the damage we are doing to the earth. The 'bad place' a person is in may not refer so much to their inner world as to the space they occupy in the outer world (Hillman 1995).

 Self-enquiry box

Harding (2006) argues that one of the best things we can do for our mental health is to reconnect with the natural world through finding our own special place where we can go on a regular basis to deepen our relationship with nature. Everyone, whether living in an urban or rural setting, will have a variety of inspiring places in their immediate surroundings they can access – a garden, a park, a wood, a river, a lane, a beach. He suggests allowing ourselves to be guided by our feeling, intuition and sensing when looking for that special place. It will be a place that evokes a profound sense of pleasure and peace. It will be a place with which we can develop a rapport and come to know in its many guises. It will be a place that restores our relationship with nature and revives our spirit as we 'suck up motherly love' and 'gleam into leaf'.

There are powerful influences at work in shaping our way of being in the world: our genetic endowment, our biology, our psychological legacy, the social and political circumstances of our lives, the sea of faith in which we swim, the health of Gaia. All impact on our level of wellbeing. The perspective of humanistic philosophy is not to see humanity as prisoners of its biology; as victims permanently scarred and weakened by past experience, or hopelessly oppressed by present circumstances. There is instead a belief in the essential freedom and responsibility of human beings to re-create themselves and their lives. If we can but begin the journey towards self-realisation, towards becoming fully functioning people, we can connect with our personal power and self-esteem, overcome adversity and find a way of being and living that is less problematic and more fulfilling.

There is a sense in which we are all on the same quest – whether we struggle with mental health problems or not – the quest to transcend the suffering that is part of every life and to find that often elusive measure of peace, happiness and fulfilment. As Victor Frankl (2004) wisely observed, this is to be found in a life that has meaning and it is the quest for meaning that draws us on into life which, when we discover it, infuses our lives with a sustained sense of wellbeing. A meaning for living is clearly not to be found where most people in contemporary Western society look – in the acquisition of status, wealth, material possession and hedonistic lifestyles. What invests life with a deeper meaning is for many people a sense of family-oriented love and duty; for others it is found in altruistic or vocational work for the greater good; for some it comes from a commitment to living ethically and spiritually in harmony with others and nature; and for those who seek meaning in the teachings of the world religions it is found through the will to live a disciplined and virtuous life according to God's purpose. The humanistic perspective would argue that the true purpose and meaning of life is to be found in the quest 'to be'; to realise our potential and be who we truly are, real and vibrant persons, aspiring to all that is noble and honourable in the human species.

The quest for sanity

Over the years the broad canon of psychiatric literature has maintained an almost exclusive focus on the nature of psychological distress, dysfunction and its treatment. Very little has been written about what it means to be sane, how we retain our sanity and how we enhance our wellbeing.

The will to be sane is often witnessed in the way people, seemingly lost in a psychotic world, can suddenly step out into what Podvoll (2003) calls 'islands of clarity'. It could be argued that what happens at those moments is the key to regaining and enhancing wellbeing. It is these restorative personal characteristics that we should be alive to and seek to strengthen in our recovery work with clients. Podvoll argues that these moments of clarity reflect a sharpening of awareness; an awakening to and a tiredness of the otherworldliness of psychotic preoccupations that inevitably lead to a chaotic life on the margins of society. There is a strengthening of the will to resist these mind excursions into a confused, fabricated world that is at odds with consensual reality. With this discrimination comes the sense that it doesn't have to be like this. When this occurs, given the presence of a healing environment, the actualisation process resumes – in other words, people begin to flourish and grow towards their potential, often after many years of arrested and distorted development.

It is frequently apparent, when people begin to emerge from an overwhelmed state of mind that may have recurred over many years, how much of a developmental lag there is – socially and emotionally – compared with their contemporaries and how ill defined their sense of themselves is. Inevitably as people begin their quest for sanity there will be uncertainties, anxieties and despairing moments as they seek to discover themselves; as they work at the task of weaving the meaning of what has happened to them into a coherent personal narrative and discover a stronger sense of self. This can for some people be an extraordinary phase in their development. It is as if their journey through a psychotic domain has opened up a level of consciousness that allows a more transcendent way of being to emerge.

We must be compassionate towards ourselves; only despair and destructive acts come from self-loathing. There needs to be a warm acceptance of our essential goodness; a forgiveness of the many times we have transgressed the grace with which the human heart has been blessed; a loving invitation to ourselves to be something more. It is in this climate of respect for ourselves that we begin the healing journey. This does not come easily to many people whose predominant experience is of being devalued and disregarded; a compassionate regard for oneself is realised gradually through the warm acceptance and unconditional positive regard found in recovery relationships, an experience that is then internalised. It is such a joy to witness how many people who navigate through their own trials of life, learning in the process compassion for themselves, then in turn are called to extend that compassion to others. For some this takes them into professional caring, or volunteering within user-led projects and advocacy programmes, vocational work to which they bring great energy and passion.

Often a desire for a more disciplined life arises in the quest for sanity; a desire to achieve a self-determined, organised way of being in the world. This may express itself in a more simplified life in which routine activity becomes an important daily structure and an antidote to the apathy, inertia and chaotic lifestyle that previously existed. It also minimises the unexpected which may threaten to overwhelm a still vulnerable mind. This extends to contacts with mental health professionals; the more regular they are and the more predictable the style of relating the better. One person I have come to know, who is emerging from many years adrift in a state of confusion and otherworldliness, has simplified his life to an ascetic degree, regulating his contacts with people so as to keep them brief and focused and resisting any attempts to orient his lifestyle towards more social engagement or towards work. Another client will only accept visits at precise times that she has agreed to and will be plunged into delusional thinking and hostility if she is not able to set the agenda for any conversation. We need to be sensitive to a client's still vulnerable mind and disciplined way of holding on to their sanity and take a non-directive stance in relation to their therapeutic care, trusting that this simplified, disciplined life is a necessary part of their recovery journey.

Podvoll also talks about the need for clarity. If we have lived a life in which an unreality has taken hold of our consciousness, then we need in a literal sense 'to come to our senses'; to 'be here now' and not drift on the swirling currents of our mind's energies which will take us off into reveries that threaten to loosen our hold on reality and disturb our equilibrium. People in recovery need to be grounded; need to anchor their life firmly in everyday realities. They need the skill of mindfulness, of dispassionate self-observation, so that attention is not so likely to be caught up in thoughts and feelings that will have a dysfunctional impact on their lives.

Finally, we need to say something about courage, an unacknowledged quality in the quest for sanity. It can take courage to overcome the distress and disturbance that has occupied your mind and disrupted your life for so long. It takes courage 'to keep on keeping on' through the setbacks, anxieties and griefs you encounter along the pathway to renewal. It takes courage to seek a different way of being and recover a place for yourself in the world after a long period of psychological turmoil. It takes courage to open the door!

It is not too difficult to see how these waymarks of sanity play a part in all our lives. To actualise more of our potential, to live a well-lived life and experience a good measure of wellbeing, we need the qualities of awareness, clarity, discipline, compassion, courage. There are moments in every life when misfortune and suffering will make the quest for sanity an urgent reality for us all. Think how we draw on what resilience we have to avoid becoming sunk in distress, lost in our troubled thoughts or defeated by an unhappy episode in our personal history. How, seemingly stuck in a lifestyle and way of being in the world that is no longer liveable, we somehow find the energy and will to change. Recognise how that takes courage and discipline, also how we can easily be distracted and confused and lose heart and give up.

A few years ago I suffered the loss of a much loved son through suicide; a loss that plunged me into grief-laden despair from which I felt I would never emerge. That I have done so has been due in no small measure to the strengths discussed above which the loving support of others helped me discover within myself: reconnecting with compassion, where there was only guilt and self-loathing; being disciplined enough to keep the everyday fabric of my life in place; avoiding dark byways of grief-stricken thought, keeping such excursions for the therapeutic space I had created for myself; and finally perhaps the hardest task of all, learning from suffering and integrating that learning into a sustaining personal narrative.

Self-enquiry box

You may like to investigate the role of these attributes – awareness, discipline, compassion, clarity, courage – in your personal history of sanity and wellbeing.

Take each characteristic in turn and draw a mind map of associations with that word. Highlight those associations that you are most drawn to, those that have particular resonance for you. Now sit quietly with those key words and phrases and ask yourself, what role they have played/do they play in maintaining and enhancing your wellbeing. Now consider how you might more fully actualise those attributes; how you can express these core values more fully in your everyday life.

Social exclusion in the experience of distress

2

The problems faced by mental health service users are often more social than psychiatric. The difficulties they face have less to do with a continuing vulnerability to disabling distress and more to do with the experience of being stigmatised, marginalised and impoverished. Poverty, unemployment, dislocated family and social networks, lack of educational and training opportunities, poor housing or homelessness, stigma and discrimination, all promote social exclusion and are both a cause of and the consequence of mental health problems. While the extreme manifestation of social exclusion seen in the appalling social eugenics programmes in Nazi Germany and in the involuntary sterilisation programme in America in the early 1900s now seem light years away, in the view of some commentators we are still living in the shadow of its ideas (Sayce 2000).

Hopton (1997) argues strongly for mental health practitioners to develop an anti-oppressive approach to practice, an approach emphasising the social, cultural and political environment as the primary source of clients' distress. It is hard to understand how psychiatry has remained so apolitical; how we continue to treat the casualties of a social system that can be so damaging to mental health without challenging social policy and working for social change! As mental health professionals, not only must we be more attuned to the social causation and consequences of disabling distress but we must review our own values to ensure that we ourselves are not perpetuating negative attitudes, discrimination and exclusion.

Stigma, discrimination and social exclusion

In the minds of many service users and mental health professionals, stigma remains the greatest problem facing people in their quest for recovery. The extent of concern about this is such that in 2004 the National Institute for Mental Health in England launched *From Here to Equality*, a five-year plan to combat discrimination. It is not stigma per se that is the problem but socially inculcated ideas about mental health problems that lead to discrimination and exclusion. The approach taken over the past three decades to change stigmatising attitudes has been to promote the idea that mental illness is an illness like any other. This seems to have had little impact in changing the widely held perception that people with severe mental health problems are likely to be 'irrational', 'incompetent', 'out of control', 'unpredictable' and 'threatening'. This perception is reinforced by the way in which deeply troubled states of mind are portrayed by the media, reinforcing an image of dangerousness in the minds of the public. Such tabloid images are also profoundly damaging to the morale and self-concept of people who have been diagnosed as having a severe mental health problem, forcing them into a reclusive lifestyle (Link & Phelan 2001).

An 'us and them' attitude exists in society towards those deemed 'mad'. In recent years there have been attempts to de-emphasise differentness and discard diagnostic labels that have such a corrosive effect on identity. Instead the discourse has shifted towards the view that distress exists along a continuum of human behaviour with dysfunctional behaviour at one end and fully functional at the other, with no discontinuity between the two. While this may go some way towards promoting more accepting and inclusive attitudes, there remains a compelling though largely unconscious motivation to alienate those who suffer severe psychological distress and disorder. Perhaps in distancing ourselves from those diagnosed as 'mad', we distance ourselves from our own madness, from the emotional tempests that threaten to blow through every human life disrupting our equilibrium and the fragile order of our lives. Until we can acknowledge our shared humanity and within that a shared vulnerability, 'alienist' attitudes are likely to persist. We need also to recognise the extraordinary contribution many people who suffer from untamed minds make to society at all levels. One only has to think of the Nobel Prize winning mathematician John Nash, the legend of popular musician Brian Wilson, and the comic genius Spike Milligan, all of whom experienced enduring mental health problems but whose work has enriched our culture.

The lesson from history is that social attitudes can take a generation or more to change. It is psychiatric system survivors and consumers themselves, supported by strong anti-discriminatory legislation, who are best placed to challenge negative stereotypes and become ambassadors of change. It calls for courage to be open about one's psychiatric history in the workplace, at college or in the context of one's social network, but that is the forge in which more enlightened attitudes can be cast. This is only likely to happen if people have been able to incorporate their experience of breakdown into a positive sense of self, from which self-esteem and confidence has grown and provided the foundation for an inclusive life. Taking a lead from the Gay Pride movement, Mad Pride events celebrate the strengths, creativity, resilience and spirit of those who come to see breakdown as a breakthrough, casting off what William Blake referred to as the *mind made manacles*. The efforts of service user organisations does not absolve those of us working in the mental health field of a responsibility for being champions of anti-discriminatory practice, for challenging stereotypical attitudes wherever we find them, for public education and for being bold enough to 'come out' about our own vulnerability to psychological overwhelm.

Poverty

Social exclusion results not just from prejudicial attitudes towards people with mental health problems but is also the result of impoverishment. While countries like the UK have experienced a relatively stable and growing economy over the last few decades which has made possible a more affluent lifestyle, this prosperity has not been distributed equitably. There is a growing underclass of which those with enduring mental illness are a disproportionately large number, with these people finding themselves in persistent poverty and separated from the rest of us (Barham & Hayward 1995).

Many users of mental health services are engaged in a daily struggle with poverty. Poverty reduces choices and opportunities. It can mean unhealthy food, cheap clothing, poor quality housing, a bleak non-sustaining living space, lack of holidays and restricted social and leisure opportunities. To feel trapped in an impoverished life is a major cause of distress. If you take any neighbourhood with a high rate of premature death and serious physical illness, then it is likely that the neighbourhood will be a poor one and that it will also show a high rate of suicide, depression, anxiety states and schizophrenia. Read (2004) forcefully argues that a circle of oppression exists in psychiatry whereby the poorest sections of the community who experience greater stress in the form of poverty, powerlessness, isolation, poor physical health, low self-esteem, violence, sexual abuse are more likely to be diagnosed psychotic and hospitalised if they experience breakdown. This further lowers self-esteem and personal power, crushing the motivation to seek a better quality life.

Many people who use the mental health services see overcoming the impoverishment of their lives as the factor that would lead to the most significant improvement in their mental health. Yet this important social dimension is often neglected by mental health practitioners. Davis & Wainwright (1996) suggest that behind this neglect is often the belief that impoverishment is, at least in part, self-inflicted, the result of the fecklessness of service users. The prevalence of judgemental attitudes is one reason why service users do not always seek help from statutory services to negotiate the benefit system and deal with debt. Instead they seek support from welfare rights advisers, independent advocates and Citizens Advice Bureaux, where they are available. There is a need for mental health professionals and service providers to become more aware of the impact of poverty and committed to anti-poverty action in their practice and provision (Box 2.1).

Employment

Work is important in all our lives and not simply for the income it provides. It gives us a valued social role and contributes to our sense of identity. The status and role work provides is critical to someone who has the 'spoilt' identity of 'psychiatric patient' (Repper & Perkins 2003). Work gives meaning and purpose to our lives, provides us with a source of satisfaction and achievement and supports our self-esteem. It also creates opportunities for social relationships and friendship. It is hardly surprising then that unemployment significantly affects mental health or that socially valued, meaningful employment can make a significant difference to the recovery and wellbeing of people with enduring mental health problems. The desire to be gainfully employed is an expressed need of most long-term service users, 85% of whom are unemployed (Office for National Statistics 2000).

Box 2.1

A charter for poverty awareness and anti-poverty action

- Recognise the social, psychological, physical impact of poverty on service users.
- Recognise the stigma and discrimination faced by service user claimants.
- Make service users aware of their rights under the Disability Discrimination Act.
- Gain sufficient knowledge of welfare rights and entitlement to provide advice and support to service users in making claims that maximises their income.
- Work with service users in an empowering enabling way in managing benefits and dealing with debts.
- Recognise the experience and 'expertise' of some service users in relation to welfare rights and benefits and utilise this in the support of others.
- Enable service users to access good quality housing, housing benefit and council tax entitlement.
- Enable service user claimants to access social funds to maintain the fabric and functionality of their home.
- Enable service users to access the means, through Direct Payments, to determine and purchase facets of their own care.
- Enable service users to access work, training and educational opportunities.
- Assist service users to negotiate the transition from benefit-based income to work-related remuneration without loss of income or rights.

Given that entry into open employment is often difficult, there is a need for more social enterprise work projects which provide meaningful, socially valued occupations, more volunteering opportunities, more empowerment-oriented educational programmes, more transitional employment schemes of the type offered by the Clubhouse movement (Norman 2006). All of these endeavours can create an empowering and supportive context in which people can gain the skills and confidence to pursue a pathway back into open employment.

Perkins & Repper argue that it is the work setting that has to change in order to accommodate people with mental health disabilities and vulnerabilities to promote social inclusiveness. Indeed the Disability Discrimination Act makes it illegal to discriminate against someone because of their mental health problems and requires employers and educational institutions to make *reasonable adjustments* to accommodate people with such difficulties. While some employers have adapted their work environments and practices to meet the needs of people with physical disabilities, few have been flexible enough to accommodate people with psychosocial disabilities. Sayce (2001) argues that mental health professionals can help make antidiscrimination legislation work by ensuring people are aware of their rights under the Act, by advocating for clients in relation to employment, training and educational opportunities, and by contributing to the dissemination of information about what *adjustments* employers and educators might *reasonably* make for people with mental health problems.

The National Health Service, one of the biggest public sector employers in the UK, has been slow to lead the way in offering employment to service users in clinical posts and support services, despite the success of such schemes in the USA.

A notable exception is an initiative by the South West London and St George's Mental Health Trust user employment programme to recruit people who have personal experience of mental health problems into all levels of the organisation. The success of this scheme has belatedly prompted a national initiative 'to enable all disabled people including those with mental health problems to work in the wider society, an initiative in which the NHS, as the largest public service employer should be making a significant contribution' (Department of Health 2000).

Housing

A high priority for service users is access to decent housing, somewhere to feel at home and secure. Studies of the homeless population of the UK suggest the proportion with severe mental health problems is between 30% and 50%, with many of this group having the additional problem of multiple substance abuse (Bird 1999). Homelessness exacerbates mental and physical health problems and in addition it can be difficult for mental health practitioners to stay in contact with clients. One of the key issues in the housing provision for vulnerable people is that it should be available with support. Tenancies may break down because of rent arrears, failure to care appropriately for the accommodation or because of disputes with the neighbours – problems which often arise in the context of relapses and which can be mitigated if housing agencies and mental health services are able to provide integrated support.

There is a clear need for more housing to be made available to people with long-term mental health problems ranging from 24-hour-staffed accommodation of the core and cluster variety, to independent tenancies with outreach support. But if social inclusiveness is to become a reality, it is important that the balance of the housing provision moves away from specialist accommodation towards providing people with enough support to maintain a place of their own in the wider community. One of the successes of assertive outreach services is in enhancing the quality of life of service users, a significant aspect of which is enabling those people with a history of homelessness to maintain a tenancy and establish themselves in a neighbourhood (Grayley-Wetherell & Morgan 2001).

Rather than see the wider community as 'another country' from which those who experience enduring mental health problems are barred from full citizenship, the neighbourhood should be seen as an 'oasis of opportunity' to be accessed with appropriate support (Morgan 2004a). To segregate people in mental health resources is to perpetuate the stereotypical attitudes that give rise to stigma and discrimination.

What are the implications of all this for the helping relationship? Clearly it is important to fully acknowledge the impact on psychological wellbeing of stigma, discrimination, social impoverishment and disadvantage. In the reality of daily practice this recognition is usually only cursory. Mental health services are dominated by models that locate the aetiology of distress and dysfunction within the individual, a condition to be put right by pharmacological and psychotherapeutic interventions, rather than seeing the origins of that distress in the social experience of the individual. Smail (1998) in a powerful argument on the limits of therapy takes the view that we cling to the 'therapeutic illusion' that a history of, for example, abuse or deprivation can be wiped away. At best therapy is only palliative. One of the lessons of history is that more can be achieved in relation to health and wellbeing by improving social conditions than through medical interventions. Davidson (1998), drawing on Smail's work, suggests that the role of practitioners is to try to understand and demystify the problems the client faces and to see that these are not the product of pathological processes but an understandable way of being and surviving, given their history and experience. A normalising stance such as this is difficult to hold on to. Firstly, a reductionist medical view of the problem is often easier both for the client and for the professional, rather than attempting to confront the deprivation and abuse that has been part of the client's experience. Facing the hurt perpetrated by others, the hurt done to others and identifying injustice and oppression does not magically cure the client, but it does place distress in its rightful context rather than obscuring it with diagnostic labels and pathologising processes and opens up the possibility of remedial social action.

Transcultural issues in the experience of distress

3

The growing ethnic diversity and multiculturalism in the UK requires mental health services themselves to be multicultural and have a workforce trained and aware of diversity issues. We must overcome the racism endemic in our psychiatric system and be more voluble in raising awareness of the impact of racist attitudes in our society on the mental health of individuals from ethnic minority groups. There is a need for better dissemination of accessible information about services to people seeking asylum and to economic migrants. Many asylum seekers, often traumatised by experiences in their country of origin, find themselves destitute on the streets of urban Britain – unable to stay and unable to return home. Amnesty International estimates that over 150 000 failed asylum seekers are living impoverished, marginalised, hopeless and fearful lives in Britain, many of whom inevitably experience a serious deterioration in their mental health and have limited or no access to mental health services (Shaw 2006).

Although many social groups in our society have experienced discrimination and oppression within the psychiatric system, it is particularly so for people of Afro-Caribbean, African and South Asian descent. It is a sad fact that racism seems to have permeated all social institutions – education, the criminal justice system, local authority services and health services. It seems only belatedly, following public inquiries such as the shaming Stephen Lawrence inquiry and the inquiry into the tragic death of David 'Rocky' Bennett in a psychiatric facility, that the existence of racism at the core of our institutions is beginning to be acknowledged and confronted.

In the preface to the third edition of their classic book on racism, psychological ill-health and psychiatry, Littlewood & Lipsedge (1997) concluded that despite the critiques of racism in psychiatry over the previous two decades very little of substance had changed. They cite the now familiar picture of continuing higher diagnostic rates of schizophrenia for British-born Afro-Caribbeans, an over-representation of black people admitted under the Mental Health Act, little or no access for them to psychological treatment, a lack of understanding of possible social determinants of mental ill-health amongst black British people, a failure to translate the personal insights and resources of service users into therapeutic care and a continued under-representation of black mental health professionals in senior positions as being indicative of endemic racism in psychiatry and wider society. Eight years on from the publication of their informed text, a Mental Health Act Commission (2005) study found little evidence of an improvement despite the priority given by NHS Trusts to diversity training (Box 3.1).

Box 3.1

Institutional racism in mental health services

Black British people are more likely than white:

- to be diagnosed as suffering from schizophrenia or other forms of psychosis
- to be admitted to a psychiatric facility
- to be detained in a locked ward or secure psychiatric unit
- to be detained in hospital under sections of the Mental Health Act
- to be referred through the courts or by the police
- to be given higher doses of medication
- to experience physical restraint and seclusion
- to spend longer in hospital
- to have less access to psychological therapies.

Source: Mental Health Act Commission (2005) and Department of Health (2005a).

A racist bias operating within mental health services does not by itself account for the statistical difference in diagnostic rates. It is the wider social experience of people from minority ethnic groups that accounts for this vulnerability. Any social group that encounters pernicious racist attitudes in everyday life, and higher unemployment, poverty and social exclusion than the general population is bound to be at risk.

The dominant discourse on severe distress is an ethnocentric Western view, which conceptualises it as a dysfunctional state located within the individual for which treatment with powerful drugs is required. So dominant is this illness hypothesis that it has achieved the status of a truth and provides the authoritative basis for professionalised care and pharmacological intervention. Western psychiatry has spread imperialistically around the world on the coat tails of Western medicine, despite the lack of any clear evidence of superiority over indigenous, traditional approaches to healing the mind (Fernando 2002). While the conception of distress as illness to be treated by health care professionals may be relevant and acceptable to many people seeking help, it is often inappropriate to people whose social experience and beliefs are rooted in non-Western cultures. Furthermore, racial stereotyping, cultural insensitivity and oppressive practices, often the experience of black and other ethnic minority users of the psychiatric system, increase the reluctance of people to access and stay engaged with services.

The idea that recovery of wellbeing requires the intervention of psychiatrists, psychologists and nurses is not a belief that is readily accepted by all cultures, and ideas of what constitutes the conditions for healing and recovery may have a different emphasis in non-Western cultures (Box 3.2; Fernando 2002). If depression is experienced more as oppression and deprivation, then it is not treatment that is required, but social action. If unusual thoughts or voice hearing relate to the spiritual realm of a person's life, then it could be the leader of their faith community that should be consulted. If the problem is perceived as a loss of harmony in a person's inner and outer worlds, then it may be that consulting a traditional healer, complementary therapist or spiritual teacher would be more advantageous. For some, the manifestation of distress may be seen as a problem requiring family care, rather than the intrusive intervention of some outside agency.

Box 3.2

Conditions for healing – a comparison of Eastern and Western beliefs

Eastern	Western
Unity of mind/body/spirit	Separation of mind/body/spirit
Disharmony	Illness
Holistic awareness	Specialist knowledge
Personal meaning of symptoms	Pathological basis for symptoms
Treatment based on indigenous knowledge/experiential evidence	Science-based medicine
Restoration of harmony/subtle energy flow/detoxification	Problem-solving
Traditional/alternative/spiritual healers	Professionals trained in science-based medicine
Conditions for self-healing created	Interventionist strategies to treat dysfunction

Source: Fernando (2002).

It is a mistake to think that the cultural identity of a client necessarily determines their conception of the problem and what needs to be done about it. Fernando argues that culture is not a fixed entity but an 'emergent' process that is influenced by the social and family context as much as by tradition. To make assumptions about an individual's mental health needs simply by reference to their cultural group leads to stereotyping. There is also a tendency to classify people whose origins are geographically similar into one group, for example South East Asians, ignoring the rich diversity of beliefs and traditions that exist in cultures rooted in that part of the world.

Training in relation to ethnicity, as with gender, often misses the essential point that the main focus needs to be raising awareness of our own prejudicial attitudes, rather than absorbing a generalised knowledge of a particular culture and familiarising oneself with relevant legislation. Individuals from ethnic minority groups, particularly those who are British born, may hold views that are divergent from the norms of their culture of origin. Taking this more fluid view of culture frees us from relying too much on having detailed knowledge of a cultural group in order to be sensitive in assessing needs and allows us to draw much more on the unique experience of the individual or family.

 ## Self-enquiry box

To split beliefs about healing into an Eastern and Western tradition does not accurately reflect today's reality. It is seldom so clear-cut in a multi-ethnic society such as Britain. Many individuals whose origins are in white Western culture have beliefs around healing that would fit more comfortably with an Eastern approach.

Continued

Self-enquiry box—cont'd

Explore your own beliefs about healing:

- What stories were you told about illness and healing as you were growing up? What effect did they have on you?
- Who was the 'healer' in your family as you were growing up?
- When you think of illness, which words and images come to mind?
- When you think of healing, which words and images come to mind?
- How have you healed yourself at times when you've been physically unwell?
- How have you healed yourself at times when you've experienced psychological hurt?
- Do you recognise messages in your somatic and psychological symptoms?
- Who have been the healers in your experiences of physical ill-health?
- Who have been the healers when you have experienced psychological distress?
- What words and images come to mind when you think of a place of healing?

Gender issues in the experience of distress

4

The experience of women

Francine's story

Theme: gender issues in vulnerability to psychosocial overwhelm

I'm 53 now and have suffered from recurrent anxiety and depression for the past 11 years. I find it difficult being on my own and get panicky. I don't really know why I should feel so helpless and worried. I know it frustrates my husband that I rely on him so much. It's not surprising he loses his temper with me. Going out is difficult as I find it hard to talk to people. I worry that everyone will know I've been in hospital and that they will be thinking I'm a loathsome pathetic person for not getting over this and looking after my family properly. I've had so much help from everyone – doctors, nurses, I'm sure they are all exasperated with me. Now they don't really talk to me much – just ask me about my symptoms, observe me, make sure I'm safe and that I look after myself properly. I've never felt safe in hospital, in a mixed ward, one woman I know was raped in a toilet by a male patient. When I'm very depressed, I get frightening thoughts that seem very real at the time, that I've done something terrible and that it's in all the newspapers. At times in the past I've been so overwhelmed with worry and just wanted it to stop, that I've tried to kill myself.

My life is quite empty really. I should have gone back to work after Julian (son) left school but I never felt confident enough or skilled enough and I didn't think they would want me. Also I wanted another baby but it didn't happen. When I look back on my life I've always had people to look after, now there's no one. My mother suffered from multiple sclerosis. My older sister and I used to look after her when she became very disabled. Then she died. I remember the house feeling very empty. My dad was good to us but he was not someone you could easily confide in or go to if you were upset. He became a strict Methodist after my mother's death and we were encouraged to look to God for comfort and guidance. I think I grew up feeling that I had to be good and that meant being nice and not making a fuss about anything. I remember being terrified by the idea that God could look into my heart and discover what a despicable child I was.

Continued

27

Francine's story—cont'd

I'm not sure what's going to happen to me, but I am feeling a bit more hopeful. It's about 18 months since I last had to go into hospital. I'm still taking regular medication although it hasn't really helped me much. I see my community nurse once a week and we work on building up coping strategies and I also have a support worker. If I begin to relapse now, I can check myself into The Moorings (a woman's respite and recovery house). I have experienced a lot of love and care there and have been able to give some in return. I remember the first time I was there, one of the women sat up half the night just holding me. It was the first time I can remember feeling safe.

An area of concern in relation to anti-oppressive practice is the frequently reported negative experience of women users of the mental health services. Much of the psychiatric literature over the past decades has reflected the patriarchal nature of mental health services. Two-thirds of the users of mental health services are women, yet the majority of key decision-makers – service planners, managers and senior clinicians – are men. This continuing gender imbalance raises the question of how sensitively aware of women's issues services can be (Payne 1998). In a reflection of the decline of feminine values in psychiatry, Kirkpatrick (2004) argues passionately that practitioners, women (and men), 'must not allow the historical goals of compassionate care of the whole individual, especially the powerless, and concern with the social and psychological context of disease, to be dismantled'. She calls for an 'integration of masculine technological thinking and feminine compassionate care in policy and practice' (p. 211). The charge is that mental health professionals have consistently failed to respond to, and in some cases have reinforced, the experience of social inequality, disempowerment and abuse that is for many women a social reality and a major factor in their distressed and disturbed behaviour. Additionally, recent reports (Sainsbury Centre 1998) have drawn attention to the dissatisfaction of many women with acute inpatient services, which often do not provide them with the privacy, sense of safety and freedom from sexual harassment that should be fundamental elements in a caring environment.

There is strong evidence that sexual, physical or emotional abuse is a major factor contributing to women's mental health problems, including those that are severe and enduring. In a review of thirteen reputable studies conducted by Goodman et al (1997), between 51% and 97% of women suffering psychosis reported being subjected to some form of abuse in their lifetime. In a further study of women with severe mental health problems, Museer et al (1998) found that 52% had been sexually abused in childhood and 67% had suffered sexual abuse in later life. These are staggering figures, way above the average for the general population and strongly indicative of the role of trauma as a precursor or precipitant of severe psychological distress in adult life. Yet psychiatry offers very little in the way of therapeutic attention to these traumatised women, many of whom show clear signs of post-traumatic stress disorder enmeshed with their psychosis (Morrison et al 2003).

Given the high incidence of abuse amongst female consumers of mental health services, it is essential that mental health workers have the sensitivity and awareness to address this issue in their conversations with clients. Not to do so is to replicate the experience of not being heard and helps to reinforce the sense of blame, shame and guilt common in the histories of abused women. There clearly needs to be not just a greater awareness of abuse, but a pool of skilled help available both within and outside the mental health services.

Social inequalities, which are more frequently experienced by women, also correlate with psychological distress and referral to the mental health services (Box 4.1). Recent reports (Department of Health 2002a, 2002b) have highlighted the need for mental health workers to recognise in their work with clients the significance of social issues and intervene in ways that seek to ameliorate these as causes of distress. The predominant experience that women have of mental health professionals is still too often of not being listened to, of routinised treatment, of high doses of psychotropic drugs and frequent admissions to inpatient units (Williams & Watson 1996). Although the use of electroconvulsive therapy (ECT) is declining in the UK, approximately 1 300 ECTs are still administered each week, of which 68% are to women (Department of Health 1999d). Recurrent

---

Box 4.1

The mental health consequences of the social and cultural realities of women's lives

- Childbirth is linked with depression for a significant number of women.
- Caring for children and dependent relatives carries a high emotional cost, particularly when associated with isolation and the low social value placed on these roles. The stress of balancing multiple roles of employee, homemaker, parent, partner, carer – largely unsupported – can have an adverse effect on women's health.
- Women are much more likely than men to live in poverty which is strongly associated with being a single parent or being divorced. The link between poverty and a higher incidence of psychological ill-health is well documented.
- Nearly twice as many women as men of working age are economically inactive and a significant number of those employed are in part-time lowly paid jobs. Unemployment has a strong correlation with mental ill-health.
- Women are more vulnerable to social isolation than men because of poverty, lone parenthood, lack of mobility, fear of street violence.
- Between 18% and 30% of women experience domestic violence sometime during their lifetime, largely perpetrated by men. Links between domestic violence and mental health difficulties are now well established. It is estimated that women on average experience 35 episodes of violence before seeking help.
- Studies indicate that between 14% and 40% of women have been victims of sexual violence. The majority of sexual assaults are likely to be perpetrated by current partners or a man a woman is acquainted with. Research shows a strong link between sexual violence and mental ill-health.
- The international literature suggests that between 7% and 30% of girls experience sexual abuse in childhood, an experience that can have a profound effect on mental health. Some studies of women using mental health services suggest that as many as 52% have been victims of sexual abuse in childhood.

Source: Department of Health (2005b).

depression in women is more likely to be seen as an internal event, unrelated to the cultural and social circumstances, to be treated by physical means.

What is crucial is that the education of mental health workers should provide an opportunity to develop a critical awareness of the experience, needs and resourcefulness of women seeking help. This learning can come from various sources: listening more to women users, by women's groups being involved in training mental health workers, from women-centred mental health projects and from the growing body of literature. An increased awareness can also be derived from our own experience of oppression and entrapment.

Self-enquiry box

Make a list of statements about yourself and your life beginning with the phrase *I must* ...

Put this list of statements out of sight and complete a second list beginning with the phrase *I choose* ...

Now compare the two lists. Consider the extent to which your way of being is a self-determined choice and how much is an expression of the internalised expectations from your family and the wider culture.

Self-enquiry box

The following exercise can be a useful way of identifying unacknowledged resentments and uncovering the unexpressed appreciations you feel in relation to significant people in your life and the various roles you play. The exercise may enable you to articulate these feelings more assertively.

Make a list of all the things that you resent:

* About the way you are treated as a man/as a woman.
* About the way you are treated as a member of an ethnic minority group.
* About the way you are treated as a gay man/lesbian.
* About the way you are treated by your parents/your partner/your children.
* About the way you are treated as an employee.
* About the way you are treated as a citizen.

When you have completed one of the above categories, think about the 'expectations' that underlie the resentments and capture them as written statements. Try and be as clear and direct as you can, as in the example below.

* Resentment: 'I resent the way you treat me like a child'.
* Expectation: 'I want you to respect my decisions and choices'.

Now using the same category, list all of the things that you appreciate.

Reflect on your lists and consider how you might use what you have learnt as a basis for personal or social action.

The experience of men

Over the past few decades much of the debate on gender has rightly addressed the experience of women. More recently the wellbeing of men has come into focus. Young men seem particularly vulnerable to distressed and troubled states of mind, reflected most strikingly in the higher suicide rates and the increasing incidence of drug and alcohol abuse (National Suicide Prevention Strategy for England 2002). Studies show a prevalence of drug misuse or dependence for young males newly diagnosed with psychosis of around 15% and for alcohol misuse or dependence of 31% (Bird 1999). There are some indications that psychosis tends to have an earlier onset and be more disabling in men than in women. It could be that the greater prevalence of cannabis and alcohol misuse in young males is a factor; also the greater social inclusiveness of women could be an influence. There is need for further research in these areas.

Tremendous changes have taken place in the lives of men over the latter half of the 20th century and continue today. The declining industrial base and the disappearance of traditional labour-intensive industries have robbed men of the occupational roles from which they once drew their sense of identity. In the process, the 'lessons in masculinity' that were absorbed from the work culture are no longer available. The 'new man' syndrome which began to emerge in the liberal culture of the 1960s, which created a social climate in which men could develop their feminine side, has left men feeling incomplete. While there is satisfaction for many men in being able to develop and express a more caring, feeling side, it has been at the expense of the positive masculine energy referred to by Robert Bly as the 'inner warrior'. When energised, this male archetype strengthens and ennobles men with boldness, fortitude, competitiveness, vigour, honour and pride (Bly 1990). There needs to be a balance; to be defined by qualities most often associated with femininity can be threatening to most men. Male aggression and sexuality has been demonised in our culture, where it has become linked with domestic violence, child abuse and criminality. It is an image that makes it difficult to accept and integrate positive masculine energy, and to allow it to infuse the personality and be expressed in constructive ways.

The 1960s also saw the emergence of a strong feminist movement, which has led to women becoming more assertive in claiming their rights and changing their role in society. Women are no longer so dependent on men.

Men are no longer the sole providers or protectors of the family. This and the high divorce rate have had a significant impact on the psychological and physical health of men. While separation and divorce can put a huge burden on women, particularly if there are children involved and little financial or practical support from an absent partner, men too show an increased susceptibility to physical and emotional problems following the breakdown of relationships.

Embedded in the national psyche is the idea that women are more vulnerable, more likely to be victims, but also more emotionally literate and socially adept than men. Men are characterised as being more emotionally constrained, tough minded and needing less emotional sustenance from their relationships. It is of course a stereotype but one that has sufficient power to make many men seek refuge in denial, reluctant to acknowledge their distress and seek help.

Men who have not found a place in society, who have no concept of what it is to be a man, are vulnerable to a desperate sense of alienation, apathy, dysphoria and anger which frequently manifests itself in antisocial behaviour, substance misuse and mental health problems. Perhaps what is missing most from the lives of many men is the positive presence of a father. There is a need for elders and mentors in the development of masculinity. What it is to be a man can only be learnt from other men, from their example and from their stories.

 James's story

Theme: gender confusion and psychosocial overwhelm

I first met Jimmy 15 years ago. He was a scrawny pubescent 20-year-old who had been admitted to an acute ward following a psychotic episode and a suicide attempt. The most striking thing about him at first sight was the aesthetic quality of his physique; he was often referred to by his family as a 'beautiful boy' and indeed he was. Jimmy had been largely brought up by his mother and had little experience of the company of men. His father had beaten him savagely as he was growing up; violent abuse which eventually led to a term of imprisonment and an exclusion order.

Throughout his secondary education Jimmy had been bullied because of his timidity and androgynous looks. He had sought refuge in a reclusive lifestyle within which a rich fantasy life evolved that gradually seemed to grade into a virtual world – an archetypal, utopian world of fiction largely populated by women and boys. It was a loosening of Jimmy's power to discriminate between this inner realm of the imagination and consensual reality that led to a referral to the psychiatric services. He had begun stalking a local woman onto whom he had projected characteristics of the 'spirit maidens' who populated his fantasy world; he had subsequently been questioned by police in relation to an unsolved local rape but was later cleared of any involvement.

The central problem for Jimmy was that he did not know 'how to be' in the real world and more specifically 'how to be' in the world of men. So much of his emergent masculine self had been a cause for ridicule and punishment and had been suppressed and buried deeply in catacombs of his psyche. The task was to help him resurrect his masculine energy which could carry him more boldly into the world. In his therapy with a male therapist he was able to confront some of his fear of men and the residual post-traumatic stress from the beatings and bullying. A significant step in his recovery journey was to discover the 'missing men' in his fantasy world. Essentially he saw them as warrior males away on a quest and their return in his imagination heralded the beginning of a change in his way of being in the real world. Jimmy seemed able to identify with and integrate some of their courage, vigour and pride into his persona; and began to be excited by, rather than fearful of, their masculine aggression, which he came to see as potentially a socially constructive energy, rather than a destructive force. It is of interest that as his identity morphed into a more masculine persona during the 18 months of his therapy so his bodily shape began to fill out into that of a mature young man.

The last time we met he had discarded Jimmy and had adopted his birth name, James.

Creative solutions to crisis 5

Crisis intervention involves brief periods of intensive support aimed at helping people through periods of high levels of distress. If early signs of increasing distress are recognised and promptly and effectively responded to, an individual can be prevented from spiralling down into a deeply troubled and troubling state of mind that may lead to a psychiatric emergency and an admission. In that sense, crisis work may be seen as preventative. From the service user's perspective, a crisis is always a frightening experience and it is the responsibility of mental health services to support people through these chaotic periods in the most sensitive and effective way possible, minimising further distress, risk, and loss of liberty (Minghella et al 1998).

Crises can occur for many reasons. They commonly occur at times of change and transition, either developmental, situational or both, when the challenges of living overwhelm or exhaust our resources. How well we cope with the challenges of living depends on three factors:

- The nature of the challenge. The meaning it has for us. The magnitude and predictability of it and the amount of control we have.
- The resources we have to draw on. Our personal coping strategies and the support we have available.
- Our sense of personal power; of being in control of our lives.

A crisis can be seen as a potential turning point in an individual's life. Although a crisis is a painful and disorganising experience, it is also an opportunity to learn something helpful about our lives and ourselves. It is an experience from which many people emerge stronger and more integrated. For people with a vulnerability to severely disorganising distress, a crisis can be an overwhelming, demoralising experience for which many seek relief in medication and admission. To seek resolution solely through the sanctuary offered by a hospital admission and through the use of medication, can limit the opportunity to learn how to be more resourceful in managing future episodes of distress in a way that reduces the tendency to spiral out of control. Recurrent crises can also be demoralising for mental health professionals, who begin to blame themselves, or the client, or colleagues and feel powerless to change the relapse–readmission cycle. If both staff and client could see crisis as an opportunity to learn how to manage the problems of living more effectively, then breakdown becomes an opportunity for breakthrough and crisis can be viewed more positively.

We also need to recognise that a crisis is by no means a turning point for everyone. Some people remain highly vulnerable to troubled states of mind and periods of wellbeing can seem fragile and transient. It can take years for people to find the hope, belief and will to change their lives. Some of the issues surrounding a protracted recovery will be looked at in Chapter 8 and it is perhaps sufficient to say here that part of the reason some people remain vulnerable and stuck in a cycle of recurrent relapses is that they have become established in a victim or sick role. The dominant and defining narrative of their life is a problem-saturated one, and a way of being and living outside the role of victim, or patient, is inconceivable. But as Ron Coleman, reflecting on his own recovery process argues, 'you have to give up being ill so you can start being recovered' (Coleman 1999). What is desperately needed is a new way of working with such clients, a way that is empowering and based more on an assessment of strengths rather than needs (Ryan & Morgan 2004).

There are phases in the development of a crisis that individuals pass through (Fig. 5.1). Resolution can occur at any stage if people are able to:

- discover the resourcefulness to bring about some change in the precipitating events

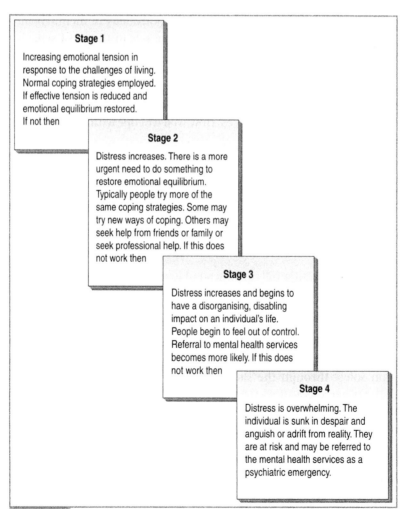

Stage 1

Increasing emotional tension in response to the challenges of living. Normal coping strategies employed. If effective tension is reduced and emotional equilibrium restored. If not then

Stage 2

Distress increases. There is a more urgent need to do something to restore emotional equilibrium. Typically people try more of the same coping strategies. Some may try new ways of coping. Others may seek help from friends or family or seek professional help. If this does not work then

Stage 3

Distress increases and begins to have a disorganising, disabling impact on an individual's life. People begin to feel out of control. Referral to mental health services becomes more likely. If this does not work then

Stage 4

Distress is overwhelming. The individual is sunk in despair and anguish or adrift from reality. They are at risk and may be referred to the mental health services as a psychiatric emergency.

Figure 5.1 ● Stages in the development of a crisis.

- bring about some change in the way they perceive those events
- bring about some change in the way they react.

People unknown to the mental health services may reach the third stage before they are referred. For those with a known vulnerability and a history of contact with the service this may happen at an earlier stage. We all have our own stress reaction pattern and express vulnerability in individual ways. For some people that reaction can be quite disabling and sometimes catastrophic in which they rapidly spiral down into deep despair or enter a confusing and threatening reality.

Self-enquiry box

Scan back over the past 10 years of your life and draw a lifeline (Fig. 5.2) representing key events both positive and negative that have happened to you during this time. Reflect on the events that caused you some distress. What did you do, what did other people do that helped you regain your emotional equilibrium? What else helped? Does this tell you anything about your coping strategies?

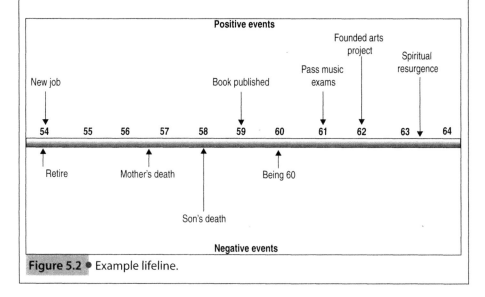

Figure 5.2 ● Example lifeline.

Early signs monitoring

Many people are extremely fearful of relapse and show a strong interest in learning about early warning signs (McDermott 1998). In fact, many vulnerable people and their carers become knowledgeably aware of signs of relapse without any help from mental health professionals. Relapse increases the probability of further crises and the likelihood of persistent disability and social dislocation (Birchwood & Tarrier 1994). It also leaves people feeling demoralised and lacking control over their lives. The early signs scale developed by Birchwood et al is a widely used, reliable assessment tool for helping clients, their carers and mental health professionals to identify a relapse signature and monitor early signs that precede episodes of disruptive distress. Signs that typically resemble anxiety and depression are frequently the earliest indicators, followed by the gradual emergence of disinhibited behaviour and intrusive, troubling thoughts (Box 5.1).

All mental health service users with complex problems are legally entitled to a coordinated care programme that should include early warning signs and a collaboratively developed crisis plan. The cognitive, emotional and behavioural characteristics of a person's relapse signature can be recorded in explicit straightforward language rather than technical terminology. Describing an early sign as 'a slowing down of speech, thought and action', is more helpful than 'increasing psychomotor retardation', 'being bothered by thoughts that people are able to see into my mind' is better than 'an increase in intrusive paranoid thinking'. Relapse prevention plans should also include information about trigger events.

Common triggers are:

- conflicts within family relationships and conflicts with others
- excessive psychosocial stimulus, which can sometimes occur as a consequence of the unrealistic expectations of professional helpers and others
- loss of key relationships, including the actual or anticipated withdrawal of support from mental health professionals
- unemployment or the lack of a meaningful way of structuring time
- social isolation
- benefit issues, poverty, social disadvantage, discrimination and oppression
- religious or spiritual alienation
- stopping medication
- use of recreational drugs and/or alcohol.

Sometimes clients are able to quantify the strength of relapse signs on a simple rating scale. For example, 'On a scale of 1 to 10, where 10 is the worst this anxious preoccupation with what people might be thinking about you has

---

Box 5.1

Frequently reported early signs

Feeling low
Difficulty in managing everyday tasks
Social withdrawal
Feeling useless or helpless
Feeling dissatisfied with self
Difficulty in concentrating
Feeling tense, afraid or anxious
Feeling irritable
Restless, unsatisfying sleep

Losing one's temper easily
Becoming more excitable
Feeling confused or puzzled
Feeling of being talked about, watched or laughed at
Talking or acting inappropriately
Intrusive, troubling thoughts
Increase in voice hearing

been, where would you put yourself at the moment?'. Continued monitoring can be a helpful indicator not only of severity but also of the timescale involved in an individual's relapse pattern. Some people spiral down very quickly into a distressed and chaotic state in a matter of days, whereas others might be able to maintain a higher level of functioning for several weeks before the deterioration begins to impact disruptively on their lives. A relapse prevention plan that includes early signs monitoring is essential for people who want to try living without long-term medication or want to reduce it and avoid a further disruptive breakdown in their personal and social functioning. However, relapse monitoring is not appropriate or helpful for every client.

Birchwood comments that for some clients the repetitive requests for information may increase anxiety about relapse and overemphasise the psychiatric vulnerability. Monitoring will also be difficult with those who have limited or fluctuating insight or who tend to 'seal over' past and incipient experiences of distress as a way of coping, avoiding conversations that focus on mental health issues. It is often not practical to use systematic monitoring continuously but it can be helpfully introduced during periods of stress or when the first early signs become evident. Mental health professionals who have worked closely with a service user, sometimes over several years, get to know an individual's early signs pattern, which can be quite idiosyncratic. Carers too will often be aware of subtle but significant early signs of relapse and justifiably complain that these observations have not always been taken seriously and responded to by mental health professionals.

 Naomi's story

Theme: early signs monitoring

Mark, my son, first became ill when he was 19. We noticed that he had become very quiet over a period of several weeks; he seemed distant and distracted as if he had got something on his mind. We thought he must be worrying about something, but he just got irritable if we asked what was bothering him, in fact he became quite abusive at times, which was so unlike him. I wondered if he was still getting over breaking up with his girlfriend or if he was upset because his father had recently remarried and moved to live closer to his work. I made him go to the doctor who said she thought Mark was depressed and prescribed some antidepressants. After I suppose about 3 months he virtually stopped going out socially and was missing more and more of his college course. He began to do odd things like wearing sunglasses in the house or turning his head away from people when they spoke to him or passed him in the street. Often he would sleep late and be wandering about the house at night. One night I heard him crying and went down to him. He told me that certain people on the television were able to see right into his mind and that when people stared at him in the street they knew that he was different. He was also hearing voices telling him that he had 'gone wrong' and would have to be 'dealt with'. When we tried to talk to him about it the next day he just got very excitable and aggressive. We had to call the doctor and a social worker and he was admitted to hospital. I suppose it must have been about 4 months from the time

Continued

Naomi's story—cont'd

we first became concerned about him till he was admitted and we were told he was suffering from schizophrenia. It was such a traumatic time. We couldn't accept it at first. No one in either of our families had had psychiatric problems and up until that time Mark had seemed just a normal young man.

This was 6 years ago and since then he has had two more admissions. We are hoping now that Mark is taking a newer drug with fewer side effects, that he'll continue taking them and will stay well. The other positive and helpful part of his recent care has been that he has been able to forge a good relationship with his CPN who monitors Mark quite closely, though not in an intrusive way, for early signs that he is breaking down again. We know what to look for now and I think Mark himself recognises when things are beginning to go wrong. Sunglasses or shutting or blinking his eyes a lot are a sign. He seems low in spirits at these times and stands around in a rather pensive preoccupied sort of way and is reluctant to go out. When we notice this we know it won't be long before Mark begins to be troubled by voices and the idea that people can see what he calls his 'impurity'. He does become quite distressed when he reaches this stage. What seems to help is being in quiet surroundings. Working in the garden or taking the dogs for a walk also seems to help. If he's around a lot of people he seems more troubled. His psychiatrist usually increases his medication and his CPN comes in more regularly and talks to him about his worrying thoughts and any current problems he has. It is difficult to know exactly what triggers off these unsettled episodes. Usually it's something to do with him feeling left behind, seeing others getting on with their lives – building careers, setting up home, getting married and having children. In many ways he is still an adolescent with all the anxieties and insecurities about finding a place in the adult world.

Crisis services

The National Service Framework for Mental Health (1999) set out as one of its main agendas the creation of crisis resolution services across the UK, available 24 hours a day, 7 days a week, providing intensive support and therapeutic care, that offered a viable alternative to admission. This followed a number of reports highlighting serious deficiencies in psychiatric inpatient care. A Sainsbury Centre survey (1998) found that much of the current inpatient care that people had access to was 'anti-therapeutic'. It often did not address individuals' psychosocial needs even though these factors were underlying the crisis. Care programmes were often routinised and limited, lacking in therapeutic focus, rather than individualised and responsive to assessed and expressed need. Length of stay for many was much longer than was needed; mainly because of a lack of accommodation and home-based support. A survey by the Mental Health Act Commission (1997) of the experience of service users admitted to over 300 acute wards highlighted the lack of meaningful activity, the absence of a relaxed environment in which people felt safe and supported, poor amenities, a lack of quiet spaces and limited one-to-one contact with ward staff. Women in particular expressed, and continue to express, dissatisfaction with issues of safety and privacy in admission units (Department of Health 2002b).

It is now widely accepted that crisis care can be delivered to people in their own homes (home treatment), or in crisis houses that can provide sanctuary and skilled support. Admissions will continue to be necessary, to provide containment, care and treatment for some people during episodes of acutely distressed and disturbed behaviour – particularly if a high level of risk is identified, but the length of stay in hospital can be considerably reduced by the presence of a home treatment service. Effective community-based crisis services have been slow to develop in the UK, but evidence of best practice is emerging and the target of establishing over 300 crisis resolution teams covering the whole of the country is well underway (Minghella et al 1998, Chisholm & Ford 2004).

Crisis resolution teams embrace an important gatekeeping role to mental health services. Their brief is to work with people experiencing acute episodes of severe mental illness of such severity that without the intervention of the crisis resolution service admission would be necessary. In practice, referrals often span the spectrum of human distress. Effective triage, brief intervention and judicious referrals to other agencies is therefore necessary if home treatment services are not to have most of their energies diverted into helping individuals struggling with less severe emotional crises and the normal miseries of everyday life. This would significantly reduce their capacity to make a difference to the relapse–readmission cycles affecting the most vulnerable and the most at risk.

It is often the fear of being hospitalised, being forcibly medicated, of being sectioned, of the stigma and loss of autonomy associated with being a psychiatric patient that prevents people seeking help in the early stages of a crisis. Crisis plans therefore need to address these issues. Respectful adherence to advance directives, setting out how an individual would like their care managed in the event of a further breakdown in their mental health, can encourage people to become proactive in the event of early relapse signs.

Crisis management

The immediate task in crisis management is to intervene in a way that brings a sense of safety and containment to the situation and reduces the level of distress. People caught up in escalating distress often feel troubled, helpless and out of control. It is important to act calmly, to listen, and to be a supportive presence. If people are not too disturbed by an experience of a confused and threatening reality, or too sunk in despair or too fearful and agitated, it is usually possible to engage them in conversation about their distress. As they begin to talk about their experience, the flow of words carries and dissipates some of the emotional pain and tension. The cathartic expression of feeling in appropriate ways can be experienced as a release and a relief. Being heard in an empathic way anchors the client psychologically in calmer waters and reconnects them with a consensual reality. Where people are too distracted by their distress or too sunk in their despair to engage in conversation, it is important to try and be an undemanding compassionate presence, leaving people feeling cared for and held psychologically. The available level of support and the assessed risk will determine whether an admission is necessary.

An early discussion of a person's medication needs will usually be necessary. People will have strong feelings based on previous experience of medication, so this discussion should be conducted in a way that acknowledges and respects an individual's attitudes and be non-coercive. The desirability of rest and sleep and the relief of anxiety and accumulated tension may be the initial prescribing goal, leaving a discussion of longer-term medication needs until later, when some calm and better cognitive functioning has been restored. People may need practical help with urgent issues such as obtaining benefits or a crisis loan, getting a meal or shopping, contacting power suppliers or topping up a meter card to get heating or lighting restored, liaising with a housing agency where there is a threat to tenancy or helping the client obtain emergency housing. Sometimes there are personal strategies that clients can be encouraged to adopt to bring their attention out of the distress – listening to music, prayer and contemplation, spending time in a place of calm, connecting with nature, exercise, reading inspirational poems or prose, doing simple practical tasks mindfully, being around others who are a calm and accepting presence, curling up on the couch wrapped in a blanket – people will know what works for them.

Often it is the family's need for support that requires some priority. If the relatives' emotional overload can be relieved, then some of the helplessness, fearfulness and exasperation that build up as a crisis deepens can be dissipated. They are then able to be a more supportive and restorative presence for the client. The accessibility and availability of the crisis resolution service is a major factor in achieving this, as is information, advice and emotional support. Increasing the flow of positive emotional energy into the family dynamic and reducing the negative undercurrents will be significant in mitigating the crisis. Of course there are often more intractable issues in family relationships which impact on mental health and these can be the focus for longer-term family work once the immediate crisis has been resolved. Much of the above could also be applied to staff teams in supported housing projects who can be significant sources of support to individuals in the recovery of their equilibrium given an accessible, available crisis resolution team.

Once some of the intensity has diminished, it is possible to engage people in problem-solving in relation to events surrounding the crisis. Gerard Egan's problem management model of helping (Egan 2006) discussed in Chapter 11 offers a framework for approaching this task in a systematic way. Within the context of a problem-solving process, it may be possible for people to take some action to change the circumstances that have led to the development of the crisis. Secondly, it may be possible for them to perceive the situation differently so that it becomes less problematic. Finally, clients may be able to change their reaction to events so that these become less distressing (Box 5.2). Through engaging in supported problem-solving to manage the challenges of everyday living, clients gradually internalise this skill and learn to be more resourceful and less crisis prone.

Of crucial importance in the management of a crisis is the level of social support to which a person has access. The recurrent and disturbing nature of a severely troubled state of mind results in many people becoming isolated from the broad stream of social life and lacking the emotional and practical support of

---

Box 5.2

Crisis management: strategies for changing

The situation
Noticing and reducing the influence of triggers; supported problem-solving; practical help with pressing social issues; conflict management; family work and carer support; solution-focused interventions; mobilising social support; accessible/available professional support; respite care; inpatient care.

The perception
Re-evaluation of experience through cognitive strategies and other therapeutic approaches; contextualising distress; crisis as a living–learning experience; information/education; encouraging realistic hopefulness; encouraging a sense of mastery over the challenges of living; encouraging a sense of being grounded in reality.

The reaction
Early signs monitoring and early intervention; coping strategies enhancement; response inhibition and wise action; verbalising concerns and appropriately discharging feelings; relaxation techniques; mindfulness; reconnecting with nature; religious support and spiritual sustenance; complementary therapies; medication; self-soothing; restorative self-care; risk management; defusing aggression.

---

family and friends. Many become attached to professional helpers as their main source of support. A therapeutic system forms within which a service user seeks to meet their dependency needs. Like family systems, therapeutic systems may not always provide an emotional climate that is conducive to recovery and wellbeing. It may, for example, hold the individual in a 'sick role' or 'victim role' if support is given in an intrusive, imposing way, or given conditionally and critically. These are the dynamics that can replicate the high emotional expression often seen in families and known to increase the incidence of relapse (Tatton & Tarrier 2000). The system then becomes part of the problem rather than the solution.

 Justine's story

Justine is a 35-year-old British-born African-Caribbean woman who has been referred to the acute psychiatric inpatient services on eighteen occasions over the past 15 years. The usual scenario is that she becomes increasingly excitable and caught up in web of unusual thoughts both of an egotistical and persecutory nature. Before too long there is a hostile confrontation with a member of the public, the police become involved and she is admitted under a section of the Mental Health Act. Admission is resented and resisted and usually exacerbates Justine's distress and delusional thinking. She frequently refuses antipsychotic drugs and because of her highly aroused hostile behaviour is given her medication by injection. After about a week Justine is usually more composed and less immersed in her delusional world, although she remains volatile and very sensitive to the behaviour of staff towards her. Periods of admission have lasted between 3 weeks and 3 months, during which time Justine becomes a subdued and compliant figure.

Continued

41

Justine's story—cont'd

Justine is divorced and has a child who lives with her ex-husband and his wife. She has not held a job for 10 years and lives by herself in a council flat. Her main source of support is her mother. Unfortunately this support takes an unhelpful form when Justine is unwell. She sees her daughter's behaviour as 'the devil having hold of her tongue' and has on occasions brought members of her local Pentecostal church to visit Justine to 'heal her through prayer'. Justine does not share her mother's faith and finds these healing invocations upsetting. She is desperate for another relationship and often she has become involved in sexually and financially exploitative relationships with men she has picked up in local pubs and clubs.

Justine has a negative view of herself, both as a person and as a woman. She often feels isolated and lonely and excluded from the mainstream of life. She feels stigmatised by her psychiatric history and as a consequence is not very receptive to the idea of becoming a member of a local resource centre for people with long-term mental health problems. She does have frequent contact with a CPN and a support worker who also has an African-Caribbean background. It is her frequent ruminations on what's missing from her life and her frustrated attempts to claim an ordinary life for herself that seem to precipitate a crisis spiral. An early sign is that she expresses more dissatisfaction and despondency with herself and her life and becomes irritable and is easily angered. She then rapidly spirals from a low mood into excitable chaotic behaviour and before long delusional beliefs begin to emerge. She believes that she is a reincarnation of an African princess and that her daughter is also of royal blood. She says she has been reborn in exile to be safe from 'all the killing' and that she receives messages in news reports on television. Often she will behave unwisely, giving all her clothes and belongings to Oxfam or buying expensive jewellery for her daughter.

The staff team involved in Justine's care have established a crisis plan with her in an attempt to minimise the distress and disruption of crisis episodes and reduce the need for such frequent admissions. Justine held a copy of this plan.

Crisis plan
- Be aware of early signs.
- Increase support. Daily contacts shared between CPN, a member of the crisis resolution team and support worker.
- Work on here-and-now feelings and frustrations, including gender and ethnicity issues.
- Strengthen self-esteem/feel more positive about myself/make use of personal history book.
- Hold on to hopefulness.
- Avoid demanding, over-stimulating social situations/precipitating events.
- Get appropriate support from mother.
- Make use of self-coping strategies.
- Increase medication.

If feeling more troubled, excitable and delusional I would prefer the following plan to be implemented:

- Seek bed in The Willows (crisis house).
- Engage in quiet activity with staff.

- Frequent opportunity for conversation with staff, focusing on here-and-now feelings and frustrations.
- Opportunity to talk about my unusual beliefs and minimise adverse consequences or unwise action associated with those beliefs.
- Aromatherapy massage.
- Art therapy.
- Maintain medication programme.
- Learn from the crisis experience, incorporate learning into my repertoire of coping skills.

Early intervention

Early intervention in first-episode psychosis has emerged in recent years as being of paramount importance in the recovery process. It is not uncommon for people to experience emotional and behavioural difficulties which are the precursors of a more serious breakdown for up to 5 years before those difficulties develop into the turmoil of psychosis (Johannesson 2004). Even then, the severity and nature of a young person's distress – we are principally talking about the 16–25 age group – can sometimes go unrecognised for a further 1–2 years before an appropriate psychiatric intervention is offered. It is important that a compassionate, recovery-oriented intervention is available and accessible in the prodromal phase or early in the psychotic phase of a person's breakdown because of what Birchwood et al (1998) have referred to as a 'critical window' for maximising the potential for full recovery. The longer psychosis remains untreated, the more entrenched and skewed an individual's self view and world view become and the more dysfunctional their behaviour.

Effective intervention at an early stage can reduce the risk of psychosis occurring (Falloon 1992, McGowry et al 2002) and where a transition to a psychotic episode has already taken place, can reduce the likelihood of further relapses (Power et al 1998). It is not only an improvement in prognosis that makes early detection and intervention an imperative but also because there is a resultant decrease in the risk of suicides, the majority of which take place in the first 6 years following the onset of psychosis (Mortenson & Juel 1993), and other damaging behaviours such as substance abuse.

What is involved in a compassionate, recovery-oriented intervention in first-episode psychosis? While a 'best practice' regime has yet to emerge from current research, some strong pointers to what is effective have come from the first wave of early intervention programmes. Most advocate an approach which combines an intensive case management model with low dose antipsychotic medication (Falloon et al 1998). The cornerstone of the approach is the development of a therapeutic relationship between the case manager and the client, a process which takes place within the client's familiar social world. Through this relationship an enormous amount of psychosocial support can be provided. Work on 'triggers', 'relapse signatures' and 'coping strategies' can take place and access to other interventions and services which the client may need to recover and pursue their personal goals can be facilitated. Interventions and services that have been shown to have an influence on recovery and relapse prevention are psychotherapeutic interventions (Gleeson et al 2003), psycho-educational family work (Mullen et al 2002), and access to vocational training or educational opportunities. Engagement with services needs to be sustained over at least 2 years (Birchwood et al 1998).

A study by O'Toole et al (2004) looked at service users' perspectives on the treatment they received from an early intervention team in the London Borough of Southwark. What emerged strongly was the importance of the person-centred relationship that developed between mental health workers and clients in the recovery process. Clients valued the availability of their case managers, felt respected, cared for, listened to and understood. They were involved in treatment decisions, actively supported in structuring their day and helped in getting their lives 'back on track'. Also seen as important was the mediation work with families.

The strong working alliance with case managers and other members of the team is undoubtedly experienced as a formative relationship during a period in individuals' lives when they feel lost, overwhelmed, confused and frightened. Through these relationships people are able to come to some understanding of their psychological crisis, are able to find themselves and reconnect in positive ways with the social fabric of their lives. Johannesson (2004), commenting on developments in early intervention services, underlines the importance of the therapeutic relationship in the following observation:

> We meet people who suffer the deepest possible anxiety, the deepest despair and depression that any human can experience. And we, being therapists, find that in this place before the psychosis and psychotic way of reasoning has tightened its grip, it is easier to talk, easier to relate and easier to re-establish a normal psychological pattern. We see that the social consequences are less devastating, the suffering person has better insight, and the families and social network are better preserved. (p. 331)

Working with risk

6

Risk assessment and management is rightly high on the agenda of mental health services. The National Service Framework for Mental Health (Department of Health 1999a) identifies service standards in which risk reduction is a core theme. The continuing problem of caring for at-risk clients has been the subject of an extensive inquiry into homicide and suicide (Department of Health 1999c). The inquiry points to inadequate communication and liaison between the various agencies involved; inadequacies in gathering a full, accurate, verified history; Section 117 aftercare procedures not being closely followed; a failure to adopt an assertive outreach approach to the delivery of care, or respond to early warning signs of a relapse; and, last but not least, a neglect of the rule that the best predictor of future behaviour is past behaviour. The result is the inadequate delivery of care to individuals involved, with the inevitable tragic consequences. While all risk will never be eliminated in mental health care, there is clearly a need for continuing scrutiny of risk protocols and for all front-line staff to have regular training in risk assessment and management. Clients, their families and the community have a right to expect the minimisation of risk through 'safe, sound and supportive care' (Department of Health 1999b).

Risk is generally defined as the likelihood of an adverse event happening. In a psychiatric context it refers to:

- harm to others
- harm to self
- neglect of self
- exploitation by others.

Not all risk should be considered adverse. Change and development is not possible if some risk is not accepted as a necessary part of living. As Joseph Berke puts it, 'Risk is part of life. No risk no life!'. Berke (2003) argues that there are dangers in systematic risk assessment: being identified as someone 'at risk' or who is 'a risk' can become another stigmatising label. It often takes risk behaviour out of its psychosocial context, linking it too readily with pathology. All too easily being assessed as 'a risk' becomes a basis for restrictive care and social control and once such a definitive assessment is arrived at, it sticks and can be very difficult to lose. Judi Chamberlin, a leading voice in the consumer/survivor movement, argues that noncompliance is a necessary element in empowerment and recovery (Chamberlin 1999a). To reclaim sovereignty over your life, to determine what is helpful and healing, to choose how to live and what personal goals to pursue is to assert the right to be at risk and to reject a life of acquiescence to a powerful social system. Similarly

Patricia Deegan, another prominent figure in the consumer/survivor movement, regards the dignity of risk as being a value that underpins all care that is truly therapeutic. She exhorts mental health professionals to 'embrace the dignity of risk and the right to failure if they are to be supportive of us' (Deegan 1996).

However, in a climate of criticism and blame, mental health services tend to retreat into defensive practice. While many practitioners embrace the humanistic philosophy of care, central to which is the right of the client to self-determination and the dignity of risk, in the prevailing climate in which provider organisations are wary of litigation and public censure, there is a very real danger of overly cautious, restrictive care practices being adopted.

O'Rourke & Bird (2001) draw attention to the fact that for most service users with severe and enduring mental health problems the community poses a bigger threat to them than they do to themselves or to others. Many service users experience:

- abuse and hostility from the public
- sexual abuse and exploitation
- domestic violence
- homelessness
- poverty
- social exclusion, isolation and loneliness
- financial exploitation
- iatrogenic harm
- unmonitored relapse
- lack of socially valued occupational/recreational opportunities
- avoidable and stigmatising involvement with the police and criminal justice system.

Assessment of risk is a continuous process. The daily care of clients involves making choices and decisions that will involve some element of risk. Risk assessment should be explicitly open and always involve the client and carers. For some individuals, particularly those who have a known history of risk behaviour or whose history reveals significant risk factors (see Boxes 6.1, 6.2 and 6.3), a more systematic assessment might be required. This may be carried out and repeated as part of a care programme approach under Section 117 of the Mental Health Act.

Box 6.1

Risk factors for aggression and violence

- A previous history of violence
- A diagnosis of schizophrenia with paranoid features
- Signs of a relapse
- Presence of positive symptoms such as delusions of persecution and command hallucinations
- Outbursts of anger
- Drug and/or alcohol misuse
- Deterioration in social/family relationships
- Threats of violence/declared intentions

- Loss of contact with the mental health services
- Non-adherence to medication programme
- Developmental history of exposure to aggression and violence
- Cultural values in relation to aggression and violent acts
- Failure to learn to delay gratification of wants
- Inability to cope with frustration and conflicts
- Failure to learn alternative strategies, other than aggression
- Unresolved conflicts
- Impulsive behaviour
- Antipathy and hostility towards authority
- Preoccupation with violent fantasies
- Denial of aggressive behaviour
- Lack of remorse

Adapted from Morgan (1998).

Self-enquiry box

You may find it helpful to reflect on a client that you are currently working with, who has a history of exhibiting aggressive or violent behaviour, who may or may not have been involved in a formal risk assessment.

Identify how many of the risk factors outlined above apply to this person. Are there others not listed?

If it seems appropriate, discuss with the person concerned their experience of managing their aggressive and violent tendencies. The following questions are offered as a guide but you will probably want to reframe them to suit your own conversational style and the client involved.

'Are there times now, or have there been in the past, when you've had thoughts of harming others?'

'How often do you have such thoughts?'

'Have there been occasions when you've acted on those thoughts?'

'What did you do?'

'What happened to the person involved?'

'What's prevented you from acting on those thoughts?'

'Have the police ever been involved?'

'Are there certain situations in which you find yourself becoming angry and have an impulse to behave aggressively or violently?'

'When was the last time? Could you describe what happened?'

'What is it about those situations that causes you to react in that way?'

'Had you been drinking or taking drugs at the time?'

'Have there been times when you've reacted differently?'

'Could you imagine yourself dealing with that situation differently, dealing with your feelings without behaving aggressively or violently?'

'On a scale of 1–10, how worried should I be about you harming others over the next week?'

A more immediate assessment of risk will of course be necessary when a client is in an aroused and hostile state of mind. The degree of arousal and control can be assessed from the client's non-verbal behaviour such as muscular tension, agitation, invading personal space, hostile silence or loud aggressive tone of speech and from verbal threats, abusive language and destructive acts to property. They may or may not be responsive to defusing calming interventions. This should be seen as an early indication of the likely course of events, either towards regaining composure or towards an escalation of hostility. This latter scenario, particularly if in conjunction with some of the above risk factors, would signify a challenging situation in which there was potentially an immediate risk to the safety of others.

Dealing with anger and hostile behaviour

- Acknowledge the person's anger and the right to their feelings.
- Allow the expression of anger in appropriate safe ways – verbalising anger, discharge of anger in non-destructive acts. Anger is self-limiting unless re-stimulated.
- Try and stay calm (use self-coaching and relaxation techniques). Provide psychological containment. Stay in the 'same gear', avoid any tendency to retaliate or appease.
- Be aware of your body language. Try not to communicate threatening non-verbal signals.
- Don't try to defend the situation or individuals the person is angry about.
- Avoid a struggle of wills, somebody has to lose. Look for compromise.
- Be aware of power issues in the helping relationship and a person's need to rebel, or the need to reclaim power and assert autonomy.
- Set limits. Encourage self-restraint. Raise awareness of response cost.
- Help the person explore the immediate cause of their anger.
- Help the client to engage in problem-solving. Be clear about what you can and cannot do.
- Accept that some anger may be projected or displaced onto you.
- Don't take unnecessary risks. Be aware of the indicators of high risk. If a person's anger is not subsiding but is in danger of escalating into destructive or violent acts, take whatever action is necessary to protect yourself and others.
- Debrief with colleagues after the incident. Decide if you need any additional support.

High profile cases of homicide involving people with a known history of severe mental health problems, such as the cases of Christopher Clunis and Jason Mitchell, set loose an unreasonable fear in the consciousness of the general public. This is reinforced by the way the media tend to sensationalise such tragic incidents with lurid headlines. The reality is that only 14% of people convicted of homicide have symptoms of mental illness at the time of their offence, a rate that has been decreasing since community care gathered momentum in the UK (O'Rourke & Bird 2001).

The National Suicide Prevention Strategy (2002) sets out an action plan for reaching the government's target of reducing death by suicide by 20% by the year 2010. At present there are around 5000 deaths every year in UK. It targets known high-risk groups such as those in current contact or who have had recent contact with mental health services – 24% of all suicides have been in recent contact with services. Also targeted are young men, who account for 1300 deaths per year, and those with a history of self-harm – 1180 people take their own life in the year following a self-harm incident (National Suicide Prevention Strategy 2002). It further aims to promote the mental health of the wider population, focusing on the misuse of drugs and alcohol; social exclusion and deprivation; the adverse social experience of black and ethnic minority groups; and the mental wellbeing of children and young people, women during and after pregnancy and the older population. Beyond these goals the National Strategy encompasses proposals for reducing the lethality and availability of suicide methods; encouraging more responsible reporting of suicides in the press and promoting research on suicide and its prevention. Many of these strategies are now in place, such as an enhanced care programme approach for all those with severe mental health problems and a history of self-harm, a care programme that addresses social needs and sets out a contingency plan for crises. Crisis resolution teams, triage services and assertive outreach teams are now established in most areas, making 24/7 care more available.

While it is to be hoped that the proposed prevention strategies when fully implemented will lead to a significant reduction in the tragic loss of life through suicide, my fear is that it is tinkering at the edges and that it is in the social sphere of life

Box 6.2

Risk factors for suicide

- Gender (more females attempt, more males succeed)
- Age – higher rates with increasing age
- Cultural component (Asian women, young males)
- Marital status (higher in single, widowed, separated, divorced)
- Strength of emotional ties with others
- Unemployment
- Family history of suicide
- Limited social support system
- Experience of social exclusion/sense of alienation
- Recent problematic life events
- History of previous suicide attempts or self-harm
- Diagnosis of depression, manic depressive disorder, or schizophrenia
- Serious or terminal physical illness
- Alcohol and/or drug misuse
- Sleep disorder
- Expressed intent
- Evidence of planning
- Evidence of preparation
- Access to the means
- Recovery phase in severe depression
- Recent discharge from hospital
- Expression of hopelessness
- Disengagement from services and not being open to emotional support
- Feeling pessimistic about recovery

Adapted from Morgan (1998).

that most can be achieved. As Camus (1955) powerfully argues in his reflection on suicide, we need a reason to live. As a society we must do something to reduce the alienated, excluded, disaffected, meaningless state of being that is the predominant experience of so many people. Only then will we prevent a significant number choosing a state of nothingness or the hope of transcendent peace in an afterlife, to continued meaninglessness.

There is an important distinction between suicidal behaviour and self-harm behaviour. In the latter the motivation is other than the wish to die, although it is true that some people who self-harm seem ambivalent about the outcome or unconcerned about the consequences. Self-harm behaviour is a coping strategy – albeit a damaging and potentially dangerous one, a means of gaining some relief from distress. Often what underlies self-harm behaviour is the desire to punish self or others, to draw attention to psychological pain or to gain relief from emotional tension. People who self-harm often experience antipathy, if not openly critical and judgemental attitudes, from professional helpers, who see their often repeated acts of self-injury as consciously manipulative and attention seeking. Self-mutilation and self-poisoning produce strong emotional reactions in professional helpers. Staff may feel baffled, helpless, let down, guilty, angry, horrified, fearful and sad in response to an individual's persistent self-harm. Once established as a distress relief pattern, some forms of self-harm, such as cutting, can be a difficult habit to break. Until some other strategy for coping with the emotional pain is found or the underlying emotional issues or current problems are less pressing, self-harm remains for many clients a means of survival or, as Arnold (1995) puts it, 'a way of bearing what would otherwise be unbearable'.

Box 6.3

Risk factors in people who self-harm

- Age: more likely in young people (15–25)
- Gender: women twice as likely as men to self-harm
- Social deprivation
- Emotional discord in significant relationships
- Previous history of acts of self-harm
- Drug and/or alcohol misuse
- Sexual abuse in childhood
- Emotional or physical abuse
- Parental neglect
- Parental loss
- Rape or sexual abuse as an adult
- Domestic violence
- Lack of emotionally supportive relationships
- Loss of a child or inability to have children
- Emotional overwhelm
- Self-hatred/low self-esteem
- Intense feelings of anger/anxiety
- Powerlessness
- Neediness
- Dissociation/numbness/experience of unreality

Source: Arnold (1995).

Self-enquiry box

You may find it helpful to reflect on a client you are currently working with who has:

a history of attempted suicide or is considered to be at risk

or

a history of self-harm behaviour.

Identify how many of the risk factors outlined above apply to this person. Are there others not listed?

If it seems appropriate, discuss with the person concerned their experience of feeling suicidal or their need to self-harm and the way they express or manage those tendencies. The following questions are offered as a guide but you will probably want to reframe them to suit your own conversational style and the client concerned.

'Have you harmed yourself/attempted to end your life at any time in the past?'

'How do you feel about what happened?'

'Do you have thoughts of harming yourself/ending your life now?'

'Have you thought about how you might do that?'

'Do you have the means to do that?'

'When you think about harming yourself/ending your life, do you consider doing it where you won't be discovered?'

'How often do you have these thoughts?'

'What's stopped you acting on these thoughts?'

'On a scale of 1–10 how likely is it that you will end your life?'

'Have there been times recently when you've felt it's worth carrying on living?'

'Could you describe the feeling you get when you experience a need to self-harm?'

'If you could draw it/paint it what would it look like?'

'When you experience this need to harm yourself are you able to resist it?'

'Are you aware of the risks you take when you self-harm?'

'What's the feeling you get after you've harmed yourself?'

'Do you talk about these thoughts to anyone?'

'Do you know why you feel like harming yourself/ending your life?'

'On a scale of 1–10 how bad are these problems that make you want to end your life?'

'Are there other ways of getting relief/some peace without ending your life?'

'What's helped you to keep on keeping on till now, despite it being so bad?'

'What was happening in your life when these thoughts started?'

'What would you do if these thoughts of harming yourself/ending your life recurred?'

'On a scale of 1–10 with 10 being very concerned and 1 being no concern at all, how concerned should I be about you harming yourself/attempting to end your life over the next 24 hours?'

'How realistic is it of me to expect you to stay safe over the weekend?'

'On a scale of 1–10 where 10 is feeling very safe, what would that look like?

'Who would be around? What would be happening?'

⭐ **Annie's story**

Theme: Managing the risk of suicide

Annie is a woman aged 43 who has a history of depression and who has recently attempted suicide by asphyxiation with a neck ligature. She is divorced and lives with her two children, a boy aged 20 and a girl aged 17. Six months ago her mother died.

Shirley is a CPN working with a crisis service and has been caring for Annie since her discharge from the acute admission ward 2 weeks ago.

Annie

I'd been depressed on and off for about 10 years. More or less since I left my husband. I didn't have a very happy marriage. He used to drink a lot and knock me about and half strangle me. I thought that I would feel a lot better about my life and myself after I left him. I've been on all sorts of antidepressants but they haven't really lifted my depression, just stopped me feeling so desperate. Depression is difficult to explain. Most of the time it's like living in shadow – you can never find a place in the sun. But sometimes the shadows seem to darken and you feel as if you've done something terribly wrong and something dreadful is going to happen to you. Once before when I felt that way, I took an overdose but more to get some relief than anything else. A few weeks ago my daughter said to me, 'You're such a drudge Mum, when are you going to get a life?'. It sort of hit me how bleak and empty my life had become. I suppose I'm afraid of life. I tend to see disasters behind every door. So I don't open any, don't take any risks. About a week before this happened I was staring at myself in the mirror and I heard my mother's voice saying, 'You'll never amount to anything. Get out of my sight'. I was frightened that I was going mad. After that I couldn't get this thought out of my head that I should get out of everybody's sight. I thought it all out. I picked a night when my children were out and wouldn't be back till late and wouldn't miss me until the morning, then drove to the coast. I knew I wanted to die by the sea.

Shirley

I've known Annie about 2 weeks now. She was discharged from hospital after 10 days' close observation. There are some risks and I am quite concerned about her safety, but her experience of hospital was not particularly helpful in reducing her distress. What helps me to deal with my anxiety about her care is being clear about my responsibilities and having the support and involvement of the multidisciplinary crisis team. She is still quite depressed and some days feels unable to go on. We have given her quite a bit of responsibility for herself. I assess the level of risk regularly and trust her to be open with me about her suicidal thoughts. I ask her how concerned I should be about her during the next 24 hours and how safe she feels. I'm getting to know when she's having a bad day, her face has this haunted look and her voice loses its power and becomes almost a whisper. I'm meeting with her four days a week at the moment. We also have an arrangement where she will phone the service if she's feeling at risk and I or someone will call and spend some time with her, or talk on the phone, then if she is still feeling unsafe she goes to a friend's house or to Beacon House (crisis house). We've also been looking at ways of managing her bad days so that she's not so vulnerable to her depressive thoughts and feelings. I think she was shocked by the frightened, angry reaction of her children to her suicide attempt. She feels guilty about upsetting her children so much and not wanting to put them through that again has given her a reason to go on living at the moment. The children are still quite angry with her and some of my work has involved helping them deal with their feelings and help them not to feel burdened by responsibility for their mother's safety. Also I think it has been a relief to be able to talk about some of the here-and-now difficulties in her life and I sense she is beginning to feel a little more hopeful about the future, perhaps seeing this crisis as a turning point. I've begun to engage her in some problem-solving around her relationship with her children. Also there were some house repairs that needed urgent attention and were a worry and I've been able to help her arrange for those to be done. Annie has experienced a lot of trauma in her life. Her mother wasn't able to give her much affection or approval and was quite harsh with Annie because of her enuresis, sometimes shutting her in the cupboard under the stairs as a punishment. Annie's also had a violent marriage which further undermined her self-esteem. She has agreed to explore some of these earlier traumas with a clinical psychologist. She has shown a lot of courage in her life – leaving her husband, bringing up the children by herself, and I'm hopeful she will be able to draw on this resolve in overcoming her depression.

Responding to self-harm and suicidal behaviour

Managing risk in the care of suicidal or self-harm clients is not just about intervening in restrictive, controlling ways in an attempt to eliminate opportunities. Sometimes strategies that rely too heavily on observation and control paradoxically increase the risk. A depressed and suicidal person's sense of worthlessness and hopelessness may be increased by a care regime that emphasises close or continuous observation but neglects pressing psychosocial needs. Self-harm clients may take greater risks in harming themselves if their need to self-harm safely, in the absence of more constructive strategies for dealing with emotional tension, is not recognised. It is not possible to eliminate all risk even in a hospital setting. Ultimately service users carry responsibility for their own decisions and actions. Engaging service users in collaborative assessment and care planning can open up the opportunity for 'positive risk-taking' (Morgan 2004b). This is not the negligent avoidance of professional responsibility for providing directive and restrictive care where a person is unsafe. It is care that respects the dignity of risk and the rights and responsibilities of individuals to confront the problems of living and to face the reality of human suffering within a supportive therapeutic system. Strategies that promote positive risk-taking include:

- Engage in an open exploration of suicidal ideas – the frequency, intrusiveness, planning and motivation.
- Assess risk factors.
- Be present with clients in calm, accepting, empathic ways.

53

- Engage in therapeutic conversation that facilitates the safe discharge of distress and the identification of underlying issues and concerns.
- Recognise the opportunity for learning, growth and change in the crisis experience.
- Work collaboratively with at-risk clients and their family/carer in assessing needs and planning care.
- Negotiate a risk minimisation plan with the client and their family/carer.
- Be clear about a person's responsibility for his or her own safety within the context of the plan.
- Accept that in the short term some self-harm may continue and a more immediate and realistic objective is minimal risk.
- Communicate the plan to all workers involved.
- Be clear about the availability of support when a person feels unsafe and the boundaries that apply.
- Mobilise social support.
- Engaging in problem-solving with clients.
- Help maximise clients' constructive coping strategies and develop others.
- Instil hope and realistic optimism.
- Be aware of your responsibility and accountability as a professional practitioner.
- Make use of support systems, supervision and training opportunities to maintain aware and responsive care.

Working with clients who represent a risk to themselves or others in positive risk-taking ways is challenging and anxiety provoking. To practise confidently, particularly within a culture of blame and litigation, requires a cohesive framework of accountability, responsibility and support, linking practitioner, multidisciplinary team and organisation. Where this is inadequately defined, defensive practice is likely to flourish.

A person-centred approach to assessment

7

By person-centred assessment, I mean gathering information and understandings about a client's inner and outer worlds from their frame of reference. It should as far as possible be a collaborative process in which the helper and client try to identify what's going on and what's going wrong (and right too). As Egan (2006) puts it, it involves helping clients

> see what they don't see and need to see to make sense of their chaotic behaviour – all in the service of helping them manage their lives more effectively. (p. 143)

Although an assessment interview may be a discrete event, building a picture of a client's world, their problems of living, their needs, their strengths, talents and resources, is often a continuing process that is interwoven with the process of recovery/change. Assessment rightly takes a holistic approach to understanding distress. How could we understand how someone has become sunk in despair, or a prisoner of their fears, or persecuted by voices unless we were prepared to be a compassionate presence in their search for meaning in the psychological, social, spiritual and bodily dimensions of their experience? But we need to approach this task with humility. To think that through an assessment process we could come to 'know' a person in all their complexity would be disrespectful arrogance. At best we can through our conversations and our developing relationship come to some shared understanding about their experience of suffering and the help they need.

There has in recent years been some recognition of the value of a strengths-oriented assessment process in mental health care (Ryan & Morgan 2004). Assessment that dwells too narrowly on an individual's problem-filled story is disempowering and undermines self-esteem and hopefulness. It can be much more helpful to focus on strengths, skills, talents, resources, opportunities and aspirations than on problems, deficits and disabilities. Recovery is not about regaining a problem-free life – whose life is? It is about living life more resourcefully, living a satisfying and contributing life, in spite of limitations caused by a continuing vulnerability to disabling distress. Unless we see a person's strengths, qualities, talents, it is difficult to value them as individuals. The way we think about them and talk about them will have a negative slant. If we can nurture people's abilities, help them make the most of their strengths, support them in their interests and aspirations, they are more likely to be able to develop an identity not dominated by a psychiatric disability and claim an ordinary life for themselves.

Veterans of the psychiatric system often have a lot of interpersonal scarring and present in uncommunicative ways. Their message is 'I've been through all this before and I know what happens if I say too much'. Other clients will readily reveal symptoms, that is express urgent needs in a psychiatric way in an interview with a mental health practitioner as a way of getting their needs met, at least partially. If the response to a person's overwhelmed mental state is a routine psychiatric one: a change in medication, a prescriptive strategy or an admission, with no attempt made to understand the distress pattern, then the experience of distress soon becomes mystified. In a short space of time a person is unable to recognise any connection between their thoughts, feelings and acts and the events in their lives. The further clients get into their psychiatric career, the more difficult it becomes to unravel events past and present that have led to persistent disabilities or current crises (Mosher & Burti 1994).

People seeking help from the mental health services often have complex problems of a personal, interpersonal and social nature – problems of living. They are in contact with the services at times when they are experiencing considerable distress and psychological disturbance. More than anything else they need to engage in a dialogue with practitioners to reach some kind of shared definition of their situation and what should be done about it (Sheppard 1993). Developing a dialogue in which people can *uncover* the problems of living they face, *discover* the meaning of disabling distress and *recover* the personal resources to live well requires the skilled use of what Heron (2001) refers to as catalytic interventions. To my mind one of the most important catalytic skills is the ability to listen and to hear the other person. The experience and therapeutic value of being heard is eloquently captured by Carl Rogers in personal reflection:

> I like being heard. A number of times in my life I have felt myself bursting with insoluble problems, or going round and round in tormented circles or, during one period being overcome by feelings of worthlessness and despair. I think I have been more fortunate than most in finding, at these times, individuals who have been able to hear me and thus rescue me from the chaos of my feelings, individuals who have been able to hear my meanings a little more deeply than I have known them. These persons have heard me without judging me, diagnosing me or evaluating me. They have just listened and clarified and responded to me at all the levels at which I was communicating. I can testify that when you are in psychological distress and someone really hears you without passing judgement on you, without trying to take responsibility for you, without trying to mould you, it feels damn good! At these times it has relaxed the tension in me. It has permitted me to bring out the frightening feelings, the guilt, the despair, the confusions that have been part of the experience. When I have been listened to and have been heard, I am able to perceive my world in a new way and go on. It is astonishing how elements that seem insoluble become soluble when someone listens, how confusions that seem irremediable turn into relatively clear flowing streams when one is heard. I have deeply appreciated the times that I have experienced this sensitive, empathic, concentrated listening of being heard. (Rogers 1980, p. 12)

To listen well we need to have our attention free. This can so easily get caught up in our own needs and concerns or be difficult to sustain because our energy is low. We sometimes need to prepare ourselves to listen – to let go of other things and refocus our attention. I want to listen in an open way not evaluating what the client says according to my own values; not trying to apply diagnostic criteria to their experience but trying to understand it from their frame of reference. I want to try and be present with people in as relaxed and receptive way as I can. I want to tune into the fullness of their experience and this means being receptive to what is communicated through non-verbal channels as well as linguistically. In other words, tuning in to what's not being said. It can be difficult to verbalise experience sometimes; everything seems confused or threatening, and the client takes refuge from the reality of their situation behind a wall of inconsequential disclosures or withdrawal. Even though someone may say very little, their body language can communicate volumes. Emotional experience may be denied verbally, but leaks out authentically in expression, posture, movement and tone of voice.

Suggestions for improving listening

- Listening is hard work. It requires energy. It requires a commitment to listen well. It's difficult to listen if you are tired or if your own needs are pressing. Know what your limits are.
- Get physically prepared to listen. Make the environment as conducive as possible. Be aware of proximity and barriers. Check your body cues.
- Get mentally prepared to listen. Acknowledge distractions, personal or professional, put them to one side for attention later. Try and be aware of any assumptions, prejudice, stereotyping in relation to the client. Remind yourself that this is the client's time.
- Try and hold back on questions, interpretations, giving information and advice. Use a mental banking system of points to come back to. Trust yourself to ask the right question or find the right response, don't try and frame it while the client is talking. Be aware of the quality of silent interludes; wait receptively if they seem meaningful to the client.
- Try to avoid blocking tactics. 'I don't think I'm the best person to talk to'; 'I can't talk now, come and see me later'; 'Try not to worry about it'. Of course at times responding in these ways can be quite legitimate. Other blocking tactics include selective listening – hearing only what we want to hear; controlling the agenda by asking a series of questions; changing the subject; and using non-verbal cues to block the conversation.

There are a number of other catalytic interventions that are valuable in building a helping dialogue. The two that I intend to briefly focus on are questions and reflections. People suffering serious psychiatric disorders may often experience what Perkins & Repper (1996) refer to as 'cognitive overload'. It can be difficult for people to process and make sense of experience, which may be communicated to others in vague, confused, disconnected, distracted ways. Conversations that are too probing or intense can overload vulnerable people and lead to withdrawal, avoidance, or the exacerbation of acute symptoms. Others may be so sunk in depression they seem difficult to engage with. Others may be troubled and distracted by unusual thoughts or voice hearing. In all these scenarios sensitivity and awareness in the use of these skills is required.

It is usually more appropriate and helpful to ask open questions (see assessment guide below). The client is better able to communicate how they experience their problems and needs and does not feel intimidated by a string of closed questions which are often related to the practitioner's agenda and perception of the presenting problems. Follow-up questions can be used to focus down on specific issues. They may be concerned with getting clarity – 'You seem to be saying that facing the day seems so difficult that you give up. Is that how it is?'. They may be used to encourage people to say more – 'So you say that in the past when you felt bad you coped better. How did you do that?'. Follow-up questions can be used to encourage the client to reconsider some aspect of their experience – 'You say you used to enjoy things but you can't now. How do you know?'. A further way in which follow-up questions are commonly used is to identify the relevance of something that's said –'You said earlier that people never listen, never take you seriously. I'm wondering if you feel you have to threaten to do something worrying before anyone will listen?'. Probes may also be non-verbal, as when we use an expression or gesture to encourage someone to say more, or they can also take the form of minimal verbal prompts. We need to be aware that there is often concern in the minds of people about how what they confide will be seen. 'Will they think I'm mad, bad or stupid? Will they understand? Will they dislike and disapprove of me? Will they put me in hospital?'

There are a number of disadvantages related to a conversational style that relies too heavily on asking questions. Firstly it tends to locate the power with the practitioner – she decides what's talked about and directs the conversation. Secondly there is a danger that questions can be asked in a routine, unthinking manner and are not responsive to the uniqueness of an individual's experience. A further disadvantage is that people will only reply to what's asked, so that significant areas of the client's experience are not discussed.

It is good practice to develop the ability to respond reflectively in our dialogues with people in care. Reflections involve restating or mirroring back what the client has disclosed of their experience. They involve feeding back what we have heard and understood of what the client has said – the content, and the affective element. We should take care that we are restating in our own words what the client has said and not constructing a reality that doesn't match the client's experience. Discerning the more subtle or suppressed emotional experience of the client can be difficult and the reflection of feeling is best expressed in a tentative way. Used skilfully, reflective responses can communicate a high degree of empathy, identified by Carl Rogers (Mearns amp; Thorne 1999) as a core therapeutic condition.

Being reflective creates a dialogue in which the practitioner is not setting the agenda and directing the flow of the conversation. There is a shared responsibility for what gets talked about. Hargie et al (1994) in a review of the research on reflective interviews conclude that they are likely to result in the development of more positive attitudes towards the practitioner and an increase in the amount and intimacy of the disclosures.

A silence that occurs in conversations between the practitioner and client can be disconcerting for both. It is more acceptable and tolerable where a comfortable, safe relationship has been established. We often feel a need to fill the silence, to say something, anything, to reduce the social anxiety we experience. Silence can have a particular quality. It can be a resentful or angry silence; an anxious distracted silence; a reflective thoughtful silence; an uncertain reticent silence; an evasive guarded silence; a deep despairing silence; an estranged isolated silence; or a submissive deferring silence. It is important to develop sufficient comfort with silences to allow them and assess their meaning. Profound feelings can be expressed in this way. Acceptance of the silence needs to be communicated through a relaxed, attentive body language. Sometimes being quietly with someone who has little energy to talk, or is too distracted by anxiety, or who needs the recuperative sanctuary of silence, can be experienced as extremely supportive. Responding sensitively to silence can lead to important issues, concerns and feelings being shared and discussed. The way we respond will depend on how we assess the silence. For example, 'It seems difficult to continue, almost too painful to talk about', 'My guess is that in your silence you are saying you feel pretty resentful about being here', or simply 'What's on your mind?' may be appropriate.

Assessment guide

The following guide is offered as a way of bringing some structure to your assessment interviews and conversations with clients. You may need to rephrase the questions to fit your conversational style. The structure is holistic and aims to engage clients in an exploratory conversation about the physical, psychological, social and spiritual dimensions of their world in a way that throws some light on their distress, the problems of living they face and the needs they have.

Some of the questions can be quite challenging and should always be asked in a respectful and supportive way. The questions are oriented towards the past, present and future. A frequent criticism of psychiatric interviewing is that it is often 'archaeological', with too much focus on digging up and exploring the past and not enough focus on the challenges of the here and now and pathways towards a preferred future. While insight into 'the past in the present' may be a catalyst for change for some people, for others it offers no solution to their present distress and no solution to their search for a different way of being in the world.

Egan argues that from an early point in our engagement with people we should be looking towards possibilities for change and seeking strategies to bring this about. Often people are already making tentative moves in the direction of desired change, or making use of positive coping strategies to manage their distress although not perhaps fully exploiting them. Bringing this future orientation and solution focus to the conversation instils a sense of hope. Some examples of future- and solution-oriented questions are included in the sections 'Creating a better future' and 'Creating strategies to move forward' in Chapter 11.

Another criticism is that assessments tend to have a medical/symptom orientation or that they tend to be too problem focused. As I have suggested elsewhere, despite the challenge of person-centred and other psychosocial perspectives on human distress, the biomedical model remains dominant in psychiatric practice. Mental health professionals frequently approach assessment from a diagnostic perspective and are principally concerned with identifying the symptoms of, for example, depression, or the positive and negative symptoms of schizophrenia. Assessment will then often become a ritual in which the person's problem-saturated story is retold. What White (1997) calls a 'thin' narrative of a person's lived experience becomes their defining story. The more often it is told, the more the person comes to see himself as a problematic person, living a problematic life.

Assessment should not be symptom focused or problem oriented – although we might engage clients in conversations about those aspects of their experience. Instead it should be person oriented and concerned with understanding their way of being in the world and how that might change in ways that would lead to less suffering. White talks about the need for conversations that bring out the full richness of an individual's lived experiences, not the edited problem-laden versions. This is where assessment and recovery become interwoven in the helping process. As we engage clients in 'thicker' narratives, or other stories of their lived experience, in which their qualities, talents, strengths, achievements, resources are visible, when nurturing, life-enhancing events occurred, a different identity can begin to emerge.

I do not much care for the term assessment. It symbolises for me the power differential in helping relationships, where one person who has the expertise and knowledge assesses a client who has limited or no knowledge of what their distress means and little expertise to help themselves. In the humanistic tradition assessment is not greatly concerned with diagnosis or an analytic interpretation of a client's troubled state of mind; it is more concerned with the client's process and the relationship process. The focus of assessment is on whether a person is able and willing to engage in a process of reflection and growth within and beyond the helping relationship and crucially whether the necessary conditions exist (see Chapter 18) within the dynamic of that relationship for that essential flourishing of the individual to begin and continue (Wilkins 2005). Setting out the structure as a series of questions gives the impression of an interview in which the agenda is set by the practitioner. I visualise it much more as a collaborative dialogue in which the client's story unfolds and is filled out in the context of a developing relationship. Often very few questions need to be asked, if mental health professionals can create a secure base from which the 'territory of distress' can be explored. If we can be an empathic presence, accept a person's reality without trying too hard to explain it, people will return from the territory of their distress having learnt something about themselves and will have begun the process of recovery. It is when experience is explained away according to this or that dogma that seekers of truth about themselves and their lives surrender to passive resignation and the spirit of recovery fades.

An overview of the problem

'Can you say a little about what's been happening to you?'

'What do you feel you need help with?'

'Can you say a little about how you see the problem?'

'What things have been troubling you?'

'How is it affecting you/others?'

'How bad is it? On a scale of 1–10 where 10 is the worst it's ever been, where are you today?'

'How have you been coping? What has helped?'

How has your behaviour changed?

'What's become difficult for you?'

'What would you like to be able to do that you don't do now?'

'What happens when you begin to get depressed/high? What do you first notice? What else?'

'How do you know when you're becoming unwell/becoming troubled again?' 'What do you first notice?'

'What changes have other people noticed in you?'

'What do you notice yourself doing more of the time?'

'Do you find yourself avoiding people/places?'

'Have you noticed any change in your level of interest in things?'

'Do you find yourself doing things because your voices tell you to?'

'Is your behaviour more worrying for you or for others?'

'On a scale of 1–10 where 10 is that you will do anything to overcome this problem and 1 is there's nothing you can do but hope, where would you put yourself?'

'Do you ever have thoughts of harming yourself/killing yourself? How often/how detailed/how persistent?'

'What's stopped you acting on these thoughts?'

'Do you ever have thoughts of harming others? How often/how detailed/how persistent?'

'What's stopped you acting on these thoughts?'

'On a scale of 1–10 how worried should I be about you harming yourself/killing yourself/harming others, over the next week?'

The response to this last series of questions may indicate a need for a further and more detailed risk assessment.

How has your mood changed?

'How have you been feeling?'

'Can you describe the feeling for me?'

'Do you find yourself getting upset easily?'

'Are there times when you feel better?'

'How bad is your anxiety/depression at the moment? On a scale of 1–10 with 10 being the worst, where are you today?'

'How are you managing to cope when it's so bad?'

'What helps when you feel like this?'

'What happens to your anger/sadness/fearfulness?'

'Where in your body do you experience it?'

How have you been affected mentally?

'What concerns you most? What's your worst fear?'

'When you are depressed/anxious in those situations, what are your thoughts?'

'How is your concentration/memory/speed of thought?'

'Do you have thoughts that trouble you?'

'How did you come to believe that? What was happening in your life around the time you first began to think that?'

'What leads you to believe that? What evidence do you have that's what's happening?'

'How sure are you that what you believe to be happening is true? On a scale of 1–10 with 10 being absolute conviction, where would you put yourself?'

'Has anything happened recently that's increased/decreased your conviction?'

'How persistent are these thoughts? Do you find yourself thinking about it most of the time/some of the time/occasionally?'

'How are you affected by these thoughts? How do you feel/react when you get these thoughts?'

'Do you ever have the experience of voices talking to you that others can't hear?'

'What do these voices sound like/what do they say/when do you notice them most/how do they affect you/can you resist them?'

'How do you explain them?'

'How do you react to them?'

How have you been affected physically?

'How do you feel physically?'

'Have you had any physical problems lately? What do you attribute that to?'

'How do you take care of your body?'

'How do you feel about your body?'

'How's your energy?'

'How have you been sleeping? If there were a reason for you to stay awake, what do you think that would be?'

'What dreams have you remembered recently? If that dream had a title, what would it be? What connections do you make with that image in your dream? What feelings were around in the dream? What part of your life do those feelings belong to?'

'How have you been eating?'

'Do you experience any pain/discomfort in any part of you body?'

'When do you experience that? How bad is it on a scale of 1–10?'

'How do you cope with it? What helps? How do others react?'

'If your pain/discomfort was telling you something, what do you think that might be?'

'Allow your attention to focus on the part of your body that experiences pain/ discomfort for a few minutes. What images/thoughts come to mind?'

'Do you have any worries about your sexual relationship. What concerns do you have about your sexual life?'

'Have you been using any recreational drugs lately?'

'In what ways have your prescribed drugs helped? Are you experiencing any troublesome side effects?

How have you been affected socially?

'How are your relationships with your partner/children/parents?'
'Have there been any changes in your family relationships/friendships recently?'
'How have your family relationships/friendships been affected?'
'What relationships are important in your life? How are these relationships?'
'What's good about your life at the moment?'
'What's missing from your life at the moment?'
'What areas of your life need attention/need to change?'
'How do you spend your time/your day?'
'What gives you pleasure/what interests you?'
'How are you managing at work? How is not having a job affecting you?'
'Do you notice any change in the way people are with you?'
'How has your life been affected by having this mental health problem?'
'What's the one single change that would make most difference to your life right now?'
'Who or what makes life difficult for you?'
'How do you feel about talking with someone of the opposite sex/a different sexual orientation/ethnic background?'
'Could you say something about your culture that would help me understand a little more about you?'
'Have you experienced discrimination/prejudice? How has that affected you?'
'What does home mean to you? Do you have that at this point in your life?'

What sort of stresses have you been under recently?

'What changes have taken place in your life recently?'
'What's been difficult in your life lately?'
'What things are a worry at home/work/school?'
'If you could change something in your life right now, what would it be?'
'What was happening in your life when you first began to have problems?'

Does this connect with your family background/personal history?

'Could you say a little about your background – whatever comes to mind?'
'Could you tell me a little about your/father/mother/siblings?'
'Could you tell me a little about your early life?'
'Could you say a little about school/college?'
'Who were the other important figures in your life? Who were your mentors/models as you were growing up?'
'Can you scan back to times when you've felt this way before?'
'If you the child was sitting on that chair now, what would you want to say to him/her?'
'If your father/mother was sitting here right now, what would you want to say?

What in your life do you find inspiring/dispiriting?

'Does your faith play an important part in your life?'

'Is prayer/contemplation/meditation important in your life?'

'What are the things in your life that give it meaning?'

'What sort of experiences have brought you a sense of joy/peace to your life?'

'Are there some things in life that lift you out of the everyday business of living and into a more exalted state of mind?'

'Are there some virtues that are important to you in the way you live your life? How difficult is it to live up to those ethical standards? How are you affected when you don't?'

'Where do you go/what do you do when you want to find a sense of peacefulness?'

'What are some of the things that have happened in your life that have given you a feeling of goodness/when you've experienced a sense of goodness in others?'

What sort of help do you think you need?

'When you've felt like this before, what has helped you most? What else? How has that helped?'

'How do you think I/we could help? How would that help?'

'What would help you most at the moment?'

'What makes it easier for you to cope?'

'Is there anything you can do to help yourself get through this?'

'What is the thing that is most difficult/worrying/distressing/urgent that you would like help with right now?'

'Is there one thing that it would possibly be helpful to work on right now?'

Could you say a little about the good things in your life, the things that are OK?

'What are the things in your life that you get pleasure/satisfaction from?'

'What are some of the things you enjoy/are interested in?'

'What are you good at? What would the person who knows you best say you were good at?'

'What are some of the things that you've done that you are proud of/get a sense of satisfaction from?'

'Who are the people that are important in your life?'

'Who do you turn to if you need help?'

'Have there been times when other people have had to rely on you/when you've helped others out?'

'Tell me about a time in your life when you felt happy/secure?'

'What's the best job you've ever had/what sort of work would you like to do?'

'How do you look after yourself/stay well?'

'How do you relax?'

'What's kept you going through all the difficult times?'

'When things have been difficult for you, what do you do/what do other people do that helps?'

'What are some of your hopes for the future?'

'If you had to overcome these problems, what would your life look like/how would your life be different?'

'If I had met you a few years back, what would I have noticed about you that's different from how you are now?'

'If I was talking to someone who knows you really well/knows all your best qualities/good points, what would they tell me?'

Self-enquiry box

As a general principle we should not ask other people questions we are not prepared to ask ourselves! You may find it interesting to consider the question, 'Which area of my life needs most attention right now?'. Select some relevant questions from the assessment framework (or frame your own) and respond to them.

You may find it useful to use a free associative writing technique in which you allow your answer to emerge in what you write. Try not to deliberate and evaluate, just write. Don't worry about spelling or grammar. Just keep your pen moving and write whatever comes into your mind.

Creating pathways to recovery

8

Recovery is a new watchword that has crept into professional discourse over the past 10 years and is now at the heart of emerging mental health services in the UK (Department of Health 2001a, National Institute for Mental Health in England 2005). It is extraordinary that it has taken psychiatry so long to rediscover recovery, a therapeutic focus lost as the dynamism of social psychiatry during the 1960s petered out. Recovery is still an alien concept to many practitioners (Coleman 1999) and if recovery-oriented services are to be based on more than mere wordplay, a seismic shift in attitudes is required.

Mental health services have created a culture of maintenance rather than recovery, a culture in which people with severe mental health problems can become trapped in a career as a psychiatric patient. An attitude of therapeutic pessimism has developed in relation to working with deeply troubled people. There is an expectation of relapse and increasing disability and a belief that the best one can hope for is symptom control, mediated by medication compliance. The disturbed psyche is still seen primarily as the manifestation of malfunctioning neurones, a state of mind which can only be remedied with expert help and powerful drugs. Distress is seldom contextualised, or if it is, is seen as of peripheral importance in the aetiology of a person's problem. Despite a new era in which 'collaborative care' and the client as 'expert by experience' are acknowledged as the cornerstones on which therapeutic care is built, all too often personal agency and an individual's sovereignty over their life is overridden. Confronted with the power of the psychiatric system it is not surprising that many people turn their faces to the wall. The missing ingredient in so many care and treatment programmes is hope and a belief in the potential of people to change and grow, to become more resourceful human beings, more fully engaged in life. In a culture of maintenance, people are offered supportive services but have little opportunity to engage in a recovery programme which is empowering, enabling and which nurtures their growth as a person. What needs to be recognised is that people are disabled not so much by their vulnerabilities as by the anguish, despair and hopelessness that build up around them (Deegan 1988), by the social discrimination and exclusion they face (Repper & Perkins 2003) and by the iatrogenic impact of psychiatric treatment and care.

Much of the research on recovery from severe and disabling mental health problems has focused on narrowly defined clinical and social recovery. The defining criteria for recovery in these studies are the absence of symptoms for 2 years, no current medication, a socially inclusive lifestyle and evidence of independent living. Using measurable outcomes similar to these, the International Study of Schizophrenia

(Harrison et al 2001), the most substantial long-term study of recovery from psychosis, shows a favourable outcome for over half of all people followed up over a period of 25 years. Interestingly it also provides evidence of late recovery in some people, thus supporting the case for continued therapeutic optimism.

The use of such exacting and objective recovery criteria has been strongly challenged by recovery stories from within the consumer/survivor movement on the grounds that they do not encompass the individual's subjective experience of wellbeing and the recovery of a meaningful and fulfilling life, despite in some cases the continuation of symptoms (Barker et al 1999, Read & Reynolds 2000). In a radical redefinition of recovery, the 'recovery movement' see it as *a process of discovering how to live and live well* sometimes *with enduring symptoms and vulnerabilities*; a reconceptualisation that opens up the possibility of recovery to all (Roberts & Wolfson 2004).

I have come to think of recovery as a process of emergence. It is not so much that what has so painfully and disruptively gripped our lives has been removed, but that we have emerged from it; transcended it. This emergence is the culmination of a journey that can take many years, an odyssey I have discussed at length elsewhere as the hero's (heroine's) journey (Watkins 2007). It is a journey during which we endure many setbacks, challenges and tests of fortitude. A journey from which we eventually return with more understanding:

> ... of our strengths, weaknesses, qualities and fallibilities; able to accept ourselves with all our imperfections, failures and triumphs, with generous self regard and good humour. We will have learnt how to live, to say yes to life. We are not the same person as the one who set out on the hero's journey. To return to that previous incarnation would be to occupy the same perilous position. We are still vulnerable – human beings are vulnerable – but we now recognise our personal power.

To enter the often confusing, disturbing, ingenious world of madness is to risk losing ourselves, but also offers the prospect of discovering our more vital selves. I realise that this may sound like psychobabble to many colleagues whose practice is rooted in the empirical world of medical psychiatry, but I take as my evidence the well-documented recovery testimonies of many prominent figures in the consumer/survivors movement, such as Ron Coleman (1999), Peter Campbell (2000), Rufus May (2006), Patricia Deegan (1997), Judi Chamberlin (1999b), Sally Clay (1999) and Peter K. Chadwick (1997), who represent only the tip of the iceberg of those who have come through.

Entrapment

Sometimes people seem stuck or lost in a world of madness. Their lives are played out within the psychiatric system on the margins of society. Periods of mental clarity when they are able to function well socially seem tenuous and short-lived. While sometimes seemingly on the threshold of beginning their recovery journey and occasionally taking a few tentative steps along the way, they seem to falter, lose confidence, self-belief and resolve and are drawn back into their enclosed world. Why is it that these individuals have been unable to find or take a pathway towards a less problematic way of being and a well-lived life?

Perhaps the first thing to say is that there is no evidence that the troubled states of mind we describe as psychosis have any intrinsic tendency to become chronic, with individuals experiencing increased disability. That there is some apparent deterioration in mental and social functioning over time is more to do with institutionalising care, the experience of social exclusion and the incapacitating effects of antipsychotic drugs than with some sinister pathological process. Recovery is hard work and the plain fact is that there is bias towards inaction and inertia in human behaviour (Egan 2006). Passivity reveals itself in doing nothing when faced with a call to action; or acting aimlessly when our life situation calls for focused action; or uncritically accepting the solutions of others, even though we have no personal investment in that course of action and therefore little commitment to following it through.

Added to innate passivity is often a layer of what Seligman (1975) has memorably called learnt helplessness, that tendency to helplessly avoid the challenges and opportunities of living even though it would be perfectly possible for us to respond positively and effectively. Learnt helplessness has its origins in formative experience, situations where we have encountered adverse experiences over which we, as a small person, had little control or influence. As a consequence we grew up with little sense of our personal power and resourcefulness. Another layer of passivity arises from what Egan calls disabling self-talk. We all possess an inner critic, which will at times render us speechless and passive in situations that call for a response. If this is a frequent occurrence it can gradually undermine our self-confidence and social skills and lead to an avoidance of life.

It is not difficult to see how passivity, innate or acquired, may be reinforced by expert-led, medical psychiatry. To be a patient is to surrender autonomy and passively acquiesce to prescribed treatment and care. Diagnosis, with its implication of the loss of reason, erroneously raises a question mark over a person's capacity for reasoned thought and wise action; as only the voice of reason is capable of self-reflection and self-regulation, the voice of the patient is therefore invalidated. As Thomas & Bracken (2004) argue, this analysis goes to the heart of why so many service users are disaffected by psychiatry. To feel in the grip of some powerful pathological disorder that can only be resolved by the use of equally powerful drugs; drugs which can dull vitality and spirit along with the distress and produce unpleasant and potentially damaging side effects and are likely to leave you feeling a helpless victim. In every way psychiatric practice, as it has evolved over the past few decades, seems set up to subdue, pacify and control. As Gergen (1990) commented, pathologising psychosocial distress is an *invitation to infirmity*. Many people who resist the power of the system are thought of as 'non-compliant' or 'disengaged', when in reality they are defending the sovereignty of their lives against the oppressive power of the psychiatric system. The sad fact is that all this energy expended in struggling against this system could be going into transcending vulnerabilities and reclaiming life.

Recovery involves accepting responsibility for one's vulnerabilities and finding ways of managing them effectively so that one may live well. It means drawing on resources and strengths we may not feel we have. There can be anxieties about further breakdowns and about social acceptance. There may be unacknowledged grief for the life unlived, for what might have been. Moving on into the future can be difficult until we have grieved and let go the past. People feel changed by the experience of distress – they do not know themselves or how to be in the world. All these are big tasks and require a lot of work on selfhood. Coleman (1999) argues that the emergence of self-awareness, self-acceptance, self-esteem and self-confidence is an essential stepping stone on the pathway to recovery. It can seem easier to give up; to surrender to hopelessness and passivity; not to care.

Tait et al (2003) in a study of engagement patterns refer to a *sealing over* coping strategy in response to troubled states of mind. This is characterised by a lack of curiosity about the distress experience and an avoidance of any active involvement in discovering ways of managing the distress symptoms and more functional ways of being. *Sealing over* is a defence against the threat to a person's identity and self-esteem posed by the experience of a severe psychological crisis; it leads to passive engagement with services and militates against recovery (Birchwood et al 2000). It can be difficult for people to feel secure enough to break free from this 'imprisoned' way of being but people do begin to emerge in time in the context of supportive and enabling recovery relationships and develop a more *integrating recovery strategy.* This involves seeing the personal meaning in the distress experience and integrating that experience into a more positive sense of self, from which confidence begins to grow and a more inclusive life develops.

Sometimes there is a seductive element to madness; it gives life some frisson, rescues it from dull convention, allowing us to indulge our eccentricities and avoid personal and civic responsibilities. Enduring mental health problems give continuing access to the 'mental health community' which for some people offers a sense of belonging and the opportunity of meeting their emotional and social needs, opportunities which are hard to find in the mainstream of community life, from which people find themselves marginalised or excluded.

It is worth reiterating that recovery is hard work. Staying within (or returning to) the bounds of sanity and staying grounded in a consensual reality is difficult, requiring awareness and will. It is all too easy to slip these bounds of sanity and drift on manic flights through psychotic reverie, or fall into listless, apathetic nothingness. A recovery culture is one in which people find the therapeutic support to be able to hold onto their sanity; a culture which calls people forward into life.

The recovery journey can only begin when we, service users and mental health professionals, have identified and addressed these barriers to change. Inherently people are enormously powerful, resourceful and creative. How could we have survived and prospered as a species if this were not so! The task of mental health professionals seeking to be an enabling companion on the recovery journey is to be the custodian of hope and optimism, to cultivate the personal power of the individual or at least not to sabotage it, to focus on an individual's strengths rather than weaknesses, to help people imagine a different way of being, reachable through achievable incremental goals. There are always anxieties involved in setting out on any journey and we need the secure base provided by the recovery relationship to explore the terrain of a renewed life.

A recovery culture

What is it that that enables people to come through, 'to restore, rebuild, reclaim and take control of one's life' (National Institute for Mental Health in England 2005)? People who are in recovery often talk of significant turning points that changed the direction of their lives from breakdown and disintegration, to breakthrough and reintegration. This often seems to involve the presence of another person who is able to relate to them in a way that is enabling. Patricia Deegan talks about 'the loving invitation to be something more' and in Ron Coleman's recovery experience the catalyst was 'someone who saw beneath my madness and into my potential'. In a similar vein, Rogers (1978) describes a humanistic alternative to the biomedical approach and conventional care. He suggests that deeply troubled individuals, who are expressing themselves in ways that are frequently described as psychotic, can be seen as going through a chaotic stressful period of growth, and in need of understanding and companionship rather than prescriptive interventions.

What emerges from the interpersonal experiences of people who are in recovery or recovered is that relationships that facilitate recovery are characterised by:

- an attitude of hopefulness when a person cannot be hopeful for themselves
- a belief in the capacity of people to actualise more of their potential
- a respect for and valuing of a person's subjective experience
- a collaborative enquiry into the meaning of the distress experience
- a respect for the personhood of the individual
- an acknowledgement of a person's strengths and qualities rather than a narrow focus on deficits and problems
- a shared search for the richer narrative of a person's life rather than a focus on the dominant problem-laden narrative
- a respect for a person's right to self-determination which encourages self-empowerment and self-efficacy
- a recognition of the normalcy and humanity of experiences rather than the pathology.

 Self-enquiry box

You may find it useful to reflect on your current practice in relation to the characteristics of recovery relationships outlined above and rate yourself using the scale below. This might be a helpful focus for peer-group supervision, individual supervision or a team review of practice. Ask yourself what specifically needs to change in the thinking/feeling/behavioural dimension of your practice for you to more fully embrace a particular competency.

5. Always hold and express this attitude in my practice.
4. Mostly.
3. Sometimes.
2. Occasionally.
1. Do not subscribe to and express this attitude in my practice.

What kind of helping, healing relationship is likely to value these attributes and allow them to flourish? In my view this is exemplified by the person-centred model of helping developed by Carl Rogers in his psychotherapeutic practice, writing and research over 40 years (Kirschenbaum & Henderson 1990). His is a philosophy of personal and social transformation that has been substantiated and advanced by exponents in the USA and Western Europe since his death in 1987 (Brazier 1993, Mearns & Thorne 2000). Rogers was not talking about a therapeutic technique but about a way of being that is compassionate, loving, empathic and accepting. A way of relating that prizes the humanity of the other, believing deeply in their potential. This is not something that can be turned on and off – that would imply a contrived, inauthentic way of relating, rather it becomes part of who we are and manifests in all our relationships. Despite its ubiquity, the person-centred approach to helping is frequently misunderstood, being often seen as the relational background against which 'real therapy' or 'problem-solving' takes place. This misses the point that the relationship is the therapy – it is the *relational depth* that provides the safety in which suffering can be faced and healing and growth can take place (Mearns & Thorne 2000).

The basic tenets of person-centred helping (discussed in detail in Chapter 9) can be summed up as:

- People are okay though they might need some help recognising it.
- People know what they need though they might need some help expressing it.
- People can discover their own meanings though they might need some help doing it.
- People can take responsibility for themselves, though they might need encouragement to take it.

I want to make it clear that I am not talking exclusively about professional relationships; many people have found inspiration and empowerment for their recovery journey in the companionship of family, friends and other service users. Ahern & Fisher (2001), drawing on their recovery research conducted for the National Empowerment Centre, identify empowerment as the necessary condition for recovery work to be successful. They argue that the healing of severe emotional distress is more effective in the empowerment culture of user-led services than in the hierarchical, expert-centred culture of the psychiatric system. An empowerment culture is one in which someone is exposed to recovery relationships that have at their heart a belief in the individual's worth and in their capacity to live through severe distress and to learn and grow from the crisis experience; relationships in which the subjective experience of the person seeking help is validated and where there is a search for meaning that has relevance to the person's lived experience. It is a culture that enables someone to reconstruct a positive identity from one that has been fragmented and supplanted by the overwhelming experience of being deeply disturbed and distressed. It is a culture that offers social inclusion and a meaningful role rather than the socially marginalised experience of many mental health service users (see Box 8.1). Coleman (1999) too puts empowerment at the heart of the recovery process:

> I am one of those who hold to the idea that personal recovery has at its very heart the reclamation of personal power. In order for the recovery journey to be successful I believe it is important to deconstruct the power of the psychiatric system and reconstruct power as a personal commodity. (p. 48)

Self-enquiry box

Use the value statements in Box 8.1 and the self-rating scale below to reflect on your own practice. This might be a helpful focus for peer-group supervision, individual supervision or a team review of practice. With some minor adaptation it could be used as a basis for a consumer audit of a recovery service. Alternatively, rate yourself on the competencies and ask your clients to give you feedback. Ask yourself what specifically needs to change in the thinking/feeling/behavioural dimension of your practice for you to more fully embrace a particular competency.

5. Always hold and express this attitude in my practice.

4. Mostly.

3. Sometimes.

2. Occasionally.

1. Do not subscribe to and express this attitude in my practice.

Box 8.1

Characteristics of a recovery culture

- Acknowledging people as experts in their own experience.
- Recognising and supporting the personal resourcefulness of individuals.
- Recognising that recovery is a unique process and that there are many roads to the well-lived life.
- Recognising the importance of social inclusion and full citizenship in recovery and seeking to promote it.
- Embracing the diversity of views on the nature of psychological distress.
- Enabling people to discover meaning in their distress experience that is personally relevant.
- Sustaining and communicating the belief in the potential of people to grow and change in life-enhancing ways.
- Recognising the positive elements in a person's vulnerability and that breakdown can lead to breakthrough.
- Accepting setbacks as an inevitable part of the recovery journey and seeing them as opportunities for fresh insights, growth and change.
- Recognising that recovering from the social consequences of disabling psychological distress and a psychiatric diagnosis can be more difficult than recovering from the mental health problem itself.
- Recognising that grieving for what has been lost as a consequence of an enduring vulnerability to psychological distress and overwhelm is a necessary part of the recovery process.
- Recognising that recovery can occur even though symptoms of distress remain. Recovery means they interfere less with an individual's pursuit of the well-lived life.

Continued

> ### Box 8.1
>
> ## Characteristics of a recovery culture—cont'd
>
> - Seeing the role as mental health professionals in the recovery process as collaborative and facilitative rather than authoritative.
> - Affirming strengths, skills, qualities and abilities rather than maintaining an imbalanced focus on deficits.
> - Sustaining the transcendent qualities of acceptance, patience, loving kindness, hopefulness and resolve in the belief that these will find an echo in the way of being of the person in recovery.
> - Accepting that people can recover without professional help.
> - Respecting the rights of individuals to self-determination and choice.
> - Understanding the importance of the family system and personal support networks in the recovery process.
> - Maintaining a culturally sensitive approach to working with people in their recovery process.
> - Supporting the role of the user/survivor movement in the development and validation of training and the reconfiguration and auditing of the service provision.
> - Understanding the importance of living the spirit of growth and recovery in our own lives and acknowledging the reciprocal nature of healing relationships.

The ways to recovery

Edward Podvoll (2003), founder of the inspirational Windhorse project, which has pioneered an approach to working in deeply human ways with people adrift in a world of psychotic confusion called *basic attendance*, describes recovery as a journey that can require 'valiant personal action and a lifelong commitment to health'. He argues that even in the midst of madness one can recognise the seeds of recovery, which he refers to as 'islands of clarity', in which the individual regains, albeit briefly, mental clarity and engages constructively in living. These moments grow as the journey of recovery begins. It is seldom a straightforward journey. Even people some way along the road can lose their psychological bearings, stumble and become lost again in a psychotic terrain. However, once people have begun their journey, these setbacks can be temporary, can be learnt from and the recovery pathway regained.

There are many pathways to the realisation of a less troubled, more enriched life. A study by the Mental Health Foundation (2000) throws some light on what people have found most helpful on their way to recovery (see Box 8.2). What is clear is that strategies for managing vulnerability, for self-realisation and building a meaningful life, have the stamp of individuality on them (Fig. 8.1).

For some the key factor in their recovery is the presence of loving, enabling relationships. For others it is finding meaning and purpose in life through family, work, helping others or spiritual practice. Some find in their use of medication, the psychotherapies or complementary therapies, sufficient release from vulnerability and distress to grow towards becoming fully functioning people and engage more in life. Many people find in nature the peace, inspiration and resolution to heal

Box 8.2

Service users' views of factors most helpful in recovery

- Relationships: with friends, family, other service users, mental health professionals.
- Safe havens; accepting communities; shared experience/identities with others; accessible/available support.
- Finding meaning and purpose through: family, work, meaningful activity, helping others, creative expression, religion or spiritual practice.
- Use of medication, psychotherapy, complementary therapies, arts therapies, exercise, communion with nature.
- Being in control of one's vulnerability to distress; being in control of one's life; finding within oneself the will to be well.
- Having enough money, having secure accommodation, finding pleasure in life. Dealing with discrimination and stigma with equanimity.
- Integrating mental health problems and missing narratives into a positive sense of self.

Adapted from Mental Health Foundation (2000).

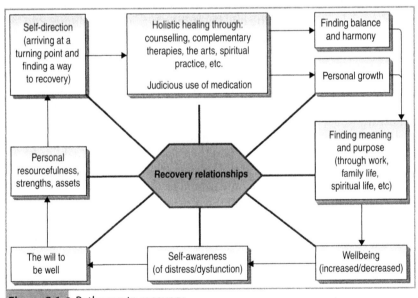

Figure 8.1 ● Pathways to recovery.

themselves and their lives. The creative process too can be immensely healing: that people feel more energised and alive when involved in some creative project should not surprise us, as creativity is linked with spontaneity, imagination, innovation, intuition, emotion, playfulness, meaning and soulfulness – the wellspring of vibrant living. Sometimes changing social circumstances become more sustaining: moving into good accommodation, having enough money to maintain a reasonable quality of life, seizing opportunities for training, education or work all draw a person on into life and away from a marginalised, impoverished existence in which the turbulent psyche seems to flourish.

None of this will work if it is part of some prescribed package of care from which the client's voice is missing and in which they have little emotional investment. Until people begin to reclaim power and sovereignty over their lives, define for themselves or collaboratively the meaning of their distress, and make choices and decisions about what will help in their recovery they will lack belief and commitment.

Steve Morgan, a leading protagonist of the strengths model in the UK, argues that working with strengths offers an empowering, enabling way of facilitating recovery. Instead of focusing so much attention on dysfunction, a person's strengths become the object of our attention – their skills, qualities, accomplishments, aspirations, interests and the sustaining elements in their life. It is concerned with what people can do, or aspire to do; with the goals that would draw people more confidently and fully into life and the resources needed to achieve them (Ryan & Morgan 2004). The originator of the strengths model, Professor Charles Rapp, defines it as an approach that sets out 'to assist consumers in identifying, securing and sustaining a range of resources – both environmental and personal, needed to live, play and work in a normally interdependent way in the community' (Rapp 1998). The strengths approach offers a strong philosophical basis for practice and has a growing evidence base to support its efficacy (Barry et al 2003).

So often, people whose lives have been lived in psychological turmoil become stuck in their problem-saturated history. The dominant narratives of our lives define us and provide the script for our way of being in the world. Our personal story can therefore be strengthening and life enhancing or undermining and life defeating. But these narratives are based not on the full text of our lives but on what White (1987) calls the thin narrative – the edited version. A key task in recovery is to help people re-author their stories so that they are no longer so problem saturated. Teasing out a person's positive attributes, abilities and potentials, discovering the growthful, gratifying moments in their lives, helping them create opportunities for success and an expression of resourcefulness, all these challenge the dominance of the problem-saturated narrative and enable the individual to begin to re-vision themselves and their lives. This is not to diminish or deny the magnitude of the adversities and traumas that many people face but to recognise that they can be overcome only from a position of reclaimed personal power, derived from the untold story and the continuing story.

 Angie's story

Theme: the recovery process

Angie is a young woman with a 10-year history of serious self-harm and frequent referrals to acute inpatient services. She has a deeply negative self-concept and correspondingly low self-esteem, which she disguises behind a thin veneer of emotional buoyancy and outgoingness. Frequently escalating psychosomatic tension and bleak feelings about herself and her life break through to the surface and capsize her mood. It is at these times that she is gripped by an urge to cut or burn herself. Over the years the frequency and seriousness of her self-harming has increased, leading to an increase in the number and length of admissions. The admissions were demoralising for Angie and seemed to be taking her in a direction away from the 'ordinary life' which she craves. It was also demoralising for the staff, who began to see Angie as a 'chronic self-harmer' with a 'damaged manipulative personality', for whom very little could be done. They experienced feelings of helplessness, guilt, anger, anxiety, distrust, sadness and perplexity in the face of Angie's continued self-mutilation.

The hypothesis about the nature of self-harming that seemed to fit for Angie was that injuring herself was both a solution and a problem. It was a solution in the sense that it had evolved as a way of externalising her inner distress and of making visible a deep sense of hurt and betrayal that had been present from her childhood onwards, connected with her mother's abandonment of her and her father when she was 4 years old. Secondly, the physical pain gave her some sense of relief by displacing emotional pain in her conscious awareness. It was a problem in the obvious sense that her self-harming had become at times life-threatening. It had also caused multiple disfiguring scars, which Angie was increasingly sensitive about and had made relationships and a working life impossible. The increasing frequency and severity of her self-injuries suggested that it was no longer a solution to her underlying distress.

A decision was made to 'appoint' Angie the expert on her own life. With the help of her key worker she was asked to construct a plan for recovering herself and her life from the grip of the problem of self-harm. The aim of this strategy was firstly to try to separate the person from the problem. This was necessary because Angie's story had become so problem-saturated that other aspects of herself and her life had been all but eclipsed. Secondly, there was a need to demonstrate a trust in her ability to tap into her innate wisdom for a change that would make a difference. A way of responding to her distress that was different to the entrenched self-harm pattern and would begin the process of healing. To encourage in her a sense that she could become an agent in her own recovery, which was not dependent on professional help for the right medication programme, the right psychotherapeutic intervention.

Angie's perspective

At first it was a shock to realise that they were serious, that I was being expected to prescribe my own care. It didn't feel like they had given up on me or abandoned me, because there was a lot of encouragement and my key worker spent time with me and was accessible. It was a relief to know that they were not going to try and prevent me from cutting myself. They recognised that for me it was a way of coping with my feelings and until I had some other way of coping, there would still be times when I would need to self-harm. They were more concerned about me doing it safely with as little damage as possible. Strangely, the fact that I could do it seemed to lessen my need to do it and I soon found that I had gone 5 weeks without cutting which is close to a record for me. Of course it didn't last. I think what was helpful in the first few months was the feeling, for the first time really, that I was being heard. Also not being treated like a 'bad girl' but respectfully, like an adult. I began to think maybe I could take better care of myself and not damage myself so much, maybe I'm worth it. That was on good days. At other times any good and hopeful feelings I had about myself were crushed by this feeling of desolation and the thought that there would never be anything good in my life, because there was nothing good in me. With my key worker I developed a schedule of strategies that I would work through if I felt like self-harming when I was at home in my flat:

Continued

Angie's story—cont'd

- Do something active and vigorous (take a walk, dance, do some hand washing).
- Negotiate with myself to postpone self-harming for 12 hours.
- Look at my therapeutic documents.
- Telephone my key worker/support worker or the crisis line.
- Paint or draw vigorously using finger paints or charcoal.
- Take an aromatherapy bath.
- Listen to guided imagery tape.
- If I need to cut, use a clean guarded blade to limit the extent of the injury.
- Take responsibility for dressing cuts and getting myself to A&E if I need stitches.

In addition I had an agreement that if I was feeling overwhelmed and couldn't cope without cutting I could go into hospital for a day or two.

As well as seeing my key worker twice a week, I joined an art therapy group and attended a support group for women who self-harm. My self-harm rate has now gone down from about five times a month to one in the last 3 months. I'm feeling a whole lot stronger emotionally and more positive about myself. I had lost sight of so many things in my life history that affirmed a different identity from the hateful person that I'd become. It's been a bit like editing a story so that the life of the central character is not so swamped by misfortune that their life can only be seen as a tragedy and end tragically.

Early steps in an individual's recovery are tentative. People can feel extremely vulnerable as they encounter their emerging selves and begin to reclaim their lives. Demoralisation and disempowerment are commonly experienced and are significant barriers to recovery. It is important that these early steps are manageable and achievable and that people do not go too far out on a limb before the limb has grown strong enough to support them. Each small step needs to be acknowledged as evidence of an underlying healing process at work and can be worked with to encourage hopefulness and self-direction and to rebuild self-esteem and confidence. Out of these therapeutic moments come turning points. For some it might be having their subjective reality understood deeply and empathetically by another person that draws them back into the world. For others it might be daring to believe that a different life is possible or alternatively the experience of an accomplishment that awakens a sense of personal agency.

Fisher (1999) emphasises the importance of reoccupying a valued social role as a key factor in recovery. Re-establishing oneself in the world of work, becoming a student, or becoming a tenant, are examples of this. Maintaining one's place within the family and community can provide the incentive and support conducive to the recovery of sanity. Evidence for this has come from the World Health Organization's comparative studies on the course and outcome of severe mental disorder in a number of countries that span the spectrum of socio-economic development. That the outcome is significantly better in developing countries which use fewer drugs and less hospitalisation challenges the view that a highly professionalised care system is the best guarantee for improving the long-term course of schizophrenia (de Girolamo 1996).

What seems to become clear from what many people say about their 'breakthroughs' and 'turning points' is the importance of autonomy and connectedness. It is when people begin to become self-determining and take responsibility for themselves and their lives that change begins. Until that step is taken, life is lived according to the conditions of others, often in the context of controlling, dependent relationships, with all the limitations which that imposes, and people will not experience themselves as agents in their own healing process. Lives are rebuilt on hope, a willingness to act and responsible action (Deegan 1988).

The legacy of disability from the era of institutional psychiatry and from institutional patterns of care in the community that replicate an institutional model should be sufficient evidence of the damage that segregated care can do. When we become disconnected from the social moorings that anchor us in the broad stream of a shared reality and the norms and values of our culture we are set adrift in a sea of madness. The WHO studies referred to above should alert us to the fact that chronicity is not the natural outcome of severe mental disorder but what Illich (1977) has called the iatrogenic outcome of psychiatric treatment and care.

 Ben's story

Theme: the recovery process

It's about 5 years since I last had to go into hospital. I still see my CPN once a month, more frequently if I'm getting too high or too low. We've got to know each other pretty well over the years so our conversations are not all about my hassles, they are about what's going on for her as well. I feel much more comfortable with that. Before, I often used to feel like I was an observed object, part of some global experiment in mind control. I was having to take a lot of prescribed drugs at that time and I suppose I would be what people call a non-compliant patient. Only to my mind I wasn't being non-compliant, I was adopting life-saving tactics. Discovering my diagnosis was a devastating experience. My first encounter with my diagnosis was seeing paranoid schizophrenic written on my case notes; it was literally soul destroying. Recently I've written to a psychiatrist asking if I can have that diagnosis rescinded. I hate the idea of being tagged for life. Now, apart from Cathy my CPN, I have no other contact with the psychiatric services and only take medication when I need to.

Things began to change when I saw a new psychiatrist who actually listened to me and I began to feel I had some control over my life. He encouraged me to write down what I was experiencing and discuss it with him if I wanted to. I had learnt in my career as a psychiatric case that you didn't say much to the doctors or nurses because they would simply write you up as disturbed, give you more medication and keep you in hospital. For me writing was the breakthrough. At first I just wrote a narrative, 'A day in the death of Benjamin Salthouse', that sort of thing. But then I found that I could write prose poems. I'd never read any poetry before but I'd always had an ear for the lyrics of music I was into at that time. I was a big

Continued

79

Ben's story—cont'd

Bob Marley fan. When I look back at some of those early poems, a lot of them were about a young black guy who didn't conform to the black stereotype. No good at sport. No good at dancing. An introvert, with glasses and a small dick! Even my self-image had walked out on me! I was in need of an image consultant, not a psychiatrist. One of the voices I heard during that time was a black angel. She used to tell me I was 'one step away from God'. I found it both comforting and alarming. When I was low I used to think I was about to die a violent death at the hands of a friendly assassin. Often I thought that the nurses were trying to kill me. When I was high, I used to think I was in some way special, that I was chosen, that I was the black envoy of God.

A lot of people encouraged me. At some level I was able to see myself held together in the ordered structure and rhythm of the poems. My chaotic unreal world seemed no more than an awakened dream that had escaped from the night. This was narcosis, not psychosis. Who I am now struggled into existence in the poems and waited for me to catch up. For me writing is therapy. There are still times when my reality becomes confusing and I get overwhelmed and may behave in unwise ways. But I'm much better at recognising that these days. I know that what I need to do is to stay out of circulation, spend time in quiet places, go back to nature, take respite from the world for a few weeks.

In the process of recovery, chemotherapy and psychotherapy can be seen as self-determined strategies the individual recognises as being a part of their holistic self-care. But we should guard against giving any therapy the status of a panacea. For recovering and sustaining our wellbeing we all need to build into our lives experiences which are nourishing, strengthening and healing. An inspiring example of this is Rene, whose life was for many years disrupted and all but destroyed by her immobilising lows and chaotic highs.

Rene's story

Theme: the recovery process

Rene is a 37-year-old woman with a history of manic-depressive disorder dating back to her early twenties. A precipitating event seemed to be the sudden death of her father who sexually abused her until her early teens. This had remained a secret in the family until his death. Over the next few years Rene was admitted to hospital several times. She attempted suicide on two separate occasions and was drinking heavily. Medication seemed to help when she became depressed or manic but was ineffective in stabilising her mood.

Rene, with the help of her CPN, was able to identify the early signs of her deepening lows or escalating highs and become familiar with her relapse signature.

Together they were able to construct a recovery plan that she could use to balance her mood. Making adjustments to her self-medication programme was just one strategy in a plan that involved switching to a quieter lifestyle when the early signs of a high were recognised and engaging in a manageable and nurturing activity schedule when she recognised a significant downswing. She also had some alcohol counselling and later some psychotherapy. This enabled her to let go of an image of herself as a flawed and worthless human being whom other people found unappealing. Instead, she began to develop a more respectful attitude towards herself and to discover the 'treasure' hidden within her unfolding self. Some pastoral counselling from a chaplain helped Rene rediscover the comfort and inspiration of prayer and contemplation and helped fill a spiritual emptiness that had enveloped her life with meaninglessness.

All of this took courage and a willingness to invest energy in discovering herself and recovering her life. It was not straightforward. There were many doubts and setbacks along the way. Perhaps a key factor was the co-creation of motivation. We tend to see motivation as goal-directed energy that comes from within. But often motivation is the product of the social system or interpersonal context of which the individual is part. In Rene's case her sustained motivation came out of a respectful, encouraging, enabling therapeutic system, a system that involved her family, her key worker, a psychiatrist and other professional mental health workers whom she chose to work with at various points in her recovery.

Recovery involves giving our attention to the four dimensions of human experience: body, mind, spirit and our social world. A sense of wellbeing is derived from achieving a degree of balance and harmony within and between our internal and external worlds. Achieving this balance has traditionally been an integral part of the healing process in Asian and African cultures (Fernando 2002). Historically in Western psychiatry and psychotherapy the mind and body have been split, the social context of distress ignored and the spirit neglected. There is evidence that this is changing in the UK as many more people are now choosing to use alternative therapies such as herbal remedies, acupuncture, homeopathy, shiatsu, aromatherapy massage and counselling, and practices such as meditation and yoga alongside conventional psychiatric therapeutic regimes.

An extraordinary young man I have come to know professionally in recent years has made holistic therapies and practices the mainstay of his medication-free recovery from a disabling psychosis. Detoxifying and rebalancing his life have been key goals – goals alien to conventional psychiatric practice – that have enabled him to stay grounded; mindful of the otherworldliness of his mind's excursions without getting drawn into them. A personal account of his recovery journey can be found in a previous publication (Watkins 2007).

People now think of themselves as consumers of the mental health services, and in the context of oppressive social and psychiatric systems as survivors. However, Deegan (1997) advises caution in thinking that new labels necessarily reflect a change in the relationship between those labelled and those not labelled. People who have experienced serious mental health problems still find a significant power difference and a lack of mutuality in their relationships with professional helpers. White (1997) describes an approach to professionalised helping, which he calls

81

de-centred care, in which a consciousness of the power difference enables helpers to stay mindful of potential abuses. Maintaining this awareness opens up the possibility of exploring the way in which other relations of power have influenced the construction of people's stories and identity; the way in which the abuse, injustice and oppression that exists in our culture in everyday interactions is reflected in the stories people hold and tell about their lives. In de-centred care the therapeutic endeavour places the client's knowledge of their lived experience at the centre of the work, rather than the professional's 'expert' knowledge. White's contention is that the therapeutic encounter should provide a context in which the stories of people's lived experience are told, both the known and the 'missing' narratives. It is in this telling and retelling that detail emerges of alternative story lines to the dominant problem-laden story which is replayed again and again in the conventional psychiatric interview. In the retelling we discover courageous struggles against oppression and disadvantage. We find acts of care and kindness towards others. We find demonstrations of responsibility and wise action. We find accounts of relationships in which the client has been the object of loving attention. The re-authoring of lives in the light of these recovered stories nurtures the growth of a different, stronger identity from the negative and limiting self-concept that exists in many people who are deeply troubled. As White puts it, the re-plotting of dominant narratives and the telling of previously untold stories become 'expressions of persistence, determination, struggle, protest, resistance and connectedness that come to represent a turning point in a person's life'.

Wounded healers

Staff attitudes are very important in creating a culture of recovery. There is an illusory belief amongst many mental health professionals that somehow they are able rise above the anguish and struggle of human existence. As professional helpers, we need to be aware of our own wounds and to live the spirit of recovery in our own lives. The dynamic healing environment is one in which staff members are vitally involved in their own growth and recovery. As Deegan suggests, it is this that allows us to deeply empathise with the woundedness and vulnerability of people in our care. Real community is not a place, it is an inclusive attitude based on the recognition of a shared humanity.

White uses the phrase 'taking it back' to describe the reciprocal nature of therapeutic relationships. He argues that in de-centred practice the therapeutic encounter can be growthful and sustaining to the helper in a number of ways. In examining the way power is held and used in the helping relationship and in the wider social context, we are challenged to reflect on our own experience of power both in the professional and personal spheres of our lives. Acknowledging the act of trust that is involved in allowing the helper into the person's life prompts into awareness the meaning of being included (or excluded) for the helper and their lives. Joining with people in the recovery of stories that lead to a change in identity and life direction can awaken professional helpers to what is being overlooked in their own lives, to neglected experience that provides a richer narrative account of their life journey and reshapes their identity. Similarly, listening to stories of the relational experience of clients' lives can reconnect the helper with significant individuals and formative relationships in their own history. The reliving and revising of these narratives can increase our knowledge of our lived experience in a way that is healing. Being with people, witnessing their aspirations and actions in their journey towards a preferred way of being can cause ripples in the helper's own life. The stories clients tell are often graphic metaphors of the struggles of the human spirit to triumph over adversity. These storied images are carried into the helper's work and life in a sustaining way. Both in humanistic and in narrative approaches to helping, the knowledge on which solutions to the problems of living are based is generated by the person seeking help. This 'solution knowledge' and the style of therapeutic conversations in which it is drawn out are learnt from the client and carried by the helper into subsequent work with others. In these and in other ways the helper is both giver and receiver in the therapeutic encounter.

A question which needs to be asked is to what extent this should be made known to the client. White's phrase 'taking it back' is an invocation to do just that. Openly acknowledging the ways in which hearing the client's story and witnessing their journey has touched and influenced our lives and work is an acknowledgement of a shared humanity. I like a degree of reciprocity in my conversations with clients. I dislike the sense of subterfuge that occurs when I hide my humanity behind a thin veneer of invulnerable expert. Many times I've found myself listening to an echo of my own sufferings in the stories of troubled minds and troubled lives and through a client's quest for a way to recovery have often been able to reconnect with what has been and what is sustaining and healing in my own life. I am not suggesting that we should burden clients with the grief and misfortunes of our personal odysseys, but the acknowledgement that we have also been helped personally and professionally by a therapeutic encounter is an affirmation of a person's worth and a powerful expression of positive regard.

Self-enquiry box

Using the recovery pathway mapped out in Figure 8.1 as a guide, reflect on a personal experience of recovery from an episode of psychological overwhelm; a time of mental suffering in your life. Consider the factors that contributed to the recovery of your mental wellbeing:

Did your woundedness remain unattended for a time?

What prompted you to attend to your psychological hurt?

What helped in your recovery?

What part did self-healing play?

In what ways did personal qualities of awareness, clarity, compassion, discipline and courage play a part (see p. 14)?

Were there turning points?

How did relationships with others figure in your recovery?

Do you bear the (half healed) scars of those wounds in your life now?

In what ways have you carried this experience into your practice?

Humanistic approaches to helping and healing

9

Humanistic helping has at its core a belief in the emergent self; that is, a tendency for our innate human potential to unfold in the direction of optimal functioning. This is not a process that happens unfailingly but is dependent on the social environment we are exposed to as we grow up and grow older. Given favourable social conditions we develop in the direction of becoming fully functional individuals able to relate to others and pursue our lives in socially constructive ways. In adverse social circumstances this development may be thwarted or distorted, resulting in distressed and dysfunctional behaviour.

Carl Rogers in his writing, research and practice over a period of 30 years argued that the *core conditions – unconditional positive regard, empathic warmth and congruity or realness in our relating* – were vital for our essential flourishing. Can it really be that simple? I believe it can. Look at how distorted the growth of an oak tree becomes in an unfavourable landscape. To grow towards maturity and mental wellbeing we need an emotional landscape in which we are loved unconditionally by people who understand our experiential world and can be real for us. In my experience individuals who find themselves in crisis, struggling to cope with a troubled state of mind, are usually people whose growth towards becoming a fully functional person has been seriously obstructed or deflected because these conditions have not been sufficiently present in their life. They have become alienated from their true self, unhappy with themselves and confused about how to be in the world. Healing is concerned with recovering and integrating that real, authentic self.

Psychotherapeutic approaches in the humanistic person-centred tradition have not found the accepted and valued place in psychiatry that more directive forms of psychotherapeutic work have. But here we are concerned not so much with formal therapy, as with the countless contacts and conversations that take place between mental health practitioners and clients as a dynamic part of the healing process. The potential of these interactions to facilitate healing has been underestimated and undervalued in the expert-led, evidence-based, world of medically oriented psychiatry, as has a client's capacity for self-healing. In a review of psychotherapy outcome research over the past 10 years, Bozarth & Motomasa (2005) conclude that changes towards desired outcomes in psychotherapeutic interventions are due not so much to specific techniques as to the relationship with the practitioner and the client's own capacity for generative self-healing, factors that coalesce in effective care. The person-centred way of working with clients is more specific about the nature of that alliance – if the practitioner is perceived as being someone who is an authentic/real presence for the client, holds an attitude of unconditional positive regard, and has an empathic understanding of the client's frame of reference, then it is likely that the client will be increasingly empowered to resolve her or his problems and dysfunction.

Relationships in the context of the psychiatric system – perhaps all significant relationships – are never neutral; they are either empowering and enabling, or they are disempowering and disabling. If we practise with awareness we can ensure that our interpersonal work facilitates the growth and healing of those whose social sphere we enter for a while. This is not an easy task; psychiatry with its legal power to enforce hospitalisation and treatment can seem the antithesis of facilitative care, which follows and supports the client's own directionality as they seek a more harmonious and meaningful way of being in the world. As professional helpers laden with multiple theories of dysfunction, it can be difficult for us to keep our eager interpretations and prescriptive solutions on hold sufficiently to enable clients to process their own meaning and find their own answers to their distress symptoms and problems of living. Neither is it easy to feel warmly accepting of people who repeatedly behave in base ways.

The key question in humanistic, person-centred approaches to mental health care is can we work with people in a way that is essentially non-directive that avoids control over, and decision-making for, the client. In one his earliest accounts of person-centred therapy Rogers challenged practitioners to examine their attitudes:

> Do we see each person as having worth and dignity in his or her own right? If we do hold this point of view at a cognitive level, to what extent is it operationally evident at a behavioural level? Do we tend to treat individuals as persons of worth, or do we subtly devalue them by our own attitudes and behaviour? Is our philosophy one in which respect for the individual is uppermost? Do we respect his or her capacity and right to self direction, or do we basically believe that his or her life would be best guided by us? (Rogers cited in Levitt 2005)

86

This is perhaps the most fundamental and important question we can ask about the delivery of psychiatric care and about our own practice; our answer depends on our way of being with people seeking help. It is a question I have wrestled with throughout my career. I find myself in harmony with humanistic and person-centred thinking yet often forced to compromise, by a duty of care, to act in ways which seem to run contrary to a person's expressed wishes. My solution has been to adopt the position taken by another humanistic philosopher, educator and practitioner, John Heron. Heron (2001) proposes that all helping interventions can be charted along a continuum, with those that are essentially authoritative at one end and those that are essentially facilitative at the other. He argues that both authoritative and facilitative interventions are equally valid depending on the context. A balanced, fluid use of both is synonymous with 'the proper exercise of power: the practitioner's power over the client; the power shared by the practitioner and client with each other; the autonomous power of the client, at the helm of their own life' (p. 7). The question for all mental health practitioners is can we judiciously and sensitively adjust our approach along this continuum without jeopardising our engagement with people whose lives have become seriously disturbed and distressed?

Underlying every intervention, whether authoritative or facilitative, should be an attitude of respect for the autonomy of the individual and the right of everyone to sovereignty over their lives. Given this foundational belief then our practice will always be alive to the need to move from hierarchical, authoritative ways of being and working with clients, towards a more collaborative relationship and finally to non-directive ways of working, in which the client's power and autonomy are pre-eminent and markers of their recovery process. Historically the hierarchical, authoritative domain has characterised psychiatric practice; autonomous power has been stripped from clients, who become the passive objects of custodial care. Even in contemporary psychiatry where collaborative care is a watchword for good practice there are still misuses and abuses of power. We should be continually conscious that however benignly or benevolently we take away a person's liberty, enforce the use of medication, interpret their experiential reality as illness, and prescribe a programme of care that is assertively imposed, we are engaging in an assault on an individual's personhood. It is a trauma that many survivors of the psychiatric system have to recover from. For many it is a trauma of sufficient intensity to cause post-traumatic stress disorder, an iatrogenic outcome which remains largely unacknowledged and untreated by mental health professionals (Morrison et al 2003).

Abusive practice, what Heron refers to as 'degenerative interventions', are more likely to come about if we have not worked on our own accumulated distresses. If we have not achieved a level of *emotional competence* then it is likely that many of our interventions will be contaminated by our own emotional needs displaced into helping, which then takes on an oppressive, intrusive, compulsive or manipulative quality. Until personal development work is seen as a requirement, alongside professional development, in the education of mental health professionals this will remain unacknowledged and unresolved – the shadow side of practice (see Part 3, Chapter 20).

 ## Self-enquiry box

Take a random sample of your current caseload, say five clients, and in relation to your work with this cohort ask yourself the key questions below and position on the self-rating scales.

- Do I authentically and openly listen to clients in my contacts with them?
  mostly   often   sometimes   rarely   never

- Do I accede to a client's decision even though it might be contrary to my professional judgement?
  mostly   often   sometimes   rarely   never

- Do I effectively share information that is needed by clients for them to make informed decisions?
  mostly   often   sometimes   rarely   never

- In my conversations with clients do I tend to determine the direction of the conversational flow?
  mostly   often   sometimes   rarely   never

- In my conversations with clients do I tend to follow the direction of the conversational flow?
  mostly   often   sometimes   rarely   never

Continued

Self-enquiry box—cont'd

- How consultative am I in prescribing, advising, suggesting a course of action?
  mostly   often   sometimes   rarely   never

- How often do clients set the agenda for our contacts and conversation?
  mostly   often   sometimes   rarely   never

- Do I engage with clients in a search for a shared meaning for their distress?
  mostly   often   sometimes   rarely   never

- Do I intervene in ways that facilitate the client's decision-making?
  mostly   often   sometimes   rarely   never

- Do I seek to supportively raise clients' awareness of dysfunctional thinking, feeling, behaviour that they are avoiding?
  mostly   often   sometimes   rarely   never

- Do I look for the personal and social resources available to the client?
  mostly   often   sometimes   rarely   never

- How effective am I at resisting the need of clients to relate to me as rescuer.
  mostly   often   sometimes   rarely   never

- Am I able to offer emotional and practical support to clients in ways that are non-intrusive and unimposing?
  mostly   often   sometimes   rarely   never

- Do I affirm the worth and value of the client's qualities and actions
  mostly   often   sometimes   rarely   never

- Do I interpret – give meaning to – the client's behaviour and experience from the perspective of my professional knowledge base?
  mostly   often   sometimes   rarely   never

- How effective am I at not relating to clients as passive victims?
  mostly   often   sometimes   rarely   never

The further your ratings are towards the right-hand end of the scale, the more indicative it is that in your practice your style of relating is more authoritative than facilitative. While you may cognitively value client autonomy and empowerment, it may be not be evident in the way you express yourself in practice, perhaps because of the traditional role-bound values you have adopted or because of blind spots linked to personal needs and feelings. You may find it useful to explore the outcomes from this exercise in supervision or in a team review of practice.

If we take as our blueprint for interpersonal practice the person-centred humanistic approach outlined above and discussed in more detail in Chapter 20, then effective helping relationships can be summed up in the following beliefs:

- People are OK (though they might need help recognising it).
- People can discover their own meanings (though they might need help doing it).

- People know what they need (though they might need help expressing it).
- People can take responsibility for themselves (though they might need encouragement to take it).

People are OK

A fundamental belief of the humanistic approach to helping is that every person is an individual of worth. Terms such as acceptance, respect and unconditional positive regard are widely used to describe the expression of this belief in the process of helping. Self-esteem is a major element in our sense of wellbeing. An inner core of positive self-regard enables us to enter life more confidently and express more of our potential. It helps protect us from the losses, failures, disappointments and rejections that are an inevitable part of life and threaten our self-concept. Without this inner core, our self-esteem would be too externally regulated and overly vulnerable to adversity. A lack or loss of self-esteem is a problem facing many people who seek help from the mental health services. It can lie at the centre of the distress and the problems in living that people face. Part of the experience of depression is an assault on a despised self, cognitively in the form of punishing and disabling self-talk and physically in the form of self-harm and suicidal behaviour. Others, particularly those with long-term or recurrent mental health problems, lose self-esteem as a consequence of becoming a patient. It can be demoralising and undermining to face the stigma, social exclusion and disadvantage that people with mental health problems regularly encounter. Professionalised helping too can add to the diminution of self-esteem, by not involving people as agents in their own care and recovery process and by focusing too much on disabilities and vulnerabilities and not enough on talents, abilities and strengths (Chadwick 1997).

Building and strengthening self-esteem is an important task in the recovery process. This can take place in the context of a helping relationship in which the helper relates to the person in care in an authentic, accepting way. People need to feel valued and validated as a person. They need to feel that as they struggle to be more fully themselves they will not be judged or rejected. Acceptance must not be conditional on the individual being compliant and passively following advice and direction in order to retain the positive regard of the helper. Chamberlin (1999a) argues that the very opposite of this, non-compliance and the assertion of autonomy, is necessary to the process of recovery. It is sometimes not easy for people to be open and receptive to the warmth and appreciation of others, so deeply embedded is their low self-esteem. They feel bad, hopeless, useless, unlovable as a person and this can only be resolved by re-evaluating the reasonableness of their negative self-concept in the light of a living learning experience that provides exceptions to that experience of themselves.

A belief in the essential worth of human beings is not to deny that we have a shadow side and that people sometimes behave in hurtful, damaging or evil ways. Humanistic thinking has, in the past, been criticised for having an overly optimistic view of human nature. The shadow side of human potential contains both negative destructive and positive constructive parts of ourselves that we are unable to own, largely as the result of the conditional love we have experienced during our development. We soon learn that to be acceptable and lovable certain behaviours are prohibited. The child whose playful exuberance is disapproved of may lose touch with their capacity to be enthusiastic, spontaneous and playful. If our distress and comfort-seeking behaviour is ignored, we may deny our emotional hurts and our need for comfort and support and express our distress in more damaging and inappropriate ways.

If our potential to be hateful, lustful, jealous, selfish, oppressive, remains an unacknowledged and unaccepted part of ourselves, there are likely to be a number of consequences. Firstly, we use up a lot of energy repressing these aspects of ourselves, energy that is no longer available for living. Secondly, the more they are denied, the more likely they are to find expression outside of our awareness in damaging, manipulative, impulsive, unwise acts. Thirdly, the opposites of those traits are likely to be shallow and false representations of the real thing, reflected in the colloquial saying, 'he's too good to be true'. There is no light without dark! The acknowledgement and acceptance of these potentials as part of our emergent self does not lead to them being expressed unrestrainedly. In fact the very opposite occurs. Carl Rogers held the view that when we are in touch with our true self, then we have an inner sense of the rightness of our conduct in any given situation. He took the view that man was essentially a social being and that behaviour emanating from the true self would be socially constructive (Thorne 1992).

It is difficult to reconcile this with the violence and inhumanity of individuals, social groups and countries towards others. It often seems as if the potential for violent and oppressive acts is in ascendance at this moment in our history. Perhaps there is a clue in the use of the term inhumanity – less than human – do we recognise that such acts are a perversion of our natural God-given way of being in the world. There is, then, an even greater need at this moment in time for a creed, whether secular or religious, that recognises and liberates the human potential for love and compassion. There is a place within the context of humanistic philosophy for the spiritual, and both Eastern and Western spiritual traditions have left their imprint on humanistic thinking. Thorne makes an interesting comparison between creation spirituality with its recognition of the divinity of all of nature and the hopeful view of human nature held by Rogers. To realise the divinity within us and around us nurtures a more reverential attitude towards ourselves, towards others and the world in which we live.

People can discover their own meaning

For most of the 20th century the biomedical model dominated psychiatry. This pathologising perspective on the experience of deeply troubled people not only depersonalises and disempowers those seeking help but also militates against humanistic practice (Joseph & Worsley 2005). At its most pernicious, pathologising human experience is an invitation to infirmity. It legitimises 'giving up the struggle' and enrols people in a 'career' as a psychiatric patient. Breggin (1996) takes up this theme, arguing that the biomedical model fails to sufficiently value the agency and personhood of service users. People can and need to be active forces in their own recovery. Approaches to helping deeply troubled people should respect as much as possible autonomy and freedom. At times it can seem as if the person has been all but eclipsed by the diagnostic label. The human qualities, talents and potentials the individual possesses have become submerged under the problem-saturated story (the psychiatric history).

We are all authors. We all construct narratives of our lives and ourselves and use these stories to organise and give meaning to our experience. The stories we carry are selective narratives in the sense that they do not represent any absolute reality or capture what White & Epston (1990) call the full richness of any life experience. Our stories can be enabling and promote a sense of wellness or they can be undermining and disabling. In effect we become the central character in our stories as we re-enact them in our everyday lives. If our story is of being overwhelmed by life's challenges and the meaning drawn from that is that we are hopeless or inadequate or ill and unable to cope, we will become passive and helpless. If our dominant narrative is of failure and rejection the meaning drawn from that might be that we are no good and we may express that in self-harm behaviour. The task of the helper is to facilitate a conversation in which people discover or co-create new meanings. The recovery process involves a shift, for example, from seeing themselves as a bad person to seeing themselves as more sinned against than sinning; from seeing themselves as a schizophrenic, a psychiatric patient and an outsider, to seeing themselves as a person with vulnerabilities (and abilities) that can be managed and lived with. This approach has its roots in social constructionism and the philosophy of Foucault. The central premise is that dominant social discourses can seem to objectify reality and lead to rigid inflexible perspectives on social experience against which we measure ourselves. These dominant social discourses, for example on gender, shape our personal narratives and influence, often in limiting and damaging ways, the way we see ourselves and live our lives. Helping relationships that enable people to begin to re-author their lives are critical to recovery.

In the context of biomedical psychiatry, a primary role of practitioners is to monitor people for symptom reduction in response to medication, for side effects of medication and for early signs of relapse, and secondly to take an authoritative role in developing care. An extension of this role is the education of clients and their families about medication and the biomedical construct of their presenting problems. This lends itself to a prescriptive, 'expert-led' approach to care and away from collaborative care as envisaged in developing services (National Institute for Mental Health in England 2003). It presupposes that we know the cause (meaning) of a person's distressed and disturbed behaviour and know what they need in order to recover without necessarily asking them. The healing potential of the caring relationship is seen, if at all, as being peripheral to the client's recovery and leads to relationships becoming depersonalised and distant, a complaint frequently made in user satisfaction surveys (MacGabhann 2000). This contrasts starkly with humanistic practice which emphasises the therapeutic use of self, is empathic to the experience of the person in care and seeks to work with them in egalitarian, empowering ways.

The dominance of the biomedical model has tended to minimise the context as a significant factor in the client's experience of distress, disturbance and recovery. Schizophrenia is still predominantly seen as a physically based, pathological entity, despite the evidence for this view being strongly challenged by those who take a more psychosocial or psycho-spiritual perspective (Breggin & Stern 1996, Bentall 2003, Read et al 2004). Depression is still primarily conceptualised as a disorder of neurotransmission despite the evidence that this common human experience of profound malaise, despondency and despair is primarily caused by psychosocial factors (Brown 1996, Smail 1999). This is borne out by research into the significantly higher incidence of anxiety and depression in women, which points to psychosocial factors as a predominant cause (Department of Health 2002a). Fernando (2002) makes a strong case that pathogenic depression is a Western concept that has dubious validity in other cultures where distress in its various manifestations is seen as arising from the trials of life. Humanistic philosophy, in emphasising the whole being of the individual – the physical dimension, the psychological dimension, the spiritual dimension and the social dimension – as important components in the human experience of wellbeing and dis-ease, challenges the reductionist biomedical view of human suffering.

Humanistic approaches to helping are rooted in phenomenology. This is a method of enquiry employed in existential philosophy, which takes the view that knowledge and understanding can only be gained by exploring the subjective experience of people. Assumptions one holds about a phenomenon being explored are suspended and the researcher avoids imposing theoretical constructs on the experience of others. In the context of therapeutic helping, the task is to enable others to report and describe their reality without interpreting it, without trying to fit it into some classification system. A shared explanatory hypothesis of what's going on and what's going wrong (and right as well) can evolve in a way that has meaningfulness for the client and is open to change in the light of further experience. Such an approach encourages trust and openness (Mosher & Burti 1994). To call the experience of voice hearing an auditory hallucination and to interpret that as a symptom of a pathological syndrome called schizophrenia tells us very little about the nature and meaning of that experience to the individual. The work of Romme & Escher (1993, 2000) challenges the view that there is a causal connection between voice hearing and specific psychiatric disorders. They suggest that for many people voice hearing may be a survival strategy, a way of coping with trauma or some other adverse life situation, rather than a symptom of a particular disorder. Chadwick et al (1996) suggest that central to understanding psychotic phenomena is the human endeavour of trying to construct a sense of self that is valued and authentic. Events which are experienced as a threat to the sense of self, that trigger negative self-evaluation or lead to negative inferences about the intentions and evaluations of others, are common precipitants of disturbed, distressed behaviour. We need to work with people in ways that enable them to be open to and communicate their experience. It is the rediscovery or reconstruction of a sense of self that is a significant component in the recovery process in severe mental health problems.

Barker et al (1997), in developing a construction of mental health care that is broadly humanistic, strike a note of opposition to what is seen as a reassertion of biomedical orthodoxy in psychiatric care. Mental health care is seen as primarily an interactive activity concerned with establishing the conditions necessary to promote the healing and growth of the person in care. It is this emergent self and the personal resources this process releases that enables the person seeking help to manage the challenges of everyday living in less problematic ways. The focus of effective care is therefore seen as being person centred rather than problem centred. This process is seen as reflexive in the sense that it also influences the helper. I cannot be empathic with the experience of clients unless I am able to show myself that same empathy. As Deegan (1988) suggests, professional helpers need to acknowledge their own wounds and to live the spirit of recovery in their own lives. 'For professionals to accept and embrace their own woundedness and vulnerability is the first step towards understanding the experience of the disabled' (p. 18). Psychiatric practice is located in the context of the client's relational world: the client's relationship with self, with others, with the material world and with the spiritual. Practitioners enter and, for a time, become part of the matrix of the whole, lived experience of the person in care.

The whole concept of psychiatric expertise is built on the erroneous belief that as reason is primarily the product of a rational process and therefore anyone who is deemed irrational or mad cannot possibly make sense of their experience, this becomes the task of mental health practitioners operating from the high ground of rationality and sanity (Thomas & Bracken 2004). It is difficult to swim against the tidal pull of didactic authoritative approaches to psychiatric care. Nevertheless all of this is possible in an age where the mandate for a medical psychiatry is, as in the 1960s and 1970s, being seriously questioned.

People know what they need

The rhetoric in mental health care frequently extols the value of a needs-led service, i.e. a service that is responsive to the identified needs of the community. If this is not to remain empty rhetoric, the voice of user groups must be influential in determining service developments and priorities (National Institute for Mental Health in England 2003). A clear picture is emerging that significant numbers of people who use the services do not find the current provision helpful. There has been particular criticism of hospital-based acute services in meeting the needs of people in acute distress. In a recent study by service users, the three most important needs identified at times of acute distress were: someone to talk to; the need to feel safe and supported; and the need for somewhere to relax and calm down (Mental Health Foundation 1997). These needs are unlikely to be met in an acute admission unit. As one respondent commented, 'When I have been ill, I have needed privacy and peace, neither of which I have had at all in hospital. I do need medication when I am in these states but I am convinced that the usual hospital environment is bad for me and when I am at my worst I am bad for other patients too.' A Sainsbury Centre survey also highlights the dissatisfaction of service users with acute services. This study concluded that 'hospital care is a non-therapeutic intervention' which often falls short of meeting the social and therapeutic needs of patients (Sainsbury Centre 1998b). There are some hopeful signs of an emerging service that is responsive to the needs of people who become acutely disturbed and distressed. In many areas of the UK, intensive community support is accessible to people 24 hours a day (Chisholm & Ford 2004) and sanctuaries (crisis houses) as an alternative to hospitalisation are becoming available in some areas. Studies show the effectiveness of these services, on a number of measures, to be as good as or an improvement on hospital care, while user satisfaction is higher (Minghella et al 1998).

It is not just acute services that fail to meet needs. Psychiatric care that is dominated by a cure-based or a skills-based approach is unlikely to meet the needs of people with enduring mental health problems. The cure-based approach that identifies either psychopathology or neuropathology as problems to be fixed by a plethora of interventions both medical and psychological is of limited help to people who have ongoing vulnerabilities and disabilities. Perkins & Repper (1996) argue that the cure-based approach can be positively damaging to both service users and staff because of the sense of demoralisation and hopelessness that so often results when people do not recover and stay well. The cure-based approach can give rise to a culture of blame. Staff may feel they have failed and blame themselves, their colleagues, the system, or the patient and soon begin to suffer from burnout. Patients blame the staff or themselves and feel increasingly helpless and hopeless. Cure-based approaches have tended to overvalue 'the therapies' and undervalue care as a potent healing factor in the recovery process.

Skills-based approaches, which are widely used in psychiatric practice, tend to see people's needs in terms of deficits. People may be assessed as lacking life skills or social skills and rehabilitation is seen as a process of increasing a person's competence in these areas. There are a number of problems with this. Firstly, it can impose the values of professional helpers on to the person in care. A person may not value the ability to prepare a meal, preferring instead to use local cafes. They may not value independent living, which for them means social isolation, preferring instead the option of communal living. Secondly, it places the onus on the person with social disabilities to adapt to the community, whereas community acceptance of differentness would allow greater social inclusion. Would it be too much to expect a little more patience and tolerance toward a person whose inwardness and distraction make communicating with others in everyday life a little more tortuous than is usual? Finally, we should not confuse not using skills with not having skills. The former is far more common amongst mental health veterans and has more to do with demoralisation than deficit. What is needed is not so much skills training as the presence of someone who can be with people in a way that is accepting and enabling. This is not a relationship that is overtly therapeutic. It does not demand anything of the person in care, it is a non-judgemental openness to wherever the person is, whether that be in a chaotic state of mind or in the first steps of recovery. Hallmarks of this relational style, which Mosher & Burti (1994) call 'letting be', are compassion, empathic understanding, validation, support and containment. There is a similarity between what is being described here as the art of being present and the Buddhist healing tradition of 'sending and taking'. Through meditation practice of sending out compassionate thoughts and taking in the anguish that is present in the world, practitioners train themselves to be with others in a way that allows them to resonate with deeply disturbed and distressed people and be with them in a way that is understanding, compassionate and restorative (Podvoll 2003). Being present with people can give way to a more active involvement and collaborative problem-solving as their psychosocial needs become known as they begin to re-engage in life. The essential element in the spirit of recovery is the courage to hope and the willingness to try. This is unlikely to be nurtured by a service that focuses solely on skills. In contrast to this, humanistic care is concerned more with an individual's growth, than with cure. It is concerned with creating a social milieu which enables people to move towards what Rogers calls becoming a fully functioning person, a journey which we all share.

A need is a lack of something that, if it remains unsatisfied, expresses itself as suffering. Mosher & Burti (1994) put identifying needs at the centre of their model for community mental health services:

> In our work we are primarily concerned with needs: we prefer to consider symptoms as communications about unmet needs that may be recognised and met rather than as expressions of hypothetical, underlying pathological processes, whose classification results in little advantage to the patient. We must understand the message in order to recognise the presenting needs; the psychological mechanisms of symptom formation are of less concern to us. (p. 19)

There have been many attempts to classify human needs. Abraham Maslow, one of the founding fathers of humanistic psychology, developed one of the best-known classifications (Box 9.1). Our level of wellbeing can be seen as a barometer of how successful we are in meeting these needs in everyday life. Mental health service users, whose vulnerabilities and social disadvantage keep them on the edge of distress, are people whose wants and needs are often frustrated and remain unmet. What service users say they want is an ordinary life, not a life that is lived within the parameters of a mental health service provision that is annexed from the mainstream of community life. Why should people with mental health problems need a health and fitness centre of their own when there are many perfectly good ones in the locality? Do they have different housing needs from anybody else? They may need support in accessing and using these resources but that is a different issue.

It is helpful to keep in mind that the needs of a person with a mental health problem are no different from our own. They may be more urgent and pressing, they may be creating more tension and anguish at that moment in time, but in essence they are the same needs that we all have.

Box 9.1

Human needs

- To be authentic – become the person we are
- To express our spiritual nature
- To affiliate and belong
- To be valued and value ourselves
- To love and be loved
- To express our sexuality
- To feel secure and attached
- To meet our physiological needs
- To express our eco-affiliation needs*

*This represents humankind's evolutionary based affiliation with the natural world, largely ignored in contemporary culture but becoming a more urgent need as the consequences of ignoring it become apparent in terms of personal wellbeing and the wellbeing of the planet.

Adapted from Maslow (1987).

Wants can be aspirations that reflect basic human needs. This fits with the stress vulnerability model of mental disorder widely used as a model for understanding and responding therapeutically to the spectrum of distressed and disturbed behaviour that people seek help with.

Of course people do not usually express their needs and wants in quite these terms. The self-assessed needs of mental health service users consistently highlight that what they want is a home, enough money to live on, a meaningful day, support and friends, relief from suffering and access to specialist help (Strathdee et al 1997). A recent user-led research survey (Mental Health Foundation 1997, 2000) identified the following needs and wants when in distress:

* someone to talk to
* help to manage my feelings
* support from someone who will listen to me
* help to relax
* somewhere to be safe
* easier access to psychiatric care when I'm unwell
* help with practical problems
* help to cope with my voices
* information about illness, treatment, services
* help with social recovery
* spiritual care
* acceptance
* privacy and peace
* to be looked after
* counselling
* medication
* complementary therapies.

It might seem that the pursuit of satisfying needs reflects an obsession with self. While narcissism is a necessary phase in development, the meeting of needs in the context of adult relationships becomes more reciprocal and altruistic (Argyle 1994). In the person-centred approach to helping, the need to feel loved and valued is emphasised as a prerequisite for growth and the unfolding of our potential. As we grow towards being more authentic, more aware and accepting of ourselves, we become more effective in meeting our own needs and become more aware and responsive to the needs of others. There is, for example, often a great deal of anger in the experience of depression. Often people will be unable to own their anger and other feelings that are related to frustrated, unmet needs. Early experience has taught people that the open expression of needs and feelings will meet with disapproval or rejection. They learn that love is conditional on not being needy, not being upset. Disowning needs and feeling becomes a pattern and people no longer know what they need or what they feel; they have become alienated from their authentic selves. For many people the experience of depression is a grey dawn that settles on the landscape of their lives, robbing it of colour and life. In the profound bleakness of that experience is the despair of ever being prized enough to have their needs and feelings accepted, and anger that this should be so. Sometimes such despair and anger becomes unbearable and the act of suicide the only solace.

Awareness of another's needs is only possible if we can be sensitive and empathic to what the client is saying metaphorically in distressed and disturbed behaviour. If we can listen to a person's experience as it unfolds, from their frame of reference, so that it is almost as if we are sharing the experience, we can get a sense of what needs underlie their presenting behaviour. For example, a young Anglo-African man was referred to the service with a history of voice hearing. In an effort to be accepted into the host culture he had anglicised his name and limited the expression of his cultural heritage in his lifestyle. His voice hearing began during a period when he had been feeling depressed following the death of his mother. The voices were sometimes abusive and taunting, sometimes validating and at times spoke to him in a Nigerian dialect he was not familiar with. He came to interpret these voices as meaning that he was 'special' and 'chosen' and that he had 'shaman's blood' and began communicating loudly with the spirit world and posting sachets of 'herbal remedies' through the doors of neighbours. This may be seen to be unusual and disruptive expressions of a need to be valued and belong, to be his authentic self in a way that honoured his ethnicity and cultural heritage.

Hildegard Peplau (1988) has written widely about needs in the context of mental health care. She argues that 'only the patient knows what his needs are and he is not always able to identify them, knowing only that he feels the tension that needs generate. Paying attention to the needs of the patient, so that personalities can develop further, is a way of using nursing as a social force that aids people to identify what they want and to feel free and able to struggle with others to find satisfaction ... Progressive identification of needs takes place as nurse and patient communicate with each other in an interpersonal relationship' (p. 84). Peplau takes a broadly humanistic view of needs, i.e. that when basic needs are substantially met – our physiological needs, our needs for security, our need for love and belonging and the need to feel valued and to value ourselves, then more of our energy is free to develop our potential as human beings. We then begin to move towards creative, constructive, productive, personal and community living.

97

Jamie's story

Theme: dysfunctional expression of need

Jamie is a young man who has had numerous referrals to the mental health services. He grew up in a family with a physically abusive father and a depressed mother who had often been hospitalised. The most nurturing relationship in his life was with his grandmother, who died when he was 11 years old. He lives a chaotic lifestyle with no structure or anchor points. He is a sociable person but seems unable to develop relationships beyond a superficial level. His life is currently punctuated by frequent crises in which he complains of unbearable tension, feels depressed and is wracked by thoughts that he is 'bad through and through'. At times he hears voices telling him

Continued

Jamie's story—cont'd

to hang himself. The tension is expressed and finds some relief in excessive drinking and drug misuse and self-harm behaviour. During the course of various psychiatric assessments, a number of diagnoses have been made: schizo-affective disorder, borderline personality disorder, drug-induced psychosis complicated by problematic drinking. He now thinks of himself as ill and has become adept at being a psychiatric patient, at getting psychoactive drugs prescribed and at gaining admission where his needs are for a time at least partially met and his tension subsides.

An alternative explanatory hypothesis of Jamie's presenting problems could be that his behaviour is a dramatic and damaging way of expressing and getting some response to his unmet needs. Adopting a needs-led approach to this scenario, Jamie's care coordinator/CPN will have a central role in helping him identify his needs, articulated in a language that has meaning for him. Through a developing relationship there would be some direct response to these needs and help in accessing other resources. It would be onerous if not impossible for any individual mental health worker to sufficiently meet all of the needs this client has and other sources of support would need to be in place. It is only when he has a secure base provided by relationships with mental health workers who are able to acknowledge and contain his distress and relate to him in a way that enables him to feel warmly accepted and valued that he will be able to move on in his development as a person and reclaim an ordinary life. Building a relationship that is different enough to make a difference requires time and commitment. It requires a team or organisational culture in which staff feel supported and have their own feelings of anxiety, despondency, failure, inadequacy, anger that can surface in the care of people like Jamie acknowledged and contained.

The focus for much of the debate on a needs-led service centres not so much on what we have been discussing so far, the individual needs of service users, but on the availability of resources in a locality to meet the mental health needs of a local population. For example, the need for a 24-hour crisis response service, activity centres, supported housing, family intervention service, counselling services, complementary therapies, intensive care beds, crisis houses, outreach services, and so on. The user movement is becoming increasingly active and influential in the planning and development of services and in setting up alternatives to the statutory and agency provision, in the form of self-help groups, drop-in centres and sanctuaries. There has been some criticism of the community provision taking shape in the UK, which is seen by some service users as the reinvention of the institution in the community in a way that does not address their real needs (Sainsbury Centre 1998a, Chisholm & Ford 2004). The experience of many service users is that their needs are not adequately assessed, particularly in relation to the social context of their distress, and as a consequence the service response is at best only partially helpful. There can be too much emphasis on neuropathology and psychopathology so that people come to believe that the problem is within, rather than being related to the social and economic context in which they live their lives. Assessment of need should be from the user perspective. They should be able to negotiate a care programme that best meets their needs. The danger with a needs-led service that focuses too much on the provision of resources is that people with mental health problems will have to fit into whatever is available. For example, it can become routine practice for someone diagnosed as having schizophrenia to be prescribed depot neuroleptics, to attend a mental health resource centre and receive fortnightly visits by a CPN, who monitors symptoms and side effects and provides support. This may fall far short of the service user's need for better housing, a socially valued way of spending their time, ways of coping with the unusual thoughts and voices that trouble them, and an improved relationship with their family. There is a need for professionals, particularly key workers and case managers, to be creative and flexible in response to individual users' needs.

One of the most damning criticisms of community care is that it has failed to meet the needs of the most vulnerable service users. Those with long-term disabilities often either slip through cracks in the service or are difficult to engage with. The recognition that the needs of this group were being neglected has led to the setting up of assertive outreach teams. Many people in this group are distrustful of the mental health service as a consequence of previous experience and actively avoid contact. The key to engaging with this group is the ability of the key worker to establish a relationship that is accepting and understanding and seeks to be of practical help (Chisholm & Ford 2004).

There has also been criticism of the inadequacy of the provision for users from ethnic minority groups. Services can be very ethnocentric, reflecting Western values of mental health and individual needs. There are concerns about the discriminatory processes in psychiatry which are reflected in the higher diagnostic rates for schizophrenia, more compulsory admissions, high doses of medication and more unmet needs amongst service users for the ethnic minorities (Fernando 2002).

People can take responsibility for themselves

A useful adage for humanistic helpers would be *less is more*! The less we can do for someone, the more they are likely to develop a sense of personal power and agency. The aim is to work with people in collaborative and facilitative ways that maximise autonomy and self-help, with the professional helper being the midwife of change, not the originator. 'At the heart of humanistic helping is a belief in the trustworthiness of the person seeking help, as someone capable of evaluating their inner and outer world, understanding himself in its context and making choices as to the next step in life and acting on those choices' (Rogers 1977, p. 382). Brandon (1976), in exploring the art of helping, highlights the damage that professional helpers can do to a person's sense of their own agency if they take over the problems of living that a service user faces and attempt to deal with human distress in a prescriptive way. Along that therapeutic route we find increasing passivity, dependency and helplessness. It is natural for us as mental health workers to want to do something to relieve distress or to change behaviour that is damaging or limiting. But we can become so impelled by our desire to help that it becomes a kind of craving that makes it difficult for us to tolerate others' distress and accept unwise behaviour. In an interesting exploration of the Buddhist philosophy of helping, Groves (1998) suggests helpers should work at developing the skilful qualities of unconditional loving kindness and mindfulness. This allows us to be with people in a way that values them, that communicates warm regard, without demanding anything in return. Mindfulness allows us to be more aware of others, to be more aware of ourselves and more aware of the effect of our presence on others. These two qualities when present in the helper can have a liberating effect on people seeking help. If we can stop hindering the recovery process, distress will run its course and the individual will begin to respond to inner prompting to find a way of being in the world that engenders less suffering. This is very similar to the claim made for the person-centred approach to psychological helping that being with people in a real, empathic, accepting way facilitates growth and resourcefulness, so that amongst other changes they will:

- show fewer characteristics normally labelled psychotic or neurotic
- become more self-knowledgeable and more accepting of self
- become more self-directing and self-confident
- become better able to cope with the problems of living more effectively and comfortably (Rogers 1967).

In his clinical practice, Rogers became convinced that it is always the client who knows what hurts and what direction they need to move in for healing to take place. The helper's task is to help people discover their inner resources, not to impose solutions, strategies, explanations and interpretations. When there is a commitment to understanding the subjective world of the client and the client feels understood, they begin to move forward in constructive, positive ways (Thorne 1992). The act of helping then is not only concerned with enabling people to deal in less distressing, problematic ways in the here and now, but should also leave people more resourceful and less vulnerable to the challenges of living they will face in the future.

Empowerment is a word that has been used to wrap professionalised care in an attractive package. But it is a mistake to think that professional helpers can empower anyone. Power has to be taken, it can never be conferred. The best we can do is not block the assertion of autonomy in the ways we relate to people in care. Helpers need to reflect critically on their practice and be watchful of actions that deprive clients of opportunities to develop or assert their autonomy and control. The helping process should be transparent. The French philosopher Foucault argues that power is bound up with knowledge. Experts, particularly experts in the psychiatric professions who claim an understanding of human distress and what to do about it, hold considerable power, power that is sanctioned by society. Psychiatric knowledge is mystifying to those on the outside, which therefore places people using the mental health services in a dependent position. It can be very difficult for an individual to exercise self-determination in an expert-led service that expects compliance. What if the dominant discourses that circulate in society about psychological distress are not absolute truths, but simply hypothetical constructions that offer a keyhole view of the nature of human distress? In recent years the edifice of Freudian psychoanalytic psychology has been exposed as a creative but flawed construction of human experience (Masson 1988). Similarly the construction of deeply distressed people as ill and in need of treatment, rather than care in a healing environment, has been called into question (Read 2004).

Self-determination, choice and self-healing are at the heart of individual recovery programmes. Psychosocial distress is not experienced passively. Most people try various strategies to cope with it, with varying degrees of success. Identifying and enhancing those strategies that have worked for individuals and teaching additional strategies can encourage a sense of control over problematic thoughts, feelings and behaviour. In a recent study (Mental Health Foundation 1997) 80% of people said that they had developed personal ways of coping with aspects of their daily life and experience that were difficult and distressing. People who use the mental health services will have their own ways of motivating themselves, getting support, managing disturbing experiences, coping with crisis and surviving, that should be recognised, respected and encouraged (Box 9.2). Some coping strategies can of course be damaging and limiting if used excessively, for example withdrawal, self-harming, or the use of alcohol. Individual care planning is concerned with helping people become less reliant on disruptive or harmful strategies through developing and strengthening their repertoire of positive strategies.

Many people with long-term mental health problems have benefited from an involvement with self-help and user groups. In most areas of the UK people will now be able to find support groups made up of people with similar difficulties and experiences to their own. Such groups operate mainly outside the statutory mental health service provision, although they may be sponsored and assisted by it. They provide an alternative to professionalised mental health care in which helping is reciprocal and takes place in an egalitarian context. Self-help and user groups are significant sources of support, self-help, empowerment and advocacy. For many people membership provides the seed from which the spirit of recovery grows. Even in consumer organisations such as Survivors Speak Out, who have a political agenda and are primarily

Box 9.2

Examples of positive coping strategies from a representative group of service users

Complementary therapies, leisure and recreational activities, yoga, physical activity, art and music, relaxation techniques, reading, adult education classes, walks in the countryside, prayer and religious contemplation, using medication, slowing down, expressing my feelings, keeping pets, keeping busy, disputing worrying thoughts, positive affirmation, talking with friends and family, talking with a mental health professional, joining a self-help group or user group, keeping a journal, finding out about my mental health problem, contacting the crisis line, helping others, having a socially valued occupation, taking respite breaks, getting enough rest, healthy eating, being listened to, understanding my symptoms, motivating myself, taking one day at a time, having a routine, having achievable goals, monitoring my symptoms, avoid overloading myself.

Source: Mental Health Foundation (1997).

concerned with influencing change within mainstream psychiatry and in the socio-political context in which users live their lives, individuals experience involvement as empowering and healing (Campbell 1996).

Recovering from long-term mental health problems requires people to be more in charge of their own lives, to become experts in their own self-care.

Of necessity this involves 'non-compliance'. When we consider what mental health service users are unmotivated about, or non-compliant with, it is usually some element in their treatment programme that they do not value for themselves, that has been prescribed by others with little consultative discussion. Until people can dream their own dreams and find their own pathway of recovery, their lives will remain circumscribed by the limited vision of others. Patricia Deegan, a psychologist and herself a service user, put it this way:

> To me recovery means that I try to stay in charge of my own life. I don't let my illness run me. Over the years I've worked hard to become an expert in my own self-care. For instance being in recovery means that I don't just take medication. Just taking medication is a passive stance. Rather I use medication as part of my recovery process. In the same way I don't just go into hospital. Just going into hospital is a passive stance. Rather I use the hospital when I need to. Additionally over the years I have learned all kinds of ways to help myself. Sometimes I use medication, therapy, self help and mutual support groups, friends, my relationship with God, my work, exercise, spending time with nature – all these things help me remain whole and healthy even though I have a disability. (Deegan 1997, p. 21)

A philosophy of care that places a high value on self-determination and self-responsibility does not mean that a person is in some way at fault for failing to recover and flourish. To do so would fail to recognise the social constraints that operate in the lives of many long-term mental health service users. It would fail to recognise the devastating impact of a serious mental health problem on the self-concept, self-esteem and personal aspirations of the individual. It would fail to recognise the need we all have for sustaining, growthful relationships in order to live out our potential.

Part 2

The working alliance

Introduction

For the past 50 years the literature on psychiatric practice has emphasised the therapeutic value of the relationship between practitioners and people using the mental health services, placing the relationship at the heart of mental health care.

In an early study of the work of psychiatric nurses, Cormack (1976) noted the resemblance between what people using the service said nurses contributed to their recovery and what Carl Rogers, the originator of person-centred counselling, identified as the necessary and sufficient conditions for change: a helping relationship in which the helper is able to be with the person seeking help in a way that is empathic, accepting and genuine. That these relational qualities are enabling and valued by service users continues to be endorsed by research (Sheppard 1993, Rogers & Pilgrim 1994, Mental Health Foundation 2000). The emphasis here is on a way of being in relationship to people in care, not what mental health professionals might know or do. It is this facilitative contact created by these relational qualities that enables people to set out and then continue on the road to recovery.

The helping relationship can take a number of forms; as Egan (2006) puts it: 'The idea of one perfect kind of helping relationship is a myth. Different clients have different needs and these are met through different kinds of relationship'. Clarkson (1995), in her perceptive analysis of therapeutic relationships, identifies five characterising elements: the working alliance, the transference–counter-transference relationship, the reparative, developmentally needed relationship, the person-to-person relationship and the transpersonal relationship. While this hypothesis has been forged in the main out of the experience of professional counselling and psychotherapy, it seems to me to have a helpful relevance to all mental health work. The relationship types are not seen as mutually exclusive but coalesce in the therapeutic process. Part 2 takes the working alliance, the basis for all helping relationships, as its central theme.

Chapter 10 is an exploration of beginnings. Connecting with clients in a way that facilitates a sense of rapport and trust is assisted by maintaining a sensitive awareness of the dynamics that commonly come into play in the beginning phase of any helping relationship.

Chapter 11 outlines a pragmatic, problem management framework within which collaborative helping can take place. It involves working creatively with clients to help them find more effective ways of managing the challenges and opportunities of living. Problems of living are part of the fabric of life. We can never eliminate them but we can learn to manage them in ways that are less problematic, distressing and disabling. The problem management framework offers people a strategy for living more fully and resourcefully. Many people, particularly those with long-term mental health problems, have experienced oppression and disempowerment. Often this has prevented them from being the architects of their own life and has inculcated a sense of helplessness, hopelessness and dependency.

Chapter 12 examines dynamics of co-creating and holding personal power. The working alliance is seen as an enabling relationship that aims to help clients connect with and express their personal power. The power balance in our professional relationships is always a product of the dialogical contact. Some clients, perhaps anxious of a potential loss of personal power and self-direction, may relate to mental health workers in aggressive, dominant ways, eroding the personal power of the individual worker. This may result in the adoption of an appeasing stance that is not helpful to the client. Conversely some clients may exude powerlessness and helplessness which dovetails with the worker's need to feel powerful. Again this is not a scenario in which power is being co-created, held and shared in a way that leads to empowered resourceful living. Some in the consumer/survivor movement would argue that it is only in user-led services where relationships are authentically equal that the empowered self can emerge and provide the self-belief necessary as a cornerstone to recovery (Fisher & Deegan 1999).

Chapter 13 broadens the parameters of the working alliance to include carers and their families. The importance of families in enhancing the wellbeing of individuals distressed and disabled by enduring mental health problems is recognised and discussed. For families to maintain a social environment in which the recovery process can take place, mental health professionals must address their needs, problems and issues.

Chapter 14 considers the issue of reluctance, resistance and non-engagement. Despite the best endeavours of mental health professionals, some clients remain difficult to engage and work with. It can take months of persistent effort to forge a tenuous alliance. This should not come as a surprise. Often the history of service users is of abusive relationships in the personal sphere of their lives and oppressive encounters with health and social services. Non-engagement should not always be viewed negatively. For some people, defending the sovereignty of their lives against the incursions of mental health professionals represents the tender shoots of recovery.

Chapter 15 explores the dynamics of the end phase of the working alliance. Issues triggered by endings can be difficult for both the client and the helper alike and need to be managed with awareness and sensitivity. While the working alliance can be an enabling presence that is a significant factor in the client's recovery process, at some point it must end if we are not to hold people in a co-dependent relationship.

Beginnings and the working alliance

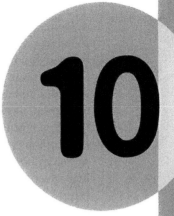

Beginnings are important. The foundations are being laid for a working alliance without which it will be difficult to help the client. This phase in the helping process can be brief or it can take some time, but it cannot be rushed. Early impressions fundamentally affect the shaping of the relationship. For instance, practitioners who create an initial impression of being controlling or insensitive may find that impression difficult to break down.

Often assumptions and expectations are present before the practitioner and client come face to face. Clients may have had a bad experience of mental health services in the past. They may have experienced oppressive or unhelpful care. They may resent their referral, which may have involved an element of coercion. They may be fearful that in becoming involved with the mental health services they will be stigmatised and their personhood submerged by psychiatric patient status. As practitioners we may be influenced by a client's reported history or diagnosis and have a prejudiced picture of them before we have even met.

It can be very difficult for some clients to trust professional carers and they may remain guarded and distant and difficult to reach out to (Fig. 10.1). This may be related to traumatising experiences of parental or statutory care in their early lives. The legacy of such an experience can be a discomfort with closeness and intimacy and a reluctance to trust others with their vulnerability. As Winship (1995) suggests, it can be difficult to accept the concern and care of staff, if caring figures in the patient's past were persecutory. Care may be perceived with suspicion and hostility. Part of the art of psychiatric care is to be able to hold psychologically these projected feelings while building a relationship with the client which is safe enough to enable them to re-own and feel less disturbed by persecutory feelings. Clearly, acting out the client's projections through oppressive action will confirm their deepest fears and undermine the foundations of a working alliance.

Where coercion, compulsion or force has been used in relation to admission or treatment, it is important to acknowledge the psychological trauma that such an experience subjects people to. It should be openly discussed with the client and their feelings heard (Campbell & Lindlow 1997). Considerable perseverance can be required to rebuild a basis of trust.

Building trust means going at the client's pace and not pushing so hard that reluctance becomes resistance. In our initial contact with a client, we need to put the emphasis on ourselves as people – the person rather than the role.

A client is much more likely to engage with you the individual than with you the social worker, nurse or psychiatrist. We need to establish a basis for collaborative relationship from an early stage by actively seeking the client's views on how they see their needs and what they need help with. Being able to offer some immediate practical help conveys a strong message that you are 'for the client', a potential ally in a world that may seem chaotic, difficult and threatening. It is, however, best to be honest about what you can and can't offer in terms of direct help and accessing resources. The philosophy of leaving clients with as much power as possible to make choices and decisions, to be in charge of their own lives, needs to come through in the initial interaction. Equally it can be important to give clients permission to rely on the mental health worker at times of difficulty and crisis.

A common concern for clients is, 'Will I be heard? Not just listened to politely but have my disclosures respected and taken seriously?'. The experience of severe psychological distress and disturbance can be very alienating and clients will feel a great need to be understood. Many people wish their experience to be understood in personal human terms and not pathologised and labelled. The fear of being labelled mad and stigmatised resides with a fear of being sectioned and hospitalised; these anxieties are at the root of many clients' reluctance to engage with mental health services. For other clients it is not their psychiatric vulnerability that is their primary concern, but the precariousness of their social circumstances – the threat of eviction or poverty and debt. This therefore needs to be heard and responded to pragmatically by the practitioner if a relationship is going to develop. Along with the concern 'Will I be heard?' is the fear 'Will I be judged?'; 'Will I be thought of as weak, stupid, mad!'.

With some clients who find it hard to engage with the service, it may be necessary to establish contact through a trusted friend, family or another service user. Sometimes the difficulty in establishing rapport can be due to a social, cultural or gender divide between the client and mental health worker and referring on to a colleague may be necessary to engage a client with the service. This should be seen as a sensitively aware, client-centred strategy and not as an admission of professional failure or inadequacy. There is some evidence that ex-service users employed as project workers within community mental health teams can be effective in gaining the trust of disaffected clients (Sainsbury Centre 1998a).

You will see from all of this that beginnings frequently require effort and sensitivity. It helps to try and get an early intuitive sense of the client's social receptivity and willingness to engage in the care process. Some clients are receptive to a warm supportive presence. Others respond better to a slightly more 'business-like' approach.

Indications that the relationship has moved beyond the beginning stage will be the sense that the client is more at ease, open and less defensive and when there is a real feeling of connecting. You are no longer meeting as strangers. The client has begun to identify you as someone who can be of help.

Self-enquiry box

You may find it helpful to reflect on your contact with recently referred clients and plot the progression of the developing relationship on the engagement scale (Fig. 10.1). As well as identifying client characteristics it can be instructive to reflect openly on your self-presentation in relation to these criteria. As in all social relations, some degree of mutuality is necessary for relationships to evolve.

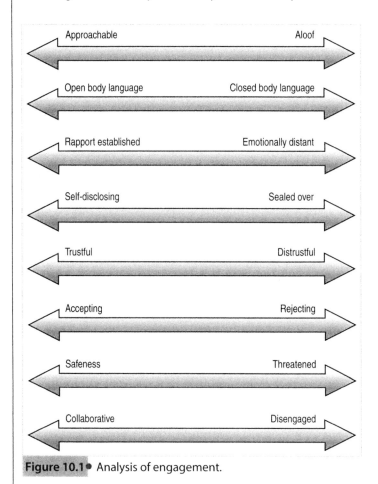

Figure 10.1 Analysis of engagement.

A framework for the working alliance

11

The skilled helper model developed by Gerard Egan over the past thirty years and widely adopted by mental health professionals in the UK offers a useful framework for the working alliance. It is a model that is at its heart person-centred, collaborative and empowering. Egan takes the view that helping is both a social influence process and a process that values client self-responsibility. Achieving this balance is important if the alliance is not to become coercive, controlling and oppressive (Egan 2006).

Democratising the helping process is encouraged if we can:

- meet people with humanity and humility so that the alliance is one of equals
- acknowledge that as helpers we are both resourceful and fallible, as is the client
- recognise that power can be shared, discovered and generated within the helping alliance
- make the helping process participative rather than directive
- share our knowledge of the helping process so that people can become more resourceful and self-supporting.

Egan's model is essentially a problem management approach to helping (Fig. 11.1). He argues that when it comes to personal, relational and social problems, we are not terribly good problem-solvers. There is a tendency to put up with difficulties, ignore them, deny them, minimise them, or attempt the same ineffective solutions over and over. Distress, disturbance and disablement build up in the wake of undealt-with problems. The helping process is concerned with enabling people to become more resourceful and creative in managing the problems facing them, in both their inner and outer worlds. The helper's task is to engage those seeking help in a process that moves through three stages:

- helping clients identify and clarify needs and problems
- helping clients create a better future
- helping clients create strategies to move forward.

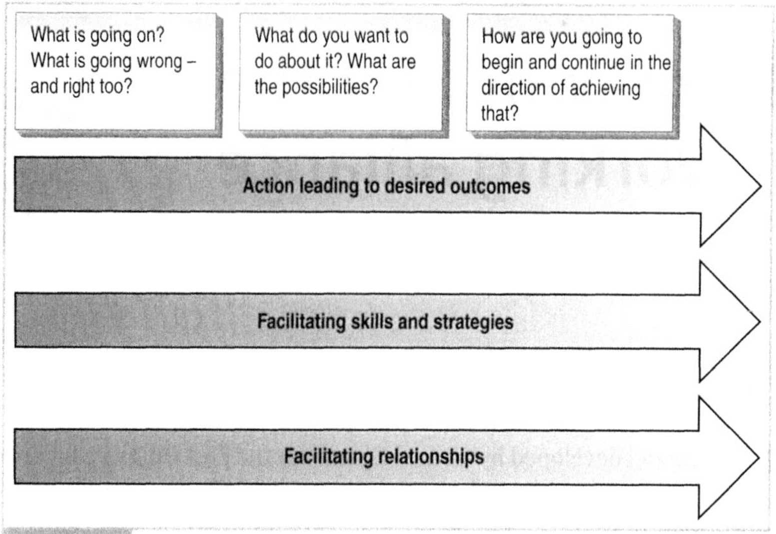

| What is going on? What is going wrong – and right too? | What do you want to do about it? What are the possibilities? | How are you going to begin and continue in the direction of achieving that? |

Action leading to desired outcomes

Facilitating skills and strategies

Facilitating relationships

Figure 11.1 ● The skilled helper model.

Helping clients identify and clarify needs and problems

The first stage of this model is to help the client tell his or her story. Some people will readily seize the opportunity to talk about what's going on and what's going wrong. To unload what might seem daunting, frightening, puzzling or painful experiences to someone who is able to listen supportively can be a great relief. But given a natural reticence in our culture and an understandable anxiety about the consequences of disclosing personal information, most people need to feel a sense of trust and safety before they are able to share and explore their problems fully. In telling their story the client is often acknowledging and facing difficult and painful issues that may have, until now, been kept at a distance. As the story emerges, the associated emotional distress may surface with it and be discharged. In the exploratory dialogue between the helper and client, the story is filled out and new perspectives can emerge. The issues and problems of living that confront the client can be viewed with more clarity or seen differently. This can mean that a problem might not seem quite so disturbing and distressing – it can be faced and coped with, opportunities can be seen.

As the client's story unfolds, we need to try to avoid assumptions and interpretations. Our task as helpers is to come to a shared understanding of the client's reality. We need to know what meaning the term depression has in relation to the client's experience of himself and his life. Words, as Wittgenstein argues, do not describe reality, but create the reality out of experience (Lynch 1997). Having expert knowledge does not give mental health professionals insight into an individual's reality; the client is the expert on that. Understanding a client's experience comes through finding a common language from which something of the client's world and its meanings can be communicated. Essentially the task of all therapeutic conversation is to find a way of co-creating a different or preferred reality.

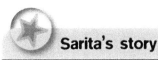

Sarita's story

Theme: identifying and clarifying needs and problems

Sarita is a 28-year-old woman who has been diagnosed as having schizophrenia. Despite trying various neuroleptic drugs she struggles to stay free of intrusive and disruptive delusional ideas. The feeling that people are watching and following her surfaces and begins to take hold, as does the belief that closed-circuit TV cameras monitor her movements. These distressing thoughts cause her to isolate herself in her flat. She also complains of hearing 'whispering', which she interprets as evidence of the close surveillance she is under.

The dialogue transcribed below took place following an incident in which the police were called to the flats where Sarita lives after neighbours heard her shouting at her persecutors. She has had three previous admissions to an acute psychiatric admission unit, during which she became very depressed and apathetic. The community team are trying to help Sarita manage this crisis episode without resorting to hospitalisation.

A key worker has established a working alliance with Sarita in which she feels safe enough to share her experience.

Key worker: To believe that you're being watched and followed must be frightening.

Sarita (crying): I can't go out now. They're always there. Did you see anyone around outside when you arrived? Perhaps I should go back to the hospital?

Key worker: I'm sorry you're feeling so upset and unsafe. I didn't see anyone suspicious in the street. Why do you think this is happening to you?

Sarita: They think I'm here illegally, don't they and they're trying to get rid of me. I've seen the cameras in the town picking me out of the crowd. Just because I've had this mental trouble they want to get rid of me.

Key worker: Are you saying that because you've had some psychiatric problems over the past few years you think the police and the immigration people have been told to get rid of you?

Sarita (nods): That's why they were here today.

Key worker: Can you think of any other explanation for why the police came? How would it seem if I said that they were called because someone here heard you shouting and they were concerned about you and didn't know what else to do?

Sarita: They couldn't give a fuck about me. I've heard them say they ought to put her in hospital or pack her off home.

Key worker: That must feel pretty hurtful.

Key worker: This worry about being watched and followed – is that something that's on your mind a lot, or just from time to time?

Sarita: They could come and get me any time. I can't sleep because they might come at night when it's quiet.

Key worker: Do you think you need to be in hospital?

Sarita: Part of me does. I'd feel safer there. They can't touch me there you see, there are too many witnesses. But I'm afraid I will lose myself if I go in again. I don't want to end up one of those empty-eyed women.

Key worker: You feel like you might, in a way, lose any chance of a normal life if you go in again? You seem a bit calmer since we've been talking and I'm wondering

111

Continued

Sarita's story—cont'd

how it would be for you if I called more frequently over the next few days and Janice (housing project worker) spent more time with you? Would that help you feel safer?

As Sarita's story unfolds it seemed that these unusual thoughts were linked in some way to her experience of discrimination both as an Asian woman and as a user of the mental health service. Her family are Ugandan Asians who were forced to leave Uganda during Idi Amin's oppressive regime. They were subjected to a great deal of intimidation prior to their exclusion and arrived in Britain as political refugees with very little. Although they had legal citizenship and have now created a new life for themselves, a legacy of insecurity and distrust has persisted in the family culture. Sarita's mother appeared to suffer from a disabling post-traumatic stress disorder for several years after the family's arrival in the UK. As a young woman Sarita's westernised values, a failed marriage to a white Englishman and in recent years her mental health problems have progressively alienated her from her family. This alienated, depressed state of mind seemed to allow persecutory thoughts to surface, take hold and take on a more extreme form. Enabling Sarita to tell her story within the context of a safe and supportive relationship relieved some of the emotional tension and distress that had built up around her disturbing thoughts and gave meaning to them. It also opened up possibilities for helping her manage this vulnerability more effectively, without the need for increasing medication or admitting her to hospital.

Sarita's story continues on page 115

Often the problems of living for which people seek help from the mental health services are quite complex. As a story unfolds, there may be a history of abuse in childhood, problem drinking, low self-esteem, volatile moods, debts, housing difficulties, suicide attempts. Egan argues that to try and work on all fronts can be overwhelming for the client and the helper. Priorities need to be identified. What is the client motivated to do something about? What would make a significant difference to their sense of wellbeing? Unless there is a shared perception about the problems and needs that the client could use help with, then the helping process will stall at the outset. This is not to say that as helpers we should collude with clients to avoid the difficult and challenging issues they face. We should make reasonable demands and encourage people to make reasonable demands on themselves. Egan identifies a number of principles for getting leverage in helping people manage their problems in living:

- If there's a crisis, first help the client manage the crisis.
- Begin with the problem that causes most distress.
- Begin with the issue that the client sees as important, which may be different from the helper's assessment.
- Begin with a manageable part of the problem. Problem management is often incremental, involving small steps rather than giant strides.
- Begin with a problem that will lead to an overall improvement in wellbeing.

Finding a different way of being that is less problematic, overcoming social disadvantage and adversity, are not easy tasks. Sometimes problems can seem to defy efforts to resolve them and create a stagnant pool of powerlessness and helplessness. At times it can be better to surrender to a problem, to stop working so hard to resolve it. Surrendering does not mean passively resigning oneself to a life limited by a problem or its negative effects, it means letting go of the tension that builds up around frustrated attempts at resolution. Sometimes this release of pressure opens up new options. A new-found acceptance of personal vulnerabilities emerges, leading to creative ways of managing and transcending them. On the other hand, many people who seek the help of mental health services readily retreat into helplessness when faced with the difficulties of living. For those individuals, the need is one of asserting some control over problem situations rather than surrendering. Their learnt helplessness needs to be replaced by the discovery of their resourcefulness. Through engaging people in a problem management process, a sense of being more in control of one's life begins to emerge, which can be both freeing and empowering.

Creating a better future

The second stage of Egan's problem management process is concerned with helping the client construct a better future. In other words, it is concerned with exploring the possibilities and setting goals, which then become a direction for wise action. The stories that people tell are often problem-saturated. This can so easily be reinforced by mental health professionals if the focus of their interest is solely on dysfunctional aspects of the client's life and does not also bring out their resources and talents. The meaning the client is likely to draw from that problem-saturated perspective is that they are ill, helpless, hopeless, inadequate or weak and have no future – a bleak picture indeed and one that can trap people in a 'career' as a mental patient or as a victim.

This can be an exciting and satisfying phase in the helping process. People begin to transcend their disabilities and regain a measure of hopefulness and resourcefulness, stepping out on the road of recovery. Step by step they begin to re-enter life and manage their lives more effectively. In so doing, their personal narratives become less problem-saturated and they begin to see themselves in more positive ways. Of course this is not an easy process – a client may well find it easier to adopt the passive role of the ill patient or the victim. Recovering or discovering a sense of personal agency, the sense of being in charge of their own lives, can perhaps be the most difficult part of all the helping process for people with long-term mental health problems, since they may have an understandable tendency to retreat from the significant and distressing problems of living into passivity, helplessness and hopelessness. Unfortunately, disempowering relationships with mental health professionals can compound this protective but ultimately limiting strategy.

This part of the helping process involves asking future-oriented questions which are intended to identify the possibilities for change. We are asking people to imagine a different life for themselves. Not a fairytale, happy-ever-after sort of life, but one in which there is more psychological comfort and social ease than there is now. In doing this we need to be careful that it is the client's wishes that are identified and not our own aspirations for the client based on our own values. It is easy to unintentionally influence clients in the direction of certain goals.

113

For some clients, greater social participation and integration may not be a desired outcome. For others, a higher level of independence may not be a valued goal, although we might value both these behavioural characteristics for ourselves.

The following are useful future-oriented questions that you may find helpful to build into your dialogue with clients. The intention is to stimulate the client's imagination in the search for possibilities, some of which then become the goals for recovery. You will notice that that they are framed in a positive, expectant way – 'When you're coping better', not 'If you were coping better':

'When you're coping a bit better, what will be happening in your life that's not happening now?'

'How will you know that some improvement is beginning to take place?'

'What will be the first thing you'll notice when you begin to get out from under this depression?'

'When you're beginning to get yourself "sorted out" what changes would others notice?'

'When you're beginning to feel a bit better, what will this enable you to do that you don't do now?'

'What do you want to happen (that would make a difference)?'

'What do you need (that would make a difference)?'

'If a miracle happened and you woke up one morning and this problem had disappeared, what would you notice that was different about you, what would other people notice?'

'Are any parts of this miracle happening already?'

'Tell me about the times when it's not so bad. What's your life like?'

'On a scale of 1–10, with 1 being the worst it's ever been, where would you say you were today? How would you need to be feeling, what would you need to be doing, to have moved up the scale a couple of points?'

'If you were able to get a pill for any characteristic, e.g. for confidence, which pills would you ask for? How would that make a difference to your life?'

Egan has suggested that for many clients it is helpful to engage in future-oriented, solution-focused talk early in the helping process. Pursuing a lengthy search of a person's history in the hope that insight and re-evaluation will lead to liberation from a problematic past and automatically enable people to create a better future for themselves is not particularly helpful. Talking endlessly with a client about the story of their disruptive highs and disabling lows gets nowhere, but if we can engage them in a dialogue about possibilities, for example 'What would be happening when you are managing this problem better?', some hopefulness, direction and motivation can return. Possible replies might then be:

'I would be able to hold a job down.'

'I wouldn't have to take so much medication.'

'I would be steadier in my mood.'

'I would have a better relationship with my family.'

'I would feel better about myself, not so useless.'

'My life wouldn't feel so empty.'

If it seems helpful, more exploratory work can be done on the story in the light of these possibilities – 'Could you say some more about how family relationships have been affected?'. From these broad statements that the client makes about his preferred future, more specific goals can be teased out – 'What would you have in your life that you don't have now if it didn't feel so empty?' 'I would like you to notice what's happening in your life on those occasions when you do feel a bit better about yourself'. Of course clients often do not find it easy to respond to future-oriented questions. They may be so sunk in their problems, feel so pessimistic and disempowered that the future is difficult to imagine. It can require considerable encouragement and an attitude of realistic optimism from the practitioner to enable some clients to become active in this part of the process. Sometimes it can help if clients notice things that happen that make life a little better and that they would like to keep on happening.

Possibilities translate into goals or desired outcomes that, when realised, would represent some positive change in the client's wellbeing. They need to be realistic and reachable. Goals may need to be broken down into smaller steps, for example obtaining a place on a supported employment programme before attempting to re-enter the job market. The client must feel a sense of commitment to their goals. It is no good if the goals 'belong' to someone else.

For some people, leaving the sanctuary of a problem-filled life can be difficult. It might seem inappropriate to use the term sanctuary in connection with enduring mental health problems that can impose such limits on a person's life. Yet it is precisely because of those imposed limitations that they are sometimes difficult to give up. To move towards becoming a fully functioning person, more engaged in living, means facing the struggles of everyday life with all its pleasures, pains and responsibilities.

It can also be equally difficult for some mental health professionals to allow people to choose that struggle. Looking openly with clients at the gains and the losses that are likely to occur as a consequence of moving towards a goal can be helpful. This process can be similar to a balance sheet – if the losses outweigh the gains, a person is unlikely to be motivated to move in the direction of a desired outcome. However, goals can be strongly motivating – many survivors have made heroic efforts to reclaim lives that have been severely damaged by long-term mental health problems and what Breggin (1993) calls toxic psychiatry. Once some goals are established, we can then think about the bridges that need to be built to help the client move from their present position to where they would like to be.

Sarita's story—cont'd

Theme: creating a better future

The following conversation took place between Sarita and her key worker after she had managed to get a good night's sleep.

Key worker: What do you feel you need at the moment that would make things a bit better for you?

Sarita: I just want it to stop. I want them to leave me alone.

Key worker: Not to be worried by thoughts that the police are going to arrive and arrest you and send you away somewhere? You need to feel safe?

Continued

Sarita's story—cont'd

Sarita: Yes. But they're not ordinary police. You can't tell who they are. I think they are like a secret force that no one knows about. I can't get any peace if they're whispering at me. I know Dr Parkes said it was because I was ill, but I can hear them.

Key worker: I'm sure they seem very real to you. One thing I notice though is that I can faintly hear people talking in the flat next door and downstairs and I can hear their televisions. I wondered if some of the time that's what you hear?

Sarita: It could be I suppose, but I hear them when I'm not here sometimes.

Key worker: So what would help you feel a good deal better would be if those thoughts about being watched and arrested were not bothering you so much and if the whispering stopped?

Key worker: When you have got these worries sorted out what will life be like for you?

Sarita: I don't know. I suppose I will go back to The Beeches (a resource centre). It's all right there, but I would like to have a job. I haven't worked since I got ill.

Key worker: What will be good about having a job?

Sarita: I would have some money and be able to get some decent clothes. It would mean having a normal life again. I would quite like to finish my business studies course as well. That would please my father.

Key worker: Would it please you?

Sarita: Yes it would, but I would probably have to start again and I haven't done any studying for years. I don't know if my mind's strong enough really.

Key worker: Are you also thinking it would be a way of reconnecting with your family?

Sarita: I would like to have more contact with them, but when I spoke to my mother a couple of weeks ago she said that I shouldn't come because my father has been unwell. He has diabetes you see and heart trouble. The doctor has said he shouldn't have any stress.

Key worker: How did you feel after that conversation with your mother?

Sarita: I felt upset at the time. A bit angry really. It was as if they didn't care about me any more. I feel like I've been banished.

Key worker: A bit like those thoughts you have about being arrested and thrown out of the country?

Key worker: It sounds as if one of the things that would make a difference to your life would be if you were able to be closer to your family again?

This conversation with its future orientation led to some realistic outcomes being identified that would, when they were in place, make a significant difference to Sarita's sense of wellbeing and the problems she experiences in living. These included:

1. Be able to deal with thoughts about being watched and followed so that they are no longer so intrusive or upsetting.
2. Be able to deal with thoughts of being arrested and deported so they no longer bother me.
3. Stop the experience of hearing people whispering.
4. Improve relationships with other tenants.
5. Explore the possibilities of getting on to a supported work project.

6. Explore the possibility of access courses to higher education.
7. Re-establish regular telephone and letter contact with my family.

These outcomes can be seen as short-term goals (1–4) and intermediate goals (5–7), which can lead to the realisation of longer-term goals: returning to full-time work; returning to higher education studies; reuniting with her family. Helping Sarita begin to imagine a better future for herself had an immediate effect on her mood and outlook, with not just her vulnerabilities being addressed in the dialogue but also her abilities and the possibilities in her life.

Sarita's story continues on page 119

Creating strategies to move forward

Many clients are already employing helpful strategies to deal with the problems they face in living. Barrowclough & Tarrier (1997), commenting on the findings of studies of coping behaviour in people diagnosed as having schizophrenia, conclude that the majority of people develop coping strategies with varying degrees of success. In a similar study of people who experience manic depression, 62% of respondents recognised the value of self-management strategies and were able to use these to some extent (Hill et al 1996). It is therefore important to recognise that people are not passive victims of their mental health problems but fight back against them in many ways. Acknowledging how people have been coping reinforces resourcefulness and encourages them to continue their efforts to manage their problems. Research into coping strategies enhancement carried out by Tarrier et al (1993) indicates the value of strengthening current coping behaviour and teaching clients new and different strategies in overcoming persistent disabilities.

Interventions drawn from solution-focused therapy can be effective in helping clients find strategies to move forward in their recovery. Clients are helped to identify current strategies by asking solution-focused questions:

'Are there times when you don't let them 'take over your mind'? How do you do that?'
'So there are some days when despite feeling bad you manage to get up and get on with the day. What happens that helps you manage that?'
'So on a scale of 0–10, with 0 being the worst you've ever been, you feel you're around 3. What's helped you get from 1 to 3? What would you need to do to move up to 5?'

Genuinely complimenting clients on their efforts to overcome their problems emphasises strengths not weaknesses, competencies not deficits, solutions not problems. The client is acknowledged as the 'expert' on their own problems in living, with the practitioner then collaborating with them to find ways of using their own strategies more effectively. Some clients may find it hard to identify helpful ways of getting to where they want to be, so that helpers may need to bring some energy to the process of searching out 'best fit' strategies just as they helped to

117

identify goals. They may often need to make suggestions or to provide information, but this needs to be done in a collaborative way that allows the client to decide if it is right for them. Exploring possible ways forward can involve asking questions such as:

'Do you have any thoughts about what helps you most when you feel particularly vulnerable like this?'

'What are some of the ways you might deal with this?'

'Have you spoken with anyone else that has this problem? How did they deal with it?'

'When you feel bothered by this idea that someone is putting thoughts in your mind, is there anything you can do that helps?'

'You say some days you cope better than others. What helps you to do that?'

'What skills do you think you need to build up to be able to get your own place to live?'

'These times when despite feeling the pressure building up inside your head you don't cut yourself – what do you do or what happens that stops you?'

'Let's think about what you might do that would help you stay OK if you reduced your medication.'

'What help would you like from me (us)? How would that support you?'

This last question is important and one that is seldom asked. We often assume that we know what clients need from us, but this may not be how they perceive or prioritise their own needs, or what they actually want from their contact with us. Asking the question encourages self-advocacy.

Like goals, strategies should be realistic, specific and owned by the client. Some people may play it safe and need encouragement to be more adventurous in choosing and using strategies. For strategies to be acted on, it may be necessary to help the client develop an action plan, identifying how, where and when something will be carried out. There is also a danger that, at times, an element of collusion may creep into the relationship between the practitioner and client, maintaining a high level of dependence. Other clients may be unrealistic or act blindly, using strategies that are unwise or beyond their present level of competence. For example, a socially isolated young man being supported by the community mental health team chose to tell people that he met in his local pub and at the filling station where he is a forecourt attendant about his psychiatric history. This led to more rejection, discrimination and a greater sense of isolation. Because of his strong need to feel included, he was inappropriately self-disclosing, so he needed to be more discreet and selective about whom he told.

Sometimes in reviewing their goals with their key worker, a client may decide they are unachievable at the present time and there needs to be an intermediate step. A client who was very keen to move on from 24-hour staffed accommodation to a flat of his own in a supported housing project realised that to achieve this goal he needed to build up his 'self-soothing' skills. He needed to deal with episodes of anxiety that increased his voice hearing so that he could avoid recurrent crises in an environment where he did not have immediate access to staff support.

Sarita's story—cont'd

Theme: creating strategies to move forward

The community team continued to work intensively with Sarita over the following week, during which time she began to feel safer and less preoccupied with her unusual beliefs. The therapeutic conversation between Sarita and her key worker is pragmatic and solution focused, concerned with establishing some strategies that will help her manage her disturbing thoughts more effectively. The intensity of face-to-face dialogue is an uncomfortable experience for Sarita, so much of the interaction transcribed below took place during some shared domestic activity.

Key worker: When you've had these upsetting thoughts in the past, what's helped, apart from medication?

Sarita: Well I usually have to go into hospital when I really get ill.

Key worker: What is it about being in hospital that helps?

Sarita: Having other people around I suppose. I feel safer. I know they won't try anything with so many witnesses. And I can just stay in the ward. I don't have to go out.

Key worker: So being with others and sort of hiding yourself away helps you feel safer and less upset. Does talking about these fears you have help?

Sarita: I was worried last time that if I talked about it too much they might give me more drugs. So I kept a lot of it to myself. I remember one nurse used to ask whether it was still on my mind. She used to say that if they were true, the police would have had no trouble in detaining me long before now. So I began to think maybe I had been mistaken and was worrying unnecessarily. She also used to let me help her write the reports in my notes. I'd got this idea in my head at that time that the reports contained coded messages about me that the immigration people would use to deport me. I felt a lot more trusting towards her after that. Do you think she was right that they would have picked me up by now if they were going to?

Key worker: I do, and maybe that's something you can remind yourself about when these ideas begin to get a grip on you. One of the things that occurs to me is that when you get these thoughts about being watched and followed, you get worried and upset and the more upset you get, the more you have those thoughts. So I'm wondering if there's anything you could do that would help you stay calm. Telling yourself that it can't be true because if the police wanted to pick you up they could do so easily and they haven't, is one useful thing you can do. But I'm wondering if it might also help to tell someone when you notice yourself beginning to think more about being watched or followed. Tell someone at an earlier stage. Not wait until it feels totally real and begins to disrupt your life. You could phone me and maybe tell Janice (housing project worker). It seems to me that you need someone to reassure you that you're safe at these times. How does that seem to you?

Sarita: I suppose part of me worries that people will think I'm mad. I mean I know it's a sort of illness but I just want a normal life back.

Key worker: I don't think you're mad but I do think you're very vulnerable to these disturbing thoughts at the moment and if we can help you find some ways of managing them better, you will be able to get your life back on track again. I seem to remember you telling me once that you had got quite good at yoga

Continued

119

Sarita's story—cont'd

at one time. I'm thinking that maybe the breathing exercises you learnt might be something else that you could make use of in helping yourself stay calm.

This and other conversations identified a number of cognitive and behavioural strategies that Sarita was encouraged to use to help manage her unusual thoughts and voices and stay in recovery:

- Remind myself that if the police wanted to pick me up that they could have done so before.
- Remind myself that surveillance cameras, rather than being a threat, increase my safety.
- Remind myself that voices whispering in the background may be other residents' televisions.
- Concentrate on my breathing exercises if I feel myself getting tense.
- Play some music that is loud enough to drown out the voices without disturbing neighbours.
- Telephone my key worker or project worker at any time if I'm feeling unsafe.

For many clients, following this problem management process through a number of times not only helps them develop strategies for managing or resolving current problems but also enables them to be more effective when faced with problems in the future. This can be a valuable asset in staying on the road to recovery. However, there will be some clients who will continue to need support in working through the process. Even though they have acquired better problem-solving skills, they become easily stressed and continue to need help and encouragement in deciding what to do and when to act on their decision. This need not of course involve a mental health practitioner. The support might more helpfully come from an independent advocate, a friend or a support worker.

The working alliance as an enabling relationship

12

Many clients who seek the help of the mental health services are strongly motivated to seek change in themselves and their lives. Their psychosocial distress urgently requires some relief or resolution. But for many others any movement towards a less problematic life is elusive and they remain immobilised by inertia. Passivity colours human behaviour in a number of ways. Most commonly we recognise it as doing nothing when faced with the problems of living. Secondly, we see passivity in compliance – the uncritical acceptance of the understandings and goals suggested by others, an attitude exacerbated by pathologising distress, characterised by Gergen (1990) as an 'invitation to infirmity'. If the vulnerabilities and disabilities the client faces are seen as a manifestation of some complex neurophysiological dysfunction, then they resign themselves to being the passive recipients of treatment, often with little hope of recovery. Thirdly, passivity is reflected in purposeless, aimless action. Finally it can be seen in withdrawn, 'shut down' or 'sealed over' ways of being.

Deegan (1996) suggests that any passivity, inertia or apathy adopted by people with serious mental health problems is often a defence against a personal view of life in which caring about themselves and their lives or being hopeful is too risky – it is safer not to care; small wonder then that there is a reluctance to emerge from a cocoon of apathy. It is important that practitioners involved with the client are able to hold hope for that person; to care about their lives for them, until they are again able to embrace life and fully engage in living. It is all too easy to give up on people when any change seems a long time coming.

The concept of learnt helplessness based on the work of Seligman (1975) has established itself in the literature. It hypothesises passive behaviour as a learnt response to the experience of being faced with life situations over which a person has no influence or control. In such situations, passivity becomes the learnt response and a fixed pattern of behaviour. Once established, even in circumstances to which a person could respond in a way that would make a difference, they do nothing. They are a prisoner of helpless passivity. Deegan (1992) argues that learnt helplessness occurs as the consequence of the cycle of disempowerment and despair experienced by many users of the mental health services (Fig. 12.1). It expresses itself in apathy, hopelessness, compliance, withdrawal, anxiety, depression and anger, characteristics that are often interpreted as negative symptoms of schizophrenia and treated with powerful neuroleptic drugs. The central issue here is the belief that a psychiatric vulnerability necessarily means that the capability of a person for reasoned thought and wise action is diminished and therefore mental health workers must take that responsibility for them. Many

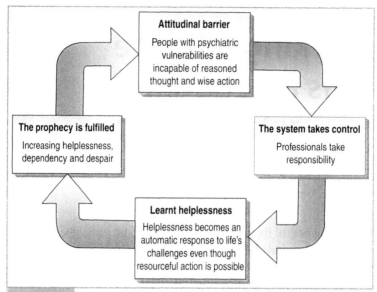

Figure 12.1 ● Cycle of disempowerment and despair.

psychiatric survivors argue that this can be more damaging than their psychiatric vulnerability. Disempowering attitudes are not simply found within inpatient services – a legacy of institutional psychiatry – but are also found within community services and in wider society. People with long-term mental health problems are not only marginalised and stigmatised by the nature of their problem, but are also excluded by unemployment and poverty. As mental health professionals, we must try to comprehend the impact on a person of such uncaring social exclusion which leaves them with one identifiable social role: that of mental patient.

The antidote to learnt helplessness requires an attitudinal shift at an individual and organisational level, so that people with disabilities can enter into true partnerships with mental health workers. They can increasingly become experts in their own care and de-medicalise their lives, instead of becoming experts at occupying a dependent sick role.

We are often very good at sabotaging ourselves with what Egan (2006) refers to as disabling self-talk. Often our inner critic will render us speechless and passive in situations that call for a response. This self-imposed impotence gradually undermines our self-confidence and social effectiveness and leads to us avoiding life. Disabling self-talk can be a particular problem for people with enduring or recurrent mental health problems. The work on cognitive approaches in the treatment of people with severe and disabling problems has been very influential in the field of mental health care over the past few decades (see Chadwick et al 1996, Chadwick 2006) and has offered many people a release from tormenting and imprisoning thoughts. The essence of cognitive behavioural therapy (CBT) is that automatic thoughts and thinking errors have a profound effect on the way we feel and act. If I think I will appear foolish to others, I'm likely to feel anxious about being in the company of others and will avoid socialising. Interventions made by the mental health professional can helpfully focus on assisting clients to identify and dispute these unreasonable thoughts, replacing them with more adaptive ways of thinking and being. What is being argued is that engaging people in an alliance that is empowering often involves overcoming disabling self-talk.

Empowerment

Power can be seen as a social construction as well as coming from within. Authority and power are invested in social roles to varying degrees. The power that an individual is able to exert in a given situation may depend on factors such as age, gender, social class, education, ethnicity, knowledge and occupational status. The implication of the social construction of power is that its shadow side, oppression, is not simply a matter of individual attitudes but that it is embedded in social systems. The therapeutic system enshrines this power difference, which can often be experienced as oppressive and disempowering by clients.

McLeod (1998) argues that there are a number of mechanisms at work in therapeutic encounters that are far from empowering in their effect. The language of psychiatric practice wraps human experience in a blanket of mystifying and excluding terminology, creating the role of expert – one who knows –and the role of client, who is the passive recipient of that expertise. Foucault, whose ideas have been influential on the thinking of psychiatric practitioners and user groups, was very interested in the relationship between knowledge and power and in particular the knowledge base of the human sciences and the power that exerts on human beings. He argued that if there is no such thing as absolute truth, then knowledge is not static and immutable but growing and changing. But often the ideas of a powerful minority are propagated as truths and become the 'dominant discourse' in society and in time accepted as truths by the majority. Those who originate those 'psychiatric truths' then have a claim to be experts on the behaviour of the rest of us. If certain human experiences are labelled depression and are understood as a neuro-transmission deficiency, we are likely to wait passively for the medication to work. If the same human experience is seen as a dispirited state, a consequence of significant loss or of social deprivation, oppression or entrapment, then reviving the spirit and assisting that person to reconnect with their personal power becomes the focus for helping. It also demystifies and de-professionalises helping and healing, locating it in the family, the community and society.

A continuing debate has taken place within the mental health professions over the last decade on the issue of empowerment (Campbell & Lindlow 1997, Barker 1999, Repper & Perkins 2003). Successive reports have emphasised the need for a partnership in care between professional helpers and clients – *Working in Partnership* (Department of Health 1994), *Pulling Together* (Sainsbury Centre 1997); yet despite this, a service that truly empowers its users still seems an aspiration rather than a reality. The legacy of institutional attitudes persists amongst many mental health professionals and the medical model still dominates the understanding and management of psychiatric illness despite the strengthening voice of the user movement and the development of an advocacy network that are challenging mental health professionals to rethink their role and philosophy of care. So disillusioned and pessimistic are some service users and survivors about the likelihood of a culture of empowerment flourishing in the statutory or voluntary services that they argue that real recovery, rather than symptom management, can only take place in user-led services (Fisher & Deegan 1999).

The term empowerment suggests that it is something that can be given. This is misleading. It is perhaps more accurate to say that we can facilitate empowerment by not putting barriers in its way through our attitudes to service users and by respecting and nurturing self-esteem, confidence and assertiveness (see Box 12.1). Ultimately mental health workers cannot empower clients, only clients can empower themselves. This means service users accepting more responsibility for themselves in facing the problems and opportunities of living. This can be extremely challenging to many clients whose self-esteem and confidence are low and who, because they have never achieved a strong sense of their own autonomy and initiative, commonly seek out 'rescuers' in the form of professional helpers when life becomes difficult; this is a dynamic that frequently dovetails with unmet needs of mental health workers that express themselves in over-solicitous care.

Box 12.1

Factors that facilitate user/consumer self-empowerment

- Allow more time for people: for listening; for talking; for doing things together.
- Normalise the helping relationship.
- Avoid mystifying, excluding jargon.
- Respect the way people experience their reality.
- Respect the expertise of people in knowing what helps.
- Provide accessible information and ensure it is understood so that people can make informed choices.
- Encourage people to take a leading role in the care planning process, such as carrying out a self-assessment.
- Enable access to resources outside the service provision in meeting needs, such as adult education, recreational facilities, complementary therapies and counselling.
- Respect people's right to choose.
- Practise judicious non-intervention.
- Respect the client's right to the dignity of risk.
- Avoid coercion and threats.
- Celebrate people's achievements, successes, strengths and abilities.
- Nurture hopefulness.
- Help people gain the skills they need to feel more empowered and be more assertive.
- Acknowledge the impact of social inequalities and impoverishment on the lives of people who use the mental health services.
- Acknowledge the impact of stigma on the lives of people who use the mental health services.
- Openly discuss experiences of compulsory supervision, admission, detention and treatment.
- Encourage the use of independent advocacy and user-led resources.
- Encourage involvement in user groups and patient councils.
- Seek users' views on the service and encourage user-led research.
- Avoid pathologising labels and deterministic explanations.
- Avoid believing mental health professionals are an omniscient presence in the lives of clients. We are not that important!
- Keep in mind that many people recover mental wellbeing without recourse to professional help.

Self-enquiry box

The 'drama triangle' (Fig. 12.2) is a powerful way of analysing a form of role-playing that commonly occurs in both social and professional relationships. These are inauthentic roles based on old script strategies that have their origins in the past, rather than the here and now. To use the language of transactional analysis, the persecutor views others as being 'one down' and 'not OK'. A rescuer also sees others as 'not OK' and 'one down' but responds by offering or imposing help from a 'one up' position. The rescuer's belief is that they have to help because others are not able to cope. The victim sees himself as 'not OK' and in the 'one down' position. Victims will search out a persecutor who will put them down, confirming their view of themselves. Other victims will search for a rescuer to confirm their view that they cannot cope on their own. All three roles involve a 'discount'. The persecutor discounts others' value, dignity and wellbeing. The rescuer discounts others' ability to think for themselves and use their own initiative. The victim discounts himself or herself, seeing themselves as deserving denigration or needing help in order to cope and survive. Although people may seem stuck in a particular role, they are also likely to switch to another role in playing out their scripts. A victim may become a persecutor; a rescuer may become a victim.

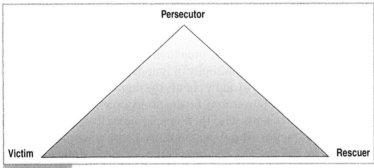

Figure 12.2 ● The 'drama triangle'.

Take a few minutes to brainstorm all the words you associate with the three roles. Consider what the differences are between an authentic rescuer and an inauthentic one. Can you make the same distinction for victims? Reflect on your own experience of occupying these roles, through being 'recruited' into one, having one imposed on you, or through acting out your own script in your personal and professional life.

125

An empowered state of being can be seen as a fluid state which ebbs and flows depending on circumstances of our lives. Sometimes, perhaps during periods of crisis, we may relinquish a degree of autonomy and retreat for a time into a more dependent state of being before regaining our inner strength and sense of mastery over the challenges of living. Heron (2001) emphasises the need for flexibility and judgement in the helping relationship between the poles of authoritative interventions at one end and facilitative interventions at the other (Fig. 12.3). He argues that in our desire to move away from a hierarchical, authoritative approach towards facilitative helping, we have thrown out

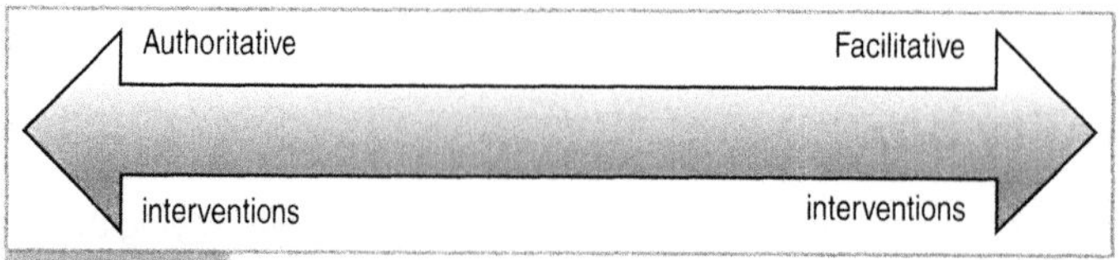

Figure 12.3 ● Heron's (2001) authoritative–facilitative continuum.

the positive elements with the damaging ones. A client so distressed by unusual and frightening thoughts that he is intent on jumping off a road bridge needs (for a time) care that is both prescriptive and supportive. There is within us all a need for dependency as well as a need for autonomy, which will fluctuate through the life cycle. As Sheehy (1997) puts it, we have a need to separate and achieve a sense of mastery in our world, which she calls our *seeker self* and also a need to merge with others and seek the security and support, our *merger self*. We will return to this theme when we consider developmentally needed relationships. Judicious flexibility is a key skill in mental health work.

Why is it that after all this debate many mental health professionals find it difficult to embrace the philosophy of empowerment? The reasons are complex. It is argued (Horsfall 1997) that many practitioners themselves do not feel empowered or supported in their role as care coordinators, or key workers, and may feel unable to assertively express their professional autonomy, particularly if that involves challenging the system. If judicious risk-taking is not supported by management, and at times the philosophy of empowerment will entail some risk, practitioners may feel unable to allow clients the dignity of risk. At a deeper level, underlying the misuse of power may be the projection of our own vulnerability and dependency onto clients who then appear more in need of prescriptive care than they actually are. Many personal needs are unconsciously met through the caring role; the need to feel powerful in order to mitigate a sense of weakness or inadequacy, the need to feel needed, valued, loved, good, can all intrude in unhelpful ways into our practice and must be acknowledged and explored in supervision if we are to relate to clients an authentic, emotionally clean way.

Young and in search of manhood, yet fearful of masculine power, I entered the world of mental hospitals at a time when the brutality of institutional regimes lingered on. Despite the presence of benevolent paternalism, what I predominately witnessed was a world dominated by alpha males who subjected patients to oppressive regimes. It was an experience that left me even more estranged from my masculine energy and gave me more affinity with feminine values. Needless to say I did not fit easily into this prevailing culture and was seen by many senior colleagues as 'not tough minded enough'. The pull to belong in this institutional world was strong and many times I compromised myself by treating people in harsh, depersonalising ways, noting as I did the seductive frisson of power that accompanied these displays of authority.

It took me many years to feel comfortable with masculine aggression, my own and others, during which time I often related in passive, acquiescent ways in my professional relationships when a more challenging stance would have been more helpful. As is often the case when we suppress and disown some personal attribute, it has a habit of expressing itself in an intensified form and many times I felt my aggression rise volcanically within me and express itself in angry, dominating, disempowering reactions to others. Gradually I came to recognise that it was not simply a potentially destructive force that had to be contained at all costs but one that could also be a positive energy released in socially conscious ways, infusing life with an enabling vitality.

Caitlin's story

Theme: a practitioner's experience of powerlessness

Introduction

We, as professional mental health workers, may at times feel powerless in our role for a complexity of reasons that may be both related to our personal history and socially constructed.

Caitlin is a recently qualified mental health nurse working in an acute inpatient unit.

Caitlin

I suppose I've never felt a very powerful person although sometimes clients will say they see me as self-assured, so I must mask it quite well. There are some situations in which I can literally feel my power drain away. Sometimes people's problems and needs seem so enormous and intractable that my contact with them leaves me feeling helpless and inadequate. It seems as if I have little to offer that will make any tangible difference. The supervision I have doesn't help me with that because my supervisor is such a capable and experienced nurse, who always seems to have the 'answers', that it leaves me feeling even more inadequate by comparison.

Meetings and case conferences are also situations in which I lose my voice and I often don't say what I want to say. I often end up feeling quite compromised and dissatisfied after meetings. I think it's partly anxiety about challenging authority figures but also not really valuing my own point of view highly enough. I suppose I tend to regard most other people as being more able and knowledgeable than I am. I trace this back to my early life and growing up in a male-dominated family in which my mother seemed to defer to my father on most things. She didn't really have an opinion of her own on anything. Although my two brothers were younger than I was, I realised at quite an early age that their achievements were always going to be valued more than mine were. I didn't bother with sixth form and gave up the idea of going to university. I got married instead and started to turn into my mother. In some ways I can identify with the powerlessness many of my clients feel, particularly the women.

Although I still do struggle to hold on to my power in some situations, becoming a psychiatric nurse has been a real emancipation for me. I am feeling more liberated and able to be myself. I do speak my mind a lot more than I used to. I think that power has got to come from within. When I first began to find my voice it sounded quite angry and I really didn't like the way I sounded. I was playing old scripts and expecting to be disregarded or put down and was already resenting it. But because people heard and respected what I had to say, I began to respect myself more. It's been an important lesson that I've tried to take into my work with clients.

Self-enquiry box

You might like to reflect on the following questions in relation to your own power/ powerlessness. They can be usefully explored in personal or peer group supervision.

- How do I disempower myself?
- What is it about this person/this situation/people like this that causes me to lose my power?
- How do I empower myself?
- How do the social systems, e.g. clinical team, professional discipline of which I'm part, influence my sense of personal power?
- How do the wider social systems, e.g. class, ethnicity, education, affect my sense of personal power?
- To what extent does the gender bias in the way power is held influence my sense of personal power?
- Are there times when it is helpful to share my feelings of powerlessness with a client?
- Are there times when the feeling of disempowerment I experience belongs to the client?
- Do I hold clients in a powerless position to increase my own sense of power?
- Do I ever abuse power to cover a sense of powerlessness?
- Can I allow myself to feel powerless sometimes?
- What can I learn from my experience of powerlessness that can help me understand my client's experience?

Self-enquiry box

You may find it helpful to reflect on your own practice in relation to the factors identified in Box 12.1. Using the rating scale below may give an indication of how characteristic of your style of relating a particular response is. Reflecting more deeply on the issues raised by your self-evaluation can usefully take place in supervision.

- I always relate this way in my contact with clients.
- I mostly relate this way in my contact with clients.
- I sometimes relate this way in my contact with clients.
- I occasionally relate this way in my contact with clients.
- I rarely relate this way in my contact with clients.

The working alliance with families and carers

13

The success of community-oriented psychiatry depends on a real partnership being forged between carers and mental health professionals. The National Service Framework for Mental Health (Department of Health 1999a) identifies caring for carers as central to the task of improving standards of mental health care. It acknowledges that carers play a vital role in the care and recovery of mental health service users, particularly those with severe and enduring mental health problems – around 600 000 people in the UK, a substantial proportion of whom either live with or have regular contact with their family. The framework recognises the demands and responsibilities of caring and acknowledges the impact it can have on carers' mental and physical health. It sets out the standards to be achieved by local mental health services, which include an assessment of needs and the formulation of a care plan for carers. The full implementation of an effective service for carers is still some way off, with too many carers still experiencing a lack of support and little acknowledgement of their significance in the process of their loved ones' care and recovery (Department of Health 2002c).

The 'great divide' that can sometimes exist between a carer and mental health practitioners can be complex. It is often historical and based on the quality of care and support experienced during a family member's initial breakdown and subsequent early episodes of distress. Families may have felt their view of the client's distress and needs were received incredulously and not taken seriously by staff. They may have experienced a slow response from services to a developing crisis and feel let down and angry that they were left in such desperate circumstances. Often people will feel shut out of the information loop and find it hard to get answers to their questions about diagnoses, treatment and care – a situation often justified on the grounds of confidentiality, even though if asked, most clients will not be averse to their psychiatric care being judiciously discussed with their closest relatives. Even where clients insist on strict confidentiality we should not forget that carers and families will have their own confusion and emotional turmoil arising from the shock of their loved one's breakdown and need a compassionate response from practitioners. Sometimes staff attitudes leave families feeling that they are part of the problem rather than the solution, a response that exacerbates the guilt and self-blame they already feel. Of course the emotional vectors that run through the family system, particularly at a time of deepening emotional crisis, can precipitate and exacerbate a state of psychological overwhelm; of course a dysfunctional family system can contribute to the evolution of severe mental health problems; but any system is amenable to change and families can become a key source of loving support in the recovery process if they are not alienated by the therapeutic team. It is quite often the case that carers have become burnt out as a result of the emotional burden of caring with little support, often over long periods of time and at some cost in terms of their emotional wellbeing and a life of their own. The recovery journey can include the whole family. It can be a period of growth and change for everyone, in which relationships are realigned, wellbeing restored and personal lives reclaimed. These issues, the legacy of past experience, have to be acknowledged, reflected on and resolved in an open dialogue with mental health professionals before any sense of trust, partnership and support can be established with carers. All this does of course point to the vital importance of early intervention services engaging fully with families in first-episode psychosis.

It is helpful, in my view, to take a systemic view of work with carers and families. As practitioners we are never working solely with the individual in isolation from his or her family or community. All of us, however insular or marginalised our lives might be, are part of a number of social systems that both influence us and on which we in turn have an influence; systems that have a significant effect on our mental wellbeing and none more so than the family. The level of mental and social functioning, or dysfunction, of clients relates as much if not more to the functioning of the family and other social systems as it does to the psychodynamics of the client's inner world. The research emphasis on the inner world of the client in recent decades, particularly on aberrant neurones, has caused the social world the client occupies to slip out of focus. It can be easier for families to see the problem in terms of psychopathology or neuropathology located within the individual, but my experience is that many families, maybe most, simply don't believe this is the full story. Intuitively they know that their way of being as a family is significant in the way a troubled state of mind manifests itself and endures. This is not to apportion blame – every family will find the best way it can of functioning as a system, a system which will inevitably go through periods of dysfunction in its history. Even if our work as practitioners is primarily with the referred client we are, albeit temporarily, entering their family system, often in quite a powerful way. If by our presence and our interventions we increase the flow of positive energy within that system – perhaps through behavioural change or relationship realignment, then the wellbeing of not just the client but of the whole family can improve.

I am mindful of a family I worked with recently in which the parents – mother and stepfather – were split about the nature of their daughter's troubled state of mind. The mother could not accept her daughter's distressed and disturbed behaviour as indicative of a serious mental health problem, preferring instead to see her daughter as a locus of suffering within the family, a family who had experienced some significant traumas and stresses during the previous year. She became more intrusively controlling of her daughter's life, desperately seeking out many alternative forms of healing, some quite esoteric, to restore her daughter's equilibrium. Her daughter's delusional world reflected her mother's watchful, over-solicitous care; she began to believe her mother could read her thoughts and insert thoughts into her mind and that she was being 'groomed' for union with some malevolent force. In family work it became clear that her mother was intuitively correct in that there was much unexpressed and unresolved grief and grievances held in the family as a whole, which everyone had to work on in order to free the daughter from the grip of the family's unacknowledged emotional turmoil.

Another focus for the work was to strengthen the parents' bond so that they could communicate more effectively, act in unison and share the care. It was also necessary to redefine the boundary between mother and daughter so that the daughter could grow towards greater autonomy and responsibility for her life.

Not only are carers and families facing the emotional strain of living with a person whose behaviour is problematic, they may also be experiencing the pain of grief. Enduring and disabling mental illness constitutes a loss for the family. It can seem as if the person being cared for has become trapped and unreachable in their troubled, perplexing world, provoking feelings of helplessness and powerlessness in those closest to them. Hopes and aspirations begin to recede, as the enduring nature of the disturbed and distressed behaviour becomes apparent. Families need time and help to accept the reality of the disability and the implications and meanings it has for them. They need time to acknowledge the pain of the loss and work through the feelings that may recur over many months, perhaps even years. Sometimes feelings of anger and protest surface; about the unjustness of what has happened; about the inexplicable behaviour that has intruded disruptively into their lives; about the inadequacy of treatment regimens to resolve the problem. Eventually grief gives way to a state of acceptance, an attitude of mind that is more than mere resignation. Resignation is a capitulation, a giving up and passively allowing events of a seemingly overwhelming nature to run their course. Acceptance is different. It means that we are able to acknowledge the reality of the situation and live with that reality without losing our emotional equilibrium. We are not oppressed or depressed by it but are able to integrate it into an essentially positive view of life. From this position it is possible to see beyond vulnerabilities, to see again a person's worth, to see their qualities and strengths, to see the possibilities and opportunities in a life that has changed. It is at this point that families can become a positive force in a loved one's recovery. It is at this point that they find the emotional energy to invest in other relationships, both inside and outside the family, and for reclaiming their own lives.

The Department of Health (2002c) guidance document on services for carers and families identifies a broad focus for the support of carers:

*   support and advice
*   information giving
*   respite
*   psychosocial interventions.

It requires services delivering this care to operate from the basis of four underlying principles:

*   Services should be positive and inclusive, involving carers in decision-making and seeing them as co-experts.
*   Services should be flexible and individualised, sensitive to the multiracial, culturally diverse nature of Western society.
*   Services should be accessible and responsive, able to offer a rapid response to crises 24/7.
*   Services should be integrated within mainstream mental health services but retain a degree of independence from it, perhaps being managed by an organisation that is separate from statutory services.

131

An evidenced-based blueprint for the most effective configuration of family services has been slow to emerge in the UK, though there are some notable examples of positive practice. In my own area, Suffolk Carers Mental Health Project provides a county-wide service offering individualised support, carer support groups, advocacy, information and training. Rethink have relaunched their well-established Carers' Education and Training Programme. The programme provides information about illness, its treatment and local resources. It explores problem-solving strategies and helps members share practical ways of managing the difficulties they face. It also aims to reduce the stress and isolation carers often experience. In the West Midlands the Meriden Family Programme has trained around 2000 mental health practitioners of all disciplines in family work through a process of cascade training.

Families are not always easy to engage. Intervention studies report that up to 35% of families refuse therapeutic help and up to 50% withdraw from intervention programmes (Barrowclough & Tarrier 1997). Follow-up studies of this non-engaged group show a higher relapse rate for referred family members. A number of factors referred to above such as negative experiences of mental health services, a sense of futility and hopelessness, and the fear of blame appear influential in determining whether a family engages in an intervention programme.

Over the last 30 years there has been a strong research interest in the link between relapse patterns and stress within the family system. Living and coping with a relative who experiences disruptive changes in mood, or becomes apathetic, withdrawn and reclusive, or is troubled by voice hearing and unusual beliefs, can create enormous tension. In families where high levels of hostility and criticism occur in response to problematic behaviour or where care is given in an over-intrusive, over-involved way, an interaction pattern referred to as 'high expressed emotion', recurrence of the disruptive distress is likely to occur. This is linked with the stress-vulnerability theory of psychosis which argues that certain individuals have a vulnerability that predisposes them to distress patterns likely to be labelled psychotic when faced with stressful social situations, particularly if their coping strategies are poorly developed.

Studies of 'high expressed emotion' families have consistently shown a relationship between emotional over-involvement, critical attitudes and the frequency of relapse and that it is possible to improve relapse rates and social functioning of clients through psycho-educational family work (Kavanagh 1992, Bebbingham & Kuipers 1994, Butzlaff & Hooley 1999). The obverse is also true: that families that are able to relate with warmth and acceptance improve the outcomes. 'Low expressed emotion' families are usually families that have developed effective coping strategies which are likely to include adequate time out from their caring role and practical ways of responding to unusual and problematic behaviour (Kuipers et al 2002).

Kuipers et al suggest that engagement and intervention with the family should aim to:

- offer education about severe and enduring mental health problems, their treatment and recovery
- reduce family criticism and increase tolerance of problems
- reduce relatives' over-involvement and encourage the client's independence

- engage the family in a creative problem-solving process to manage problematic behaviour
- defuse emotional tension and encourage a sense of realistic optimism
- improve the client's coping skills and social functioning.

NICE recommend a minimum of ten family work sessions over a period of at least 6 months (National Institute for Health and Clinical Excellence 2002). Often such a programme will follow or run concurrently with a structured educational programme that explores themes such as the nature of psychosis, the meaning of symptoms, relapse signatures, treatment including antipsychotic medication and psychological therapies, the recovery process and creating a healing environment.

Reducing negativity

Some aspects of a client's distressed behaviour can generate strong feelings in family members. There may be high levels of irritation, annoyance, resentment and hostility in the family environment. Often intolerance is linked with ineffective coping and negative attributions associated with the problem behaviour. For example, apathy and inertia may be seen as laziness and perversity. Preoccupation with unusual ideas or behaving in unusual ways may be seen as foolishness. Sharing information about the nature of a person's vulnerability and disability and their treatment and care aims to increase tolerance and reduce criticism. Families, it is hoped, are then able to develop a more informed perspective on the problem behaviour and hold more realistic expectations.

In reviewing studies of the effectiveness of brief education, Barrowclough & Tarrier (1997) conclude that it is worthwhile, in that it increases relatives' knowledge of the disability and improves the wellbeing of carers, at least in the short term. It can also 'prepare relatives for changing their behaviour' in response to longer-term family intervention. However, brief education by itself seems to have little effect on the way carers and families cope with problem behaviour or on the outcome of the client's vulnerability. They argue that education is best started early in the course of the disability, before a family's personal explanatory theories and strategies for coping have had time to become established. Where a relative's disability has existed for some time, education needs to be seen as long term and part of the total family intervention package. Education is best approached in an involving way. While a practitioner's educational input can be structured around relevant themes and given in conjunction with information booklets, relatives need the opportunity discuss their own understandings, anxieties, practical difficulties and their adopted solutions.

Reducing over-solicitous care

Over-involvement is a term used to describe the kind of relationship in which there is an inappropriate level of dependence and over-protectiveness. It is most often seen, although not exclusively, as a feature of the relationship between a parental carer and an adult son or daughter who has an enduring mental health problem. Although troubled individuals may require considerable assistance in dealing with the challenges and opportunities of everyday living, too much care can hold people in a dependent state and block the recovery process. Often dependent relationships predate the emergence of the disability and reflect the emotional needs of the carer and the organisation of the family system. Underlying over-solicitous care may be feelings of guilt and a desperate need to rescue a loved one from their madness. The task of the professional may be to enter the family system in a way that allows some realignment of roles and relationships to take place. Bringing about some change in the relationship can be a lengthy process and finding the right lever is important. It can be helpful to emphasise the client's adulthood and the need for appropriate age-related functioning. It can be helpful to discuss the need for positive risk-taking and the low probability of the carer's worst fears being realised. Emphasising the carer's need for an independent life and as it were 'giving permission' for this to happen can initiate change. Sometimes an acknowledgement of the fact that the carer will not be able to fulfil that role forever can lead to recognition of the importance of the client preparing for a more independent lifestyle.

Limit setting can be difficult for carers but is essential if they are not to be exploited and abused. Often demanding or aggressive behaviour has become an established pattern and relatives may go on suffering this unreasonable behaviour because a person is 'ill'. It is important that carers are helped to see that the person they are caring for is able to take adult responsibility for their behaviour despite their disability. Limits should be negotiated with the person being cared for that recognise carers' rights and needs and these should be held to consistently. It can be very difficult to persuade clients with over-involved relationships to engage in a planned programme aimed at strengthening their life skills and building their confidence and independence. Some of the worries that exist around separation and individuation for the carer and client may have to be addressed first, otherwise attempts to help the client move towards more independent living will be blocked.

Creative problem management

Successful family intervention involves engaging families in collaborative problem-solving. This can be helpful not only in changing their response to problematic behaviour but also in dissolving some of the hopelessness and resignation that may have built up over years of unsupported caring. Engaging families in problem-solving may not be easy. Kuipers et al (2002) comment that some resistance from relatives may derive from them seeing an implicit criticism in the mental health professional's optimism. The possibility that some difficult aspect of a client's behaviour is reducible by dealing with it differently, or applying a strategy more persistently or consistently, may imply that they have not been making enough effort. It is important for carers and relatives not to feel the problem behaviour is being minimised or that their way of coping over the years is seen as 'wrong'. Behaviour that carers and families may find difficult and distressing typically includes apathy and inertia, withdrawal from the world outside and within the family, excessive dependency, aggressiveness, odd behaviour, voice hearing and the presence of disturbing delusional ideas in the client's conversation. It is also important to keep in mind that suicide has an increased incidence in seriously troubled people with enduring problems and families may be burdened by worries about the safety of the person they are caring for. The problem behaviour should be identified as specifically as possible. Problems which are most pressing, which are amenable to change and can be worked on, should be given priority. Often desired outcomes can be broken down into smaller achievable goals, each of which represents a tangible improvement in the situation. You may find it helpful to revisit the framework for managing problems discussed earlier in this part of the book (Chapter 11).

 Simon's story

Theme: family work in enduring mental health problems

Simon is a 32-year-old man who became extremely troubled when he was 17 and was subsequently diagnosed as suffering from schizophrenia. He has remained very vulnerable to episodes of disabling distress, during which he is disturbed by troubling thoughts and accusatory voices. Over the past 15 years he has been admitted to the local psychiatric unit on nine occasions. Many of his admission experiences have been distressing events, which have left Simon feeling very wary of the psychiatric services. He often says that he feels diminished and degraded by his psychiatric status and, as a consequence, will sometimes deny his continuing vulnerability, refuse medication and express a reluctance to have any further contact with mental health professionals. There are times when he is depressed and discouraged by the emptiness of his life and at these times he will often ask his GP for 'euthanasia', which is indicative of the hopelessness and despair he feels.

There have been attempts to accommodate Simon in supported housing, but his tenancy has broken down owing to his refusal of support and his threatening behaviour towards fellow tenants and project staff. He lived in a hostel for the homeless for a while, but for the past 7 years has lived at home with his mother and stepfather. He has two married stepsisters, one lives locally, the other abroad. His own father committed suicide when Simon was 4 years old. While his mother and stepfather have a sense of duty towards their son and are deeply concerned for him, the burden of having him live with them has been considerable and has undermined the warmth of their affection for him. Simon is a chaotic presence in their lives, which have become disrupted and strained. His stepfather gets angry at what he sees as Simon's 'nonsense' and 'laziness' and feels he could 'make more of an effort'. Simon's mother, who is his main carer, has an appeasing attitude towards him and finds it difficult to set limits. She carries a sense of guilt about Simon's problems and blames herself when he refuses medication and 'sacks' mental health staff involved in his care. Both his parents find it very difficult to deal with his persecutory, deluded thinking that emerges at times of stress and his demanding and apathetic behaviour has 'defeated' them. Simon's presence in the house has made it difficult for his parents to have a social life, to go out and leave him, or to invite people in. His mother has become particularly isolated in her role as Simon's carer and is currently taking antidepressants.

Continued

Simon's story—cont'd

Despite the somewhat gloomy overview there is a continuing desire to help Simon to move forward in his life. Simon himself recognises that he should have 'spread his wings' by now, but enjoys the comfort of home and the company, feeling that he would be quite lonely if he lived by himself.

Family intervention

The family: Simon, his parents and his stepsister were seen as a group and at other times the parents were seen alone. It was explained that caring for people like Simon, with a vulnerability to troubled states of mind, can be stressful and burdensome for all families and that sometimes the stress that builds up can aggravate the disorder. Therefore it made sense to look at ways of trying to reduce the difficulties and the amount of stress the family experienced. The family was invited to meet with the family worker and co-worker over a period of about a year, first at weekly intervals, then monthly. This was accepted readily by the parents. Simon was reluctant to agree, but had no objection to his parents attending the meetings.

The first two sessions were attended by the parents and sister and were spent talking about the nature of Simon's vulnerability. Because the term schizophrenia can be such a frightening label to many people and has such a pervasive impact on identity, it was not a term that was used. Instead the stress-vulnerability model was explained, indicating that for some people the stress reaction could be quite extreme and disabling as in Simon's case. It seemed important to release Simon from the power of the label and emphasise that the problem is the problem not the person! Like anyone else Simon had faults and failings, but also strengths, abilities, hopes and aspirations that can easily become obscured by disabilities. The family was invited to identify some attributes or characteristics that they valued and appreciated about each other before the next meeting. The intention was to help the family reconnect with some of the more positive feelings they felt towards Simon. This brought up more than liked characteristics, setting off a discussion on Simon's abilities and interests, past and present. The fact that he used to swim for a swimming club, that he is interested in classic cars, that he likes and is good with dogs, that he is knowledgeable about films.

In the wake of this discussion, feelings of sadness, anguish and bitterness about the loss of the life not lived began to emerge. His mother spoke about feeling in some way to blame for his affliction and acknowledged that she 'did too much for him' and 'gave in to him' too often to mitigate this guilt. She also talked about her anger and guilt at the time of her first husband's death and the fear that the same thing would happen to Simon. Simon's stepfather talked about how he had never felt able to act as an authoritative parent. It was agreed that the family worker should write to Simon, bringing him up to date with what had been talked about so far and inviting him to the next meeting.

An early focus in the work was to look at how 'the trouble' as it came to be called had a grip on their lives and on Simon's life. They were asked to describe how the trouble got them down, how it interfered with life, how it caused them to react. Following on from this they were asked about the ways in which they were able to influence 'the trouble'. The task set for them was to notice how they loosened its grip on their lives so that it wasn't so restricting, upsetting and difficult; how they reacted to 'the trouble', what they said or did that made a difference. This yielded some useful strategies that both the family and Simon were already using to cope with difficult behaviour. These coping strategies were reinforced and other suggestions made about what they might try. One aspect of this was emphasising the reasonableness of setting limits and the right to a life of their own. A key part of this discussion centred on re-evaluating the parents' fears about what would happen if Simon was at home alone and the need for positive risk-taking.

Finding a way of enabling Simon to become more independent proved difficult. Although he agreed that at his age he should be 'in charge of his life', he did not show any inclination to take responsibility for managing it. There was some discussion with the parents about their own experiences of growing towards independence and they both reflected that leaving home and 'having to look after yourself because there was no one else to do it for you' was the spur. Some realistic self-care goals were agreed, the parents recognising that Simon needed a similar spur in order to become more resourceful and autonomous.

A particularly significant event took place in one session when Joanna (Simon's stepsister) talked about a time when she had been involved in an accident and had to spend weeks in bed recovering. She described how her 'big brother' had spent a lot of time with her and made her laugh at a time when she was in discomfort and upset. The whole family then engaged in some enjoyable reverie about 'Simon the joker', an aspect of his personality that had become submerged beneath the dark pools of distress that had flooded his mind since his late teens. This created an opportunity to strengthen the sibling bond and led to Joanna becoming a more active and supportive presence in Simon's life.

The work continued for 18 months. During that time the emotional tension that had been a constant feature of family life eased and Simon's troubled, chaotic behaviour diminished.

Reducing the emotional labour of caring

Caring for a person with an enduring mental health problem is an emotional labour. Members of the family may experience a wide range of powerful and upsetting emotions. As discussed above, these may be associated with the experience of grief. In addition, many parents experience feelings of guilt, thinking that they are in some way to blame for the problem. There may be intense feelings of irritation, resentment and anger at the demands and difficulties posed by the client's behaviour. Fearfulness about the risks posed by a relative's behaviour and anxiety about the possibility of relapse are also commonly experienced. There is also the additional burden of living with the stigma of long-term mental health problems and the isolation that may cause. There may be frustration and disillusionment with the mental health services because of lack of consultation and support, failure to respond promptly to early signs of relapse or to crises, and the lack of continuity owing to frequent staff changes. The failure of psychiatry to cure the problem adds to a sense of disillusionment and despondency. High levels of distress over a long period can cause carers to burn out and no longer be able to provide care conducive to recovery. Sometimes, a family unable to cope any longer with the stress of continuing care may reject the client.

Helping carers and the family manage their distress is an important component of family-centred care. It is important not only from the point of view of the wellbeing of carers and other family members but also a high degree of emotional tension in the family environment may lead to a greater likelihood of relapse occurring. Barrowclough & Tarrier (1997) outline the rationale for stress management in the following way:

- Living with a person who suffers from schizophrenia can be very difficult and it is usual for relatives to feel stressed or upset at least some of the time.
- When a patient is living with the family, a lot of the day-to-day help and rehabilitation is carried out by family members. Hence it is important to make sure they in turn have help in managing their own feelings in coping with difficult situations if they are to go on helping the patient effectively.
- People who suffer from schizophrenia are unusually sensitive to the stress of others; therefore by feeling more in control of themselves, relatives are indirectly helping the patient.

Care should be taken in making this last point to families as it can easily be heard as blame. The positives of stress management should be emphasised rather than the negative consequences for the client of the carers' stress.

Reducing the family's experience of distress can have a twin focus. Firstly, if other more effective ways of responding to difficult behaviour can be found, or if that behaviour can be modified by some other intervention, for example by a change in medication or by helping the client develop a more effective coping strategy, then their distress levels should be reduced. Secondly, carers and others in the family can be taught how to manage their stress levels, including the use of respite opportunities, in a way that prevents the build-up of distress and exhaustion. It is important for professionals to accept and contain the ventilation of feelings and to normalise these feelings, particularly the negative ones, emphasising that they would be expected in any family faced with experience of caring for a relative who has become deeply troubled. A useful strategy when working with negative feelings is re-framing (Kuipers et al 2002). It is usually possible to point out the positives in the painful feelings that surface in families. Underneath the angry accusation 'you do nothing but sit around all day' is a real concern about a son or daughter losing out on life. 'I wish you'd stop behaving so stupidly, we'd get on a lot better' can be re-framed as, 'Much as I want to, it's difficult for me to feel close to you and be around you when you behave in that way'. Talking about feelings either on an individual basis or in the family group can help reduce tension and discord. When the person being cared for is present, it is important that the emotions expressed are linked with specific behaviours and not seen as a rejection of the whole person. 'I can't trust you any more' is better expressed as, 'When you wander around the house at night and leave the fire and the grill on, it leaves me feeling I can't rely on you'. Where relatives' groups exist, they can offer a useful forum for sharing feelings in an atmosphere of mutuality. The fact that other people have experienced the same distress reduces carers' worries about the unreasonableness of their feelings and offers ways of coping more effectively.

It can be useful to ask family members to keep a journal of situations that arise that result in them becoming emotionally upset. Self-monitoring requires relatives to record the situation, how they felt, what they thought and what they did. Barrowclough and Tarrier emphasise the need for interventions that aim to help carers and families to manage stress in response to their specific experience rather than in the form of generalised techniques and strategies. This approach to managing stress involves three possibilities. Firstly, the family and practitioner can look at the situation that the carers find distressing and consider ways of changing it. That might involve changing the client's behaviour or changing the relatives' behavioural response to it. Secondly, it could involve changing the way the situation is perceived: often the distress people experience arises not so much from the situation itself as from the way they see it. Thinking errors may be present, for example anxiety about going out and leaving someone in the house alone may be based on unreasonable fears about what might happen. Finally, people can learn to change the way they react internally through learning relaxation techniques, having periods of respite, removing themselves from situations that trigger distress, comforting themselves and building 'comfort zones' that offer an oasis of calm into their life.

Enhancing coping and social functioning

While family interventions are aimed at the family system, the approach we are discussing here also focuses more directly on improving the social functioning of the vulnerable family member. This allows others in the family to become involved in helping to develop constructive behaviour. Any positive change in the client's behaviour can promote a feeling of hopefulness and reduce the sense of burden and stress experienced by the family. Barrowclough & Tarrier (1997) suggest an approach that aims to build up constructive behaviour through goal setting. A helpful starting point in this process is for the client and family to identify strengths, which can later be drawn on in setting goals and action planning. Strengths may include interests, abilities, talents, personal qualities, aspirations and resources. For example, a client's paranoid anxiety and reclusive lifestyle was reduced by exploiting his interest in films and sport to create opportunities to pursue those interests in ways that involved an increasing level of 'safe contact' with others.

Problems and difficulties that are identified by carers, the family and the client in the present scenario can lead to a discussion about the preferred scenario, out of which achievable goals emerge. Asking the client and the family future-oriented questions such as, 'If a spontaneous improvement were to take place and things were 10% better than they are now, what would you notice that would be different?' or, 'What needs to be different for you to feel better about this situation?'. Once clear goals, desired outcomes have been established, strategies can be devised with the client and family to achieve them. Sometimes it can be helpful to ask about 'exceptions', times when the problematic behaviour has not occurred or occurred less, times when the preferred scenario has, if only partially and briefly, occurred. This more future-oriented, solution-focused, optimistic problem management approach counteracts gloomy, pessimistic, problem-saturated reviews of the family's experience. Rather than focusing too much on the problem of, for example, a client's apathy, inertia and social withdrawal, it is more helpful to look at ways in which the client and the family can influence the problem. Can they begin to have some influence on this 'retreat from the world', this 'immobility', rather than the problem having such a dominating and adverse influence on their lives. Similarly, the problem of stigmatising, disruptive verbalisation in response to persistent voices can involve the client and the family in finding strategies for managing the voice hearing in more socially adaptive ways. You may find it useful to revisit the framework for managing problems discussed earlier in this part of the book (Chapter 11).

 Nick and Beth's story

Theme: the impact of the carer's role on marital relationships

Nick and Beth are a couple in their early thirties who have been married for 8 years and have a daughter aged 6 and a son aged 4. Beth became very troubled and distressed following her daughter's birth and was diagnosed as suffering from puerperal psychosis. Since then her vulnerability has continued to express itself in three further episodes of acute distress which have required a period of hospitalisation. During these episodes she is troubled by somatic sensations and thoughts that her body is changing, she complains that she is not real or that she is no longer in her body. At these times she has inflicted injuries on herself to prove 'I'm still alive'.

Around the time of Beth's second breakdown, Nick was made redundant from his job as a laboratory technician and decided to stay at home to bring up his children and become Beth's primary carer. They have considerable support from Beth's mother, who provides respite for Nick by having Beth and the children to stay once a month.

Recently the family asked for help because Beth was showing early signs of another relapse. There has been continuing tension in their relationship, with frequent, sometimes violent, rows. Some of the tension centres around the way their respective roles have evolved. Nick has taken over most of the responsibility for managing the home and caring for the children, leaving Beth with what she sees as a subsidiary role. Her conception of herself as a capable parent is further diminished by her mother who 'takes charge' of the children during respite weekends. Beth is feeling like a third child and resents it. She has found it quite difficult to express her frustration because of the powerful coalition between her husband and her mother and because she fears that Nick might leave her and that she then might lose the children altogether. She resents the fact that there is little of the tenderness, affection and playfulness he shows towards the children in his relationship with her.

Nick feels that Beth's talents have never been in running a home. He argues that she seldom does things properly and the house would be in chaos if he left it to her. From his perspective both he and his mother-in-law are trying to protect her from the demands of being responsible for two lively, 'difficult' children. He says Beth is often overly anxious about the children and has at times visited the school several times during the day to reassure herself that her daughter was alright. He gets angry with her over her preoccupied state of mind and her unusual beliefs, which appear when she is stressed. He is often frustrated by her lack of motivation and indolence. Nick feels guilty about his impatience, intolerance and loss of temper; he says 'I should be big enough to accept that Beth is different'. He recalls that one of the things that attracted him to her in the first place was her 'oddity' and dreaminess. He recently experienced a family bereavement and felt unable to share his feelings with Beth, which confronted him with the emptiness in their relationship and with his own loneliness.

The family intervention, which at various times involved Nick and Beth together and separately and Beth's mother, continued weekly at first and then monthly over a period of a year. It centred on the task of strengthening the relationship between Nick and Beth by creating opportunities for them to have time for themselves and on building up Beth's parental role and her conception of herself as a capable parent. It emerged that Beth had been carrying a deep sense of guilt and resentment about not being able to care for her daughter in the early months of her life because of the onset of her psychosis. She had as a result never really felt that her daughter 'was hers' and worried that she may have 'damaged her' by not being a 'proper mum'. There was also some work with Nick around managing stress and dealing with the strong feelings that his caring role triggered. An important factor to emerge in relation to Nick's caring role was that he had grown up in a family in which his father had left his alcoholic mother when he was 6 years old. As he grew up, he increasingly took on the responsibility of 'parenting' his mother. It seemed that a repetition of this earlier script was being played out in the relationship between Nick and Beth. It was helpful to Nick to relocate some of the intense feelings he was experiencing in the 'here and now' of his relationship with Beth back into their rightful place of the 'there and then' relationship with his mother.

Self-enquiry box

A genogram is a graphic and succinct way of organising family history. The problems facing the referred family can be seen in the context of a wider family system. It can highlight patterns and themes that have recurred through successive generations and are influencing the present and can draw attention to significant events and transitions.

Nick and Beth's genogram is given in Figure 13.1.

141

Continued

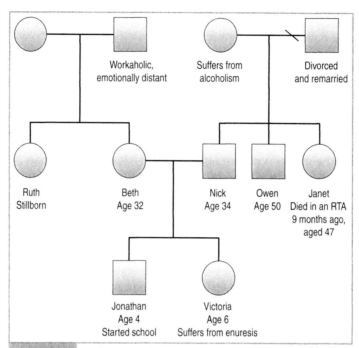

Figure 13.1 ● Nick and Beth's genogram.

What questions might the genogram prompt?

Complete a genogram for your own family. What patterns, themes, significant events and transitions are brought into relief? What arouses your curiosity?

Complete a genogram for a family you are currently working with.

While engaging and working with the whole family is the ideal, some clients are not willing to have their family involved. This raises a difficult ethical issue. Can a carer be seen as a co-worker with rights to information about the client and to be involved in care planning? Can carers and families be seen as co-clients with rights to professional help? In the model of care we have been discussing above, there are elements of both positions. Part of the difficulty lies in the changing family role, from the family as a natural source of care to the more designated role of 'primary carer'. This subtle shift can have significant implications for the relationship, between marital partners where one is the carer or between a parent and an adult child and with any other permutation. It is not difficult to see how strategic interventions or early signs monitoring might be resented. Or how the loss of reciprocity of care between spouses where one has a long-term mental health problem could undermine the relationship.

Much of what we have been discussing above in relation to family carers could also be applied to professional carers in other settings. Elements of 'high expressed emotion' may be a feature of the interaction between staff and clients in residential and ward settings. Critical, negative perceptions of residents may develop and cynicism and therapeutic nihilism creeps in. Overbearing, directive, over-solicitous care can become the norm in the culture of a staff group whose anxieties are not being heard and contained, so that it is difficult to allow residents the dignity of risk and to nurture self-determination and self-reliance. Staff face high levels of stress and can become seriously depleted, with a risk to their own wellbeing, in organisations where the emotional labour of providing therapeutic care is not openly acknowledged and mitigated through supportive, replenishing structures.

Reluctance, resistance and disengagement

14

Some reluctance, resistance and disengagement should be seen as a healthy response to professional interventions that may involve surrendering some sovereignty over one's life to others. Not adhering to a prescribed care plan may be indicative of the spirit of recovery. It can be an expression of an individual's personal power, a willingness to take some responsibility for themselves and their lives, to claim an identity different from the one 'assigned' to them by mental health professionals and to seek an alternative way to healing and wholeness.

Reluctance to engage often has to do with the conception of a person's problems in living as illness. To have one's living and being, however distress filled, problematic and perplexing that may be, interpreted as mental illness can be perceived as an assault on personhood. People take flight from labels and from the stigma associated with them. The message in their reluctance, resistance and disengagement is 'I am not mad'! Therefore if we want to engage with people we must find another way of conceptualising their problems in living. We must seek a shared understanding of the distress and disorder that has erupted in their lives through dialogue – a dialogue about their lived experience, which is not a search for pathology but an empathic search for meaning.

These are some of what we might call the macro-dynamics of reluctance, resistance and disengagement. But there are always less visible micro-dynamics at play (Fig. 14.1). Helping relationships are invariably pale reflections of the past relationships in which care was given and received. Fears of intimacy, dependence, powerlessness, rejection, abandonment present in those earlier relationships may be restimulated. Transference and counter-transference issues may be played out, disrupting the development of a working alliance. The practitioner's own wounds and undealt-with distress may get woven into the developing relationship in a way that undermines engagement.

One client known to me was very resentful of the 'successful lives' of staff. It seemed to exacerbate her sense of failure, inadequacy and inferiority. Her resentment made engagement difficult. It took the transparent humanness of those practitioners working with her for her to see that nobody's life is perfect, that they too had known suffering and failure. This led on to her being able to accept herself a little more; to see that she habitually gave away her own strengths, always seeing others as more able. She came from a family where success in the arenas of academia, work and relationships were the conditions for love and approval, conditions which she seldom met and which left her with what almost became an end-of-life report of 'not good enough'. To *fall ill* and *fail at life* was the

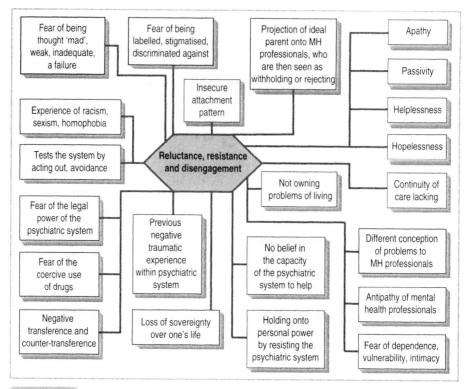

Figure 14.1 ● The dynamics of disengagement.

ultimate failure. It was not until these issues were explored that an alliance based on equality and collaboration could begin.

In the case of another client, engagement floundered on his sense of invisibility. His maternal care had been nurturing in the physical sense but he had never felt prized as a person. This dynamic became woven into his relationship with his case manager, who gave him much practical help and support but did not meet his emotional need to be seen and valued as a person. Once this dynamic was known, the case manager was able to balance care more effectively between the practical and psychological. This raised issues for her, as she recognised her tendency to skew her work more towards the practical needs of clients, avoiding the emotional terrain of her work with clients.

While engagement issues can present a challenge to the establishment of a therapeutic alliance in all facets of the mental health care, they are most clearly played out in the work of Assertive Outreach (AO) teams.

A key component of the National Service Framework for Mental Health (Department of Health 1999a) was the development of 220 Assertive Outreach teams throughout the UK to work with difficult-to-engage people living in the community. AO services are configured to work not only with people who are difficult to engage but also with those who have severe and enduring mental health problems, complex needs, a history of frequent inpatient care, a dual diagnosis involving substance or alcohol misuse, a history of housing problems, social exclusion, and are considered a high risk. The numbers of people falling into this category suggest an average caseload of 90 per 250 000 of the adult population (Department of Health 2001b).

AO services are intended to improve engagement, reduce hospital admissions or length of stay, improve the stability and quality of the lives of people using the service and of their families, reduce risk and improve social and mental functioning (Chisholm & Ford 2004). These are quite challenging aims and it is perhaps not surprising that the UK evidence for the effectiveness of AO in achieving these targets is far from conclusive. In a helpful review of research, Ryan & Morgan (2004) suggest that while AO services are received positively by service users and their families and there are demonstrable improvements in quality of life, there is no consistent evidence that AO improves rates of engagement, reduces admission rates or lowers risk. However, it is a service in its infancy and the expectation is that teams will learn from experience to become more effective in meeting these targets through practitioners becoming more skilled in the intentional use of self in growthful, healing ways.

Engagement is a beginning not an end in itself; it is the possibility for recovery work that engagement opens up that is important and it is this dimension of AO work that needs to evolve. Recovery is long-term, emotionally demanding work. It needs the continuity which AO provides through a team approach. While recovery work may be facilitated by an individual case manager, it is likely the client will have significant contact with other members of the team – there is a reciprocal psychological knowing, which results in less disruption to the recovery process if the case manager leaves.

In an influential report on AO, the Sainsbury Centre (1998a) identified one of the main reasons for clients disengaging from psychiatric services as psychiatric services! Sadly many people have been traumatised by their contact with mental health services, by the manner of their admissions and detention, by the enforced use of medication, by experiences of restraint and seclusion, all happening at a time when their capacity to make sense of what was happening to them was diminished (Morrison et al 2003). Another factor in disengagement from services is the dominance of a biomedical approach in which authoritative experts reduce a person's existential distress to malfunctioning neurones and prescribe powerful psychoactive drugs that have unpleasant, sometimes serious side effects and blunt a person's capacity to viscerally engage in life. People take flight from a system that would circumscribe their lives with drugs and detention, preferring to endure lives of chaos and confusion rather than submit to it.

We have to fully embrace these facts if we are to engage meaningfully with people. Negative experiences in past contacts with services at best leave a legacy of distrust and at worst disabling anxiety in the form of post-traumatic stress disorder (Morrison et al 2003). This must be acknowledged and worked with if we are to overcome resistance and reluctance. We must listen and hear! Traces of the origins of a person's disturbed and distressed state of mind can still be witnessed as that person becomes known, and it is important to demystify the cause of their troubled psyche by locating it in the adversity and suffering they have encountered rather than in malfunctioning neurones. Only then can people begin to free themselves from powerlessness and victimhood, from the brutality of their past, from the tyranny of discordant neurones, from the iatrogenic effects of the psychiatric system, from discrimination, disadvantage and social exclusion, and start to reclaim their life.

For many people referred to AO, life has often become chaotic, empty, impoverished and marginalised. People need help to rebuild the social fabric of their

147

lives. They may not be getting their full benefit entitlement; housing may be of poor quality or their tenancy at risk; they may be unable, for a variety of reasons, to access resources in the community that add quality to life; opportunities for training and education, paid or voluntary work may seem beyond their reach. Relationships with family and friends may have broken down, resulting in a life of isolation. Helping people break free of this cycle of impoverishment, to regain a life that has some meaning and a measure of the satisfactions and pleasures we all seek, is where the process of engagement often begins and strengthens.

It seems to me that often a new approach is needed for people to want to engage with services. Most service users are tired of their problem-saturated lives, tired of stigmatising psychiatric labels, of being defined by past disabilities, failures, inadequacies and misdemeanours. Most of all they are tired of being undermined and infantilised by 'expert'-led care. They are ready for something different. It can be hope inspiring and strengthening to have your positive attributes, your potentials, your aspirations acknowledged and at the centre of your care plan. It can be empowering to be approached in a truly collaborative way, to feel that you have the freedom and the responsibility to take decisions about your care and treatment and about your life. It is important that mental health workers fully embrace the implications of this and intervene in a way that countermands the client's self-determination only when there is clear risk to the safety or welfare of that person and/or others.

Strengths approach to engagement and recovery

Conventional approaches to care and treatment focus on problems, deficits, disabilities and dysfunction, often defined in relation to the medical model. This view of mental disequilibrium as neuropathology or psychopathology sees problems in living as arising from a malfunction in neurotransmission, faulty cognition and other psychological complexes – conditions to be treated and cured. If the condition is treatment resistant and the problems remain despite a battery of therapeutic interventions, the individual joins the cohort of people with severe and enduring mental health problems – people whom psychiatric services have failed to help. But what if we are approaching recovery in the wrong way? How would it be, if instead of giving so much attention to dysfunction, we looked more at people's assets, at their qualities, skills, accomplishments, aspirations, potentials, interests? How would it be if we looked at what they can do, or aspire to do, at what it is that draws people more fully and confidently into life? So often, people struggling to live in an enduring psychological turmoil become mired in their problem-saturated history, which in some cases submerges their identity altogether. Yet I have not met anyone, even those whose minds and lives have been all but wrecked by psychological turmoil, whose positive attributes and potential to be something more than a victim of misfortune did not shine through.

Trying to help someone overcome the seemingly intractable apathy, lethargy and dysphoria that has settled on their lives with changes of medication and carefully conceived psychotherapeutic strategies can often be fruitless. What is missing is something to feel aroused, energised and uplifted about. A pathway back into work, training or education that fits with an individual's aspiration and dreams can be more motivating. Having our lives infused with meaning is what enables us to live purposefully and vitally.

In recent years there has been a growing interest in what has become known as Positive Psychology. Until now clinical psychology has chiefly occupied itself with understanding and resolving distress and disturbance and has virtually neglected positive feeling, whereas this new and exciting field of research is concerned with identifying and maximising what it is that promotes happiness and fulfilment and sustains wellbeing. Martin Seligman, a leading figure in the Positive Psychology movement, argues that what underpins *authentic happiness* is the expression of our *core values and signature strengths* in our everyday lives (Seligman 2002). By core values he means those virtues that have been universally endorsed by the world religions and schools of philosophy, namely wisdom and knowledge, courage, love and compassion, justice, moderation, spirituality and transcendence. Our signature strengths are those traits that characterise our behaviour through which we express these core values. So, for example, kindness and generosity might be a characteristic trait which expresses the core value love and compassion; similarly integrity, honesty and genuineness displays moral courage; and playfulness and humour or the appreciation of beauty communicate our transcendent nature. Seligman believes that we all have a unique personal profile of signature strengths and the more integrated they are into our way of being in the world the greater our sense of happiness and wellbeing. Identifying with this hypothesis is not difficult – most of us recognise that we feel good when we have done something honourable or loving; have satisfied our wide-eyed curiosity about something previously little understood; or shown moderation in response to some self-gratifying urge. Positive Psychology offers mental health practitioners a potentially powerful focus for recovery work through working alongside clients helping them to identify and find ways of expressing more of their signature strengths in everyday life.

The strengths approach to mental health care offers a strong philosophical basis for practice and has a growing evidence base to support its efficacy (Barry et al 2003). With its emphasis on the realisation of potentials and aspirations and the fulfilment of needs, it is at the heart of recovery. The model does not deny the existence of the psychological and social problems which can have a devastating impact on people's lives, but attempts to help people live and live well, sometimes in spite of those continuing vulnerabilities. If we can help people identify their goals and recognise their strengths and resources, if we can believe in the ability of everyone to grow and change and be a supportive presence to people in that process, then problems that seemed insurmountable become less so. Professor Charles Rapp, the originator of the strengths approach, puts it this way: the strengths model sets out 'to assist consumers in identifying, securing and sustaining a range of resources – both environmental and personal needed to live, play and work in a normally interdependent way in the community' (Rapp 1998). This moves the work of practitioners away from problem-solving towards a more facilitative role, a role that is concerned with the client's personal growth and social inclusion.

Many of us spend our lives 'waiting for Godot'. Waiting for that moment when life will miraculously change for us and we will leave the stultifying disappointment of our spoilt lives and find ourselves on those sun-filled uplands fulfilling

> ## Box 14.1
>
> ### Strength-based principles
>
> - The focus of the helping process is on service users' strengths, interests, abilities and capabilities, not upon their deficits, weaknesses, problems.
> - All service users have the capacity to learn, grow and change.
> - The service user–practitioner relationship becomes a collaborative partnership.
> - The service user is the director of the helping process.
> - Continuity and acceptance are essential foundations for promoting recovery.
> - The helping process takes on an outreach perspective.
> - The local neighbourhood is viewed as a source of potential resources rather than as an obstacle. Natural neighbourhood resources should be considered before segregated mental health services.
>
> *Source: Morgan (2004a).*

our true destiny. What we fail to be fully cognisant of is that life is here and now – this is it – and no one but ourselves has the responsibility or the will to change it. Yet we wait – for that something or someone who will sprinkle fairy dust on our lives and in waiting fail to seize the moment to set off in the direction of a life well lived. The strengths approach (Box 14.1) is an exhortation to set off on the road to recovery, where we will realise more of our potential and find more of the life satisfactions we seek.

It is not enough to pay lip service to this way of working. We have to weave it into the very fabric of our practice, make it the *raison d'être* of our service. The perception of someone using mental health services viewed from the strengths perspective is very different from that of a person seen from a problem-oriented viewpoint, with the focus being on the resources a person already has or that are available to them in their community which can be utilised to help them move towards a life with the measure of the joy and satisfaction we all seek. It is about defining goals: 'What are the things that give you a sense of satisfaction and pleasure in your life?'; 'What is it that gives a sense of meaning and purpose to your life?'. Responding to these questions can be hard, particularly when one's life has been impoverished and marginalised for some time. Nevertheless in a continuing dialogue which is strengths-focused, aspects of life that bring pleasure and purpose emerge.

Ethics of engagement

Finally I want to briefly turn to the ethics of engagement and an individual's right to refuse. Working compassionately with clients who are a potential risk to themselves or others, or who seem to be adrift in a troubling, confusing reality, or imprisoned in a distress-filled inner world, yet who still refuse help from services, is a central dilemma in day-to-day practice. To simply discharge a person who has refused or avoided a psychiatric intervention is frequently not an option. However loosely defined, psychiatry has a duty to society to offer protective care to people who would harm themselves or others as a consequence of their disturbed and distressed state of mind. No system charged with such responsibility will be 100% successful. With or without psychiatric intervention some people will find life untenable and choose to end it. With or without psychiatric supervision some people will become prey to intrusive persecutory thoughts and take the life of another. To penetrate the heart of darkness in the human psyche is a difficult undertaking. Risk screening is at best an imprecise methodology that will never unfailingly predict behaviour. Nevertheless, as several inquiries into homicides by psychiatric patients have shown, those of us working on the front line of psychiatric services must be more persistent and diligent in our attempts to engage with and come to know more deeply those troubled people who are a potential risk.

When people disengage or refuse services we often make the mistake of assuming that these individuals lack insight and are incapable of reasoned judgements about their immediate needs. In my experience it is more often the case that people are not necessarily refusing help but are saying no to the pathological interpretation of their troubled minds and to the unhelpful, invasive interventions they have experienced before. In the case of newly referred clients it can be the fearful unknowns of a psychiatric intervention that leads to avoidance. I sometimes feel we switch off our empathic antennae at these times and are persuaded by our own anxieties and the anxieties of families to intervene decisively and authoritatively, in a way contrary to a person's wishes. How frightening it must be to have your perceptions, thoughts and feelings diagnosed as a manifestation of madness and to be faced with custodial care in a psychiatric ward. How alarming it must feel to be compulsorily or coercively given powerful drugs that have unpleasant side effects and dull not just the mental suffering but the feeling of being fully alive. Small wonder people resist! It is sometimes possible to collaboratively seek a shared understanding of a troubled state of mind that avoids clinical labels; we can find an acceptable alternative to admission and to drug-oriented treatment, although this can take time, which only AO services with their smaller caseloads have. Often family and neighbourhood fears can be allayed by the presence of accessible, responsive services and family-centred interventions. Continuity of care can be vitally important; case managers, and by extension the AO teams, with established relationships and knowledge of a person's relapse signature and distress pattern can intervene early to prevent a marked deterioration in mental health and the escalation of risk. Advance directives in which a client identifies what they wish to happen in the event of further breakdowns in their mental health can be valuable in providing timely interventions that respect a client's needs and wishes.

All that has been said above hinges on compassionate presence. Reaching people caught up in a perplexing, disturbing, anxiety-provoking reality, or those trapped in anguished affective states full of self-loathing and despair can only be achieved through the authentic expression of warmth, caring, comfort, kindness and empathy. Only then will trust, safeness, engagement and collaboration begin. As Gilbert (2005) suggests, 'safeness is co-created in relationships and when adults feel safe they are more creative in their problem solving, more integrative in their thinking and more prosocial'. Dispassionate authoritative professionalism may coercively persuade someone to accept treatment or hospitalisation but does little to further the engagement process.

In the final analysis we are each of us – whether caught in a web of troubled thoughts and feelings or not – ultimately responsible for our own lives, for our asocial and antisocial behaviour, for our chaotic existence, for the devastating acts of harm we commit. While mental health services or individual practitioners may be culpable of neglect or incompetence and must accept the consequences of their shortcomings, they should not in my view carry the ultimate blame. Each of us charts our own destiny.

 Ryan's story

Theme: disengagement

Ryan

I've been in and out of hospital eight times since I was 17. Once they kept me in about 6 months. I know that I'm not right if I don't stay on my medication and I know that I'm not right if I do. That's all they seem to worry about – whether you've taken your medication or not. They want me to go to Parkside (a local mental health resource centre) – I won't because it's full of older people and nutters. I think hospitals and nurses and doctors make you worse. I pray to the Lord Jesus and I believe in guardian angels … There is a place called Arcadia, it's over the mountains somewhere, perhaps it's in the Himalayas.

I've had enough of schizophrenia, I've been in hospital eight times, I've had injections and tablets and it's made me worse. So I don't want to see psychiatrists or CPNs any more. You can't get a girlfriend if you've got a mental illness. The woman who reads the news on Anglia TV used to send messages to me. She didn't say my name but she was thinking it. I wrote to her asking her to meet me in Vagabonds Café. It's like all these mobile phones, the air's full of people's voices. You can hear voices all around you sometimes so I have to put on my personal stereo to drown out the noise of people talking … This nurse, she was staring at me and after that I couldn't get an erection and I kept thinking I had abused someone. When I was 10 this bloke made me jerk him off. I've never been violent or abused anyone. I try not to look at people because I know they will put thoughts in my head … This room is alright but I would like a flat. You can't have a dog here. I wanted to paint the walls blue and green which are my favourite colours but they said I couldn't. I spend a lot of time in the park. I think I could get a gardening job. I wrote to the hospital telling them I didn't need to see the psychiatrist any more and that I would go and see my GP. I've sacked my CPN. He was asking me about how I spent my benefits. He hasn't got a clue what it's like living on benefits.

Harry (mental health nurse with an Assertive Outreach team)

I've been working with Ryan for about 6 months now. It has been difficult for the service to engage with him for several years. Every so often he likes to give you 'the sack' and refuses to see you. It's Ryan's way of asserting his power and having some control over his life, which must seem at times to be ruled by others. What I'm trying to do is to have a different kind of contact with him, trying to normalise it as much as I can. His life had become so dominated by his illness that it's become difficult to see anything else. I've been trying to relate more to the Ryan that has dreams, interests, strengths and talents. He does get quite thought disordered and hears voices a lot of the time. But he usually manages to retain some coherence despite his thought excursions, and he deals pretty well most of the time with the voices. When they are particularly bad, he has in the past come up to the hospital and asked to see a doctor but now he's afraid of being admitted again and doesn't go there. In total he's spent about 3 years of the last 8 in hospital; the longest was 6 months. Over that time he's just become more and more exiled from an ordinary life, which is what he desperately wants. He often talks about these utopian mythological places like Arcadia. It's as if he believes he can step out of his world and into a promised land where all is well. It's usually these times that he 'sacks' us and goes into denial about his vulnerability.

Often people who have their first episode of schizophrenia in their late teens lose out on a lot of important development. This is true of Ryan – he's 25 but often he seems more like 17. I see my relationship with him as being more like a mentor than a psychiatric nurse. I'm trying to persuade him to use his local health centre for his fortnightly depot and to see his GP if he needs additional medication to help him through a crisis. What he needs at these times more than anything is someone accessible to talk to and help him deal with any current difficulty. He knows how to contact me and has done this when there have been problems. Last time was when he had gone to the police station complaining about people accusing him of abusing children. Which hadn't happened. He does sometimes suffer threats and abusive comments from people when he behaves oddly in public places and this can precipitate these paranoid anxieties about being accused of sexual abuse.

I try and respect his wishes when he sacks me and step back but usually I can arrange to meet him in a local café. We have a mutual interest in dogs and I will take my labrador up to the park and walk him with Ryan. What I'm hoping to do is to persuade Ryan to get involved in one of the nature conservation projects going on in the area and also help him pursue an application for a flat in a supported housing project. It's often these efforts to help in some practical way that lead to a willing engagement with the service, rather than one that is coercive.

153

 Dawn's story

Theme: the working alliance and engagement in case management

Dawn is a 37-year-old woman who has a long history of referrals to the psychiatric services. The central experience of her early life was of abusive parenting and emotionally impoverished statutory care. She negotiates life in her own chaotic way, but is crisis prone, periodically becoming distressed and disturbed and unable to cope. She lives alone in a small council flat. An earlier marriage failed and a long-term relationship with an older man ended with his death from pancreatic cancer 2 years ago. Dawn has two children from her earlier marriage (aged 18 and 16). Both grew up in foster care and now have no contact with their mother.

Continued

Dawn's story—cont'd

She has been variously diagnosed as suffering from a personality disorder or schizo-affective disorder. During periods of crisis she becomes emotionally volatile, self-injuring and has a confused experience of herself and the world. Over the years she has got better at recognising the early signs of her crisis spiral and will now contact her case manager. Dawn currently takes no medication and refuses to attend a local resource centre. She did agree to attend a closed therapeutic group for women with long-term mental health problems, which ended 3 months ago.

Dawn

I've been on my own a lot since Rolly died. They wouldn't let me in to see him when he went back into St Francis the last time. Said I was upsetting him and other patients, the bastards. Irene (case manager) got it sorted out for me. She helped me with the funeral and everything, because he had no family to speak of you see, except his bitch sister, who didn't want to know. I was there when he died. He gave my hand a squeeze, then he died. It may have been just a spasm or something I suppose but I think he was saying goodbye. I thought I saw him in the town once, it made my heart pound. It couldn't have been him though, could it? I'm not well again at the moment. I've got this pressure in my head. I can't seem to sleep either. I get worried that if I go to sleep something will happen to me. Irene comes two or three times a week at the moment and I can call her if I get really upset. She listens to me and I calm down and get my head straight again. She helped me unblock my sink. They're not going to stick needles in me and call me mad. She knows I hate hospitals. I used to cut myself a lot and one time they put me in a side-room and these male nurses held me down while a nurse strip-searched me. One of the women in the group said to me you've been abused all your life, Dawn – she's right I have. I get really depressed sometimes and I get this idea in my head that I'm sort of responsible for all the bad things that happen.

Irene (case manager)

I've been working with Dawn for about 2½ years now. We didn't really have a relationship for a long while. She didn't want anything to do with the mental health services and was quite resentful and at times verbally abusive towards me. She would never let me into her flat. I was really only able to engage with her through Rolly, her boyfriend. The breakthrough came when he became ill and died. I was able to help her through his death practically and emotionally. I don't think she had experienced someone just being there for her before. Most of her life she's experienced abuse and abandonment. In a way that's been replicated by the way health and social services have treated her over the years. She's had all sorts of people involved in her care at one time or another. To have a consistent relationship with one person has helped her a lot. I think she trusts me now, although she still tests me out from time to time – being unpleasant or unresponsive to me to see if I care about her enough. I have had to be quite careful with my boundaries. At one time she became very curious about my personal life and was quite possessive and demanding, making out she was a lot worse than she was.

When she started being more open with me about her problems, she let me into her flat. It was very chaotic, not at all homely. It made me realise that home is a concept that doesn't really mean much to her. One of the things we've been working at together is home-making, as well as her home management skills. At the moment I'm going in three times a week. She's going through an unsettled phase again. I think it's partly that Christmas is getting close, which is always a bad time for her, but also it's the anniversary of Rolly's death. She's also having a bit of hassle with the housing department who she feels want her out. Apparently she's been putting rubbish down the toilet and sink rather than using the dustbin. The problem was that a neighbour had told her off for using the wrong bin. There has been a bit of prejudice toward her in the flats, which is one of the reasons why she didn't want me calling round initially.

If Dawn feels rejected she starts cutting herself or smashing things; her arms are road maps of scar tissue. The worst thing is that she feels bad and that she deserves to be neglected and abused. There have been times in the past when she's gone out and picked men up and had casual sex with them, partly because of her need for human contact and partly because she has little respect for herself. The group has helped her a lot with her self-esteem. I think that she felt able to give something of value to others, which is a new experience for Dawn. It was important the group was a positive experience because it could open the door to other resources that she's refused to consider in the past.

I know she hates the thought of having to go back into hospital. Dawn's behaviour has been quite challenging in the past and she has found the care oppressive. I've tried to be open with her about what I would and wouldn't do.

Endings and the working alliance

15

There will for every client and mental health professional be endings to negotiate. The way in which this final phase of the working alliance is managed can be of great psychological significance. As Clarkson (1989) says, 'Every goodbye which is well done in the present can re-evoke and retrospectively help heal incomplete goodbyes in the past'. It is not uncommon for previous experiences of separation and loss to emerge in the end phase. Feelings of rejection and abandonment that have their origins in earlier relationships are transferred onto the present relationship. Strong feelings of anger, fear or sadness may surface: I recall one rather abrupt, insensitive ending which resulted in my car being sprayed with engine oil and the sides being badly scored by a hurt and angry client.

With longer-term relationships, a planned, phased withdrawal from a working alliance, keeping the door open and making sure the client knows how to contact the service again, can make the transition easier. This transition from professionally oriented support to social support can be difficult for many clients. Some will seek to meet their needs for affiliation through continued contact with an ex-patient subculture. This can feel less challenging socially – there is no requirement to account for an important part of their experience and there is less risk of rejection. It can also be of positive benefit to be with people who share your psychiatric experience and to know something of the struggle that may be needed to stay in recovery. But for others, maintaining contact with other users and ex-users is a threat to their self-definition and they prefer, at the risk of painful social isolation, to integrate into the wider community.

It is important to allocate sufficient time for endings. One of the issues that may arise in the end phase of the working alliance for both client and helper is a difficulty in letting go. There may be regression into helplessness, neediness and uncertainty. Symptoms and problems may reappear. The helper may collude in this process if the relationship meets an unacknowledged need to be needed, so that the client is not allowed to reclaim adult autonomy and independence. It may be that the helper's own deeply held fears about standing alone in the world will be projected onto the client, who is then not allowed the dignity of risk. There are echoes here of separation issues in parent–child relationships. The reverse of this can also happen where clients withdraw prematurely to avoid the emotional discomfort of endings. Mental health professionals too may end relationships abruptly, 'pushing clients out of the nest before they can fly' on the pretext of avoiding the client's entrapment in a dependent relationship, but at a personal level as a defence against their own anxieties around dependency issues.

For some people, ending their contact with a professional helper can be experienced as a relief. There is for many people a stigma about being helped that can undermine their self-esteem and sense of their own adequacy. As Barham & Hayward (1995) put it, 'For a person to ask for help, even to admit to himself that help is needed, is to confirm feelings of incompetence and humiliation'.

Andrew's story

Theme: endings and the working alliance

By the time I came out of hospital the second time, my relationship with Justine had finished and I had to find somewhere to live. A social worker helped me get a council flat. He was nice enough, used to call and ask me how I was doing. He was concerned about how I was spending my day. I was spending most of my time in the flat, just going to a local café for my meals, not meeting many people. I got so I didn't bother to tidy the flat or myself very much. I felt demoralised and humiliated really, being on benefits with no prospect of work. In a way, him visiting made things worse. I needed to turn over the page on that chapter of my life. Being ill had really shaken my confidence and I needed to prove to myself I could manage. Prove to myself that I was not a mental wreck or a psychiatric case. I got so I rather resented the visits and resented him for being so damn capable and having it all.

There is a need to acknowledge and deal with the feelings and unfinished business that endings evoke, to acknowledge regrets, disappointments, resentments or guilt, as well as any feelings of satisfaction and appreciation. If important feelings are left unexpressed, it can be hard to let go and move on. This can be as true for helping relationships as it is in personal relationships. During the end phase clients will often look back on their journey through a period of distress and disruption in their lives. There may be a feeling of having 'got somewhere', of improvement in their sense of wellbeing, in relationships and life skills, in their self-esteem and confidence. Reinforcing what the client has achieved can be a helpful counterbalance to self-doubts that often emerge about their readiness to cope. Allowing time to do this is also important to the helper's sense of competence and worthwhileness.

Therapeutic stocktaking at the end of the working alliance can also be about accepting the 'good enough'. No therapeutic intervention offers a panacea for all life's trials and tribulations. This does not mean that people should abandon cherished dreams and aspirations; however, it is worth noting the prayer attributed to St Francis of Assisi:

God grant me the serenity to accept the things I cannot change

The courage to change the things I can

And the wisdom to know the difference.

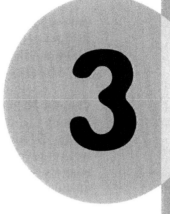

Part 3

The therapeutic use of self

Introduction

Part 3 of the book goes beyond the working alliance to examine the other characterising elements of therapeutic relationships identified by Clarkson (1995). What is being proposed in this part is not that mental health professionals should all become therapists, but that we should all be more aware and intentional in how we engage and interact with service users, if we are to be able companions on their recovery journey.

Chapter 16 looks at the psychodynamics of helping relationships and in particular explores the phenomenon of transference and counter-transference. Relationships with mental health professionals often provide a blank screen onto which clients project feelings and unresolved issues from other significant relationships in their lives. Similarly, professional helpers bring their own unacknowledged emotional legacy to the relationship, which also becomes part of the unfolding drama. An awareness of what is being acted out in the helping relationship can be important, both in developing and sustaining the relationship and in providing a fulcrum for change.

Chapter 17 explores the reparative, replenishing role of mental health professionals in long-term relationships with service users, a role analogous to parenting. It is argued that through working awarely with this dynamic in the relationship, healing and personality development can take place.

Chapter 18 examines the significance of person-to-person interactions as a catalyst for constructive change and some of the ethical dilemmas that working in this way can raise. Working in person-centred ways with service users involves developing helping relationships in which there is more mutuality and equality than in conventional 'expert-led' relationships. It is a relationship characterised by being real in the relationship rather than role-bound.

Chapter 19 considers the nature of spiritual care and psycho-spiritual overwhelm as a source of distress. Many people, ordinary individuals as well as health care professionals, are able to relate to others in a way that is infused with spirituality. By this I do not mean to suggest some pious act of caring but rather the ability to communicate deeply in warm, accepting, understanding ways; ways that transcend barriers such as disability, ethnicity, culture, education, class and poverty.

Chapter 20 throws some light onto the shadow side of helping. We would like to think that it is primarily an altruistic motive that draws us into professional caring. Yet it is often our own unmet needs and unresolved issues that prompt us to engage in such work. If we are to work in ways that help people in their recovery, we need to be aware of how our own needs and distress distort our attempts to help others.

The dynamics of therapeutic care

16

Transference

Transference is a psychoanalytic concept that describes a key dynamic in helping relationships. It is a phenomenon in which one person, the client, unconsciously experiences the helper as if they were someone else – a significant figure, such as a parent, from their past. What is transferred are the feelings and fantasies that belong to this previous relationship, which may be of a positive or negative nature. There may be feelings of love, affection, pleasure, admiration, concern, desire; or feelings of anger, resentment, bitterness, mistrust, guilt and envy. What distinguishes these feelings from everyday emotional transactions is that they are inappropriate and too intense. As a helper you have a sense of being responded to 'as if' you were someone else (Perry 1991).

It is important, however, not to interpret every intense emotional transaction as transference. The client's response might be a very valid reaction to the helper's attitude or behaviour. For example, the client may feel understandably angry when faced with a helper's authoritative, superior attitude, or experience envy and resentment towards a helper who appears to have all the things in life which the client most desires, but which seem beyond their reach. It is entirely reasonable that a client might feel love and affection and sometimes sexual desire for a helper who has supported them in a warm, concerned, understanding way through a challenging period in their life.

The helping relationship provides an ideal screen on which to project these feelings, the caregiver often becoming a significant temporary attachment figure (Byng-Hall 1995). How these are managed has importance for the helper, whose sense of self can be inflated or deflated by the buffeting of these projections, and for the outcome of the therapeutic alliance, which may be undermined. Transference is not, however, a phenomenon that is exclusive to the therapeutic process. It occurs in everyday life between one person and another, between an individual and a group and between an individual and an institution. The script for our ways of relating is laid down in our early formative relationships. Insecure attachments to caregivers during those early years may lead to these insecure attachment patterns being played out in adult relationships.

If transference is not too strong and does not disrupt the relationship and interfere adversely with the helping process, then it may be sufficient to simply acknowledge that some transference is likely to be taking place. Rogers (1986b) takes the view that interpretation of transference is unnecessary and unhelpful. He argues that if the helper is able to demonstrate accurate understanding and acceptance of what the client is experiencing in the here and now, with no interpretation or evaluation, then 'the transference attitudes tend to dissolve and feelings are directed towards their true objects' (p. 133). Rogers seems to be suggesting that what we project defensively is what cannot be faced and accepted as part of ourselves. If the helper can contain and accept the projections without getting caught up in them, then they can be taken back and owned by the client who relates them to their true source.

Sometimes, however, in order to deal with a difficult dynamic that has arisen from the client's transference, it may be necessary to engage with the client in a more challenging way – what Egan (1994) describes as immediacy. Immediacy involves focusing on and exploring what is happening here and now in the relationship between helper and client – in the relationship as a whole or in some segment of dialogue. An awareness of a replicative script being played out can be a starting point from which the client can begin to recognise this as a pattern that tends to disrupt their relationships. At a deeper level, a connection may be made with the origin of that behaviour in early experience. The relationship with the helper may, for example, be idealised by the client, who surrenders all autonomy and seems to expect the helper to magically intervene to make life better. Alternatively the relationship may be one where the worker is experienced as detached, preoccupied and not to be bothered. The client always waits for the worker to initiate contact and expresses guilt about making demands. In another scenario, a client complains about other mental health workers, seems jealous of other clients and has a need to know about the nurse's personal relationships. Unaddressed, these situations would all make it difficult to work effectively with the client in an adult-to-adult way. Failure to recognise and work with transference is thought to be a common reason for unsuccessful treatment (Watkins 1989).

There is some risk in transferential relationships with people who become distressed and disturbed in a psychotic way. Transference is rather like a personal drama being played out with the helper cast in a role. As in the theatre, the client needs to appreciate the 'as if' quality as the unfolding drama. There is a danger that this may be lost in people who are very psychotic with the helper becoming confused with the object of the transference (Brown & Pedder 1991).

It is not possible to avoid transference completely but it can be minimised. This can be achieved by refusing the parent role and engaging with the client in an adult-to-adult way that reasserts the working alliance. Reality testing is also a way of reducing the distortion of reality that transference induces. Raising the client's awareness of the here and now – 'Is it true that no one listens or cares about you?' – helps achieve this. Dis-identifying from the transference object is also sometimes a necessary intervention – 'You seem in a way to be confusing me with your father. I am not your father and it might be helpful to remind yourself of the ways in which I am different'. This can help realign the relationship so that a more adult–adult transaction is possible rather than parent–child.

Withdrawal and the inability to engage in social or therapeutic relationships may also be seen as transferential (Clarkson 1993). Sometimes what the client is transferring is the experience of invasive, neglectful or abusive parenting. Building up trust with such clients can take a long time but it is through the experience of a caring relationship in the here and now that they learn how to be open to nurturing relationships in everyday life while protecting themselves in more appropriate ways.

Joanna's story

Theme: transference in the helping relationship

Joanna is a 19-year-old unmarried woman with a 5-month-old baby daughter called Rebecca. She has spent the last 2 months in the Mother and Baby Unit at her local mental health unit being treated for puerperal psychosis.

Joanna's early life was characterised by two key losses. Firstly, her parents separated and divorced when she was 10 months old, since when she has only seen her father intermittently. Secondly, her mother had to work, which meant she and her 2-year-old brother spent much of their early life with a succession of child-minders. Her mother struggled on with very little support and was treated by her general practitioner for depression. When Joanna was 4, her mother began a relationship with another man. Her mother was 'captured' by that relationship and became less accessible to Joanna and her brother.

When Rebecca was born, Joanna seemed to project all her own neediness onto the baby, providing it with over-solicitous mothering. In the months that followed, Rebecca became increasingly fretful and difficult to satisfy, confronting Joanna with her fear that she was an inadequate mother and at a deeper level, with the fear that she would never find the love and care she needed for herself. This seemed to precipitate a profoundly hopeless and troubled state of mind in which she developed unusual ideas about the baby and herself. It seemed to Joanna that Rebecca was not her child and she withdrew from her, on one occasion referring to her as the cuckoo. Her belief was that her baby had been given to a childless couple by social services. She showed no distress about this, believing that they would be able to give the baby everything. She became preoccupied with the ideas that she was 'bad inside', that all her 'goodness' and strength had gone into the baby.

During her hospitalisation, Joanna has developed a transferential relationship with Hannah, her primary nurse, who is about the same age as her own mother. She has found it difficult to cope with Hannah's shift patterns and days off, frequently thinking that she must be to blame in some way for her absences and seeking reassurance that she hadn't done anything wrong. She tended to idealise Hannah, seeing her as kind and caring and other staff as hurtful and unpleasant. Often she would try to stay in proximity to Hannah and to other staff when Hannah was not on duty and would often 'collapse' on to staff as if wanting to be held.

The nursing care Joanna received created a scenario on which she projected and played out some of the undealt-with issues from her own childhood. Hannah found it helpful to give portions of boundaried time, when she could give free attention to Joanna. She was conscious of feeling drained by the demand of being constantly needed. She was able to challenge Joanna's elevated view of her and the contrasting negative view of other staff, helping her to see that this represented how she thought about herself and Rebecca. Slowly Joanna began to re-own and affirm her own 'goodness'. From this more integrated, if fragile position, she was able to accept Robecca's contentment and demands and reconnect with her maternal feelings.

Counter-transference

Counter-transference is concerned with the helper's feelings and fantasies about the client. There is no general agreement about the nature of counter-transference which, like transference, is part of the social transactions of everyday life. One way of talking about it is to think of it as being proactive – what the helper transfers onto the client from their own past, or reactive – the responses the client induces in the helper.

In its proactive form, the helper relates to the client in a way that is reminiscent of a previous, significant relationship. An example of this is seen in a helper who finds difficulty in being sufficiently assertive in working with clients. In supervision, the helper is able to link this with his need for parental approval, which was conditional on being 'nice' and 'compliant'. Another example is of a helper who, in supervision, acknowledges strong feelings of anxiety and guilt towards a client who has recurrent mental health problems. These were feelings she was able to connect with her own 'parentified' childhood where she had to care for a chronically ill mother.

In reactive counter-transference helpers might find themselves experiencing feelings of anxiety, helplessness, despondency or anger for which there were no identifiable reasons in their life. These feelings may be what the client has difficulty in acknowledging and expressing in himself, which he excludes by putting them out onto the helper – a process called projective identification in psychoanalytic psychotherapy. This ability to resonate with the client's emotional world, communicated in largely unconscious ways, is clearly a useful window onto the client's inner emotional world, if helpers can stay sufficiently aware of what belongs to them and what to the client.

Another example of reactive counter-transference can be seen in a helper's tendency to project their own vulnerability or helplessness onto a client, seeing them as more dependent than they actually are and in the process denying their own neediness. Meeting a need for power or esteem may also be a hidden motive in the helper's over-caring and overbearing approach to working with clients.

Sometimes as helpers we may over-identify with clients and avoid areas that are similar to our own problems or avoid feelings that are difficult for us to acknowledge and deal with in ourselves. The other side of the coin to this is that we work on issues we ourselves need to work on vicariously through the client. So, for example, the client may be asked to carry and work on our own losses as well as their own.

Counter-transference is also seen in our reaction to the transference of a client, for example by taking criticism to heart, or being seduced by a client's expressions of love or sexual desire. Perhaps more commonly this form of counter-transference is seen in the reaction to a client who gives out dependency signals with the helper becoming the protective, nurturing parent. This is of course not necessarily an unhelpful complementary role, but if the role is occupied in an unaware, fixed way it can limit the client's opportunity for personal growth.

We need to guard against any tendency to label every feeling we have for a client, whether positive or negative, as counter-transference. Sometimes strong feelings are the authentic here-and-now responses of one person to another. Rogers (1967) regards 'the full experience of an affectional relationship' as being an important element in the helping relationship for some clients, which may lead to significant learning about the self and others.

This brief section on counter-transference underlines the value of both personal development work and supervision as part of the training experience of professional helpers working in the mental health field. It is only through this experience that we can minimise what Heron (2001) calls contaminated helping – that is, helping that is adversely affected by our own agendas. The mental health professions have until recently failed to recognise the duality of the personal and the professional in the helping role and have neglected to make provision for this in training and support. It is precisely because personal needs and feelings are denied at a personal and organisational level that we attempt to deal with them vicariously in caring for others. Hawkins & Shoet (2000) make the challenging observation that effective helping arises out of our willingness to examine our own motives and that in doing so, there is less likelihood of 'the psychiatric client having to carry our own craziness'.

 Tony's story

Theme: counter-transference in helping relationships

One of the things I noticed quite early in my relationship with Adrian was that he often made reference to similarities between his father and me. I think this made it difficult for him to trust me enough to let me into his life initially. I suspect he must have been wondering whether I would be another critical and ultimately abandoning 'parent'.
I was putting in a lot of time with Adrian helping him to open out his life but even so I found myself feeling guilty that I wasn't giving him enough time and leaving him at the end of one of my visits often felt like a small betrayal. I also felt annoyed because I thought he was expecting too much of me and seldom showed me any appreciation. The other thing was I found myself feeling quite anxious about confronting him verbally about his behaviour or encouraging him to take risks in facing situations I knew he would find challenging. We were tending to stay in fairly safe territory.

Taking this to supervision I began to see that some of these feelings had relevance for me and my life. It seemed as if I was accepting his transference, trying to be the 'good father' that he wanted, but could of course never be. I was also picking up his resentments about how his father used to come, stay for a short while, then go, just like me. Not seeing the bigger picture, Adrian's resentment was leaving me feeling both guilty and annoyed.

My uneasiness about challenging Adrian is partly that I am aware of his vulnerability to quite overwhelming paranoid anxiety and I don't want to go too far too fast. But I think this gets overlaid with my own fear of criticism and ridicule that I experienced in my relationship with my father. This causes me to hold back from making interventions.

What I feel now is that we deal with these undercurrents more of the time. If I find myself avoiding, I will look at it with Adrian and explore whether we are colluding. I've tried to dis-identify from Adrian's father by getting Adrian to identify some of the ways I'm different from him. I've also encouraged Adrian to acknowledge the feelings that arise in the 'here and now' of our relationship more of the time and to relocate some of those feelings in the 'there and then' of his past, where that has been appropriate.

Self-enquiry box

You might find it helpful to reflect on the following questions. How might these reactions impose limitations on the process of helping?

- Do I require affection, approval, appreciation, regard, to be liked, in my relationships with clients?
- Do I need to take charge, be authoritative, feel important, be protective, be prescriptive, in my relationships with clients?
- Do I find it difficult to allow closeness in my relationships with clients?
- Do I see people as individuals or do I have a tendency to label and stereotype people?
- Do I feel uncomfortable with certain issues and feelings that arise in my conversations with clients? Are these issues and feelings I need to deal with myself?
- Do I catch myself being over-solicitous in my care of people?
- Do I feel resentful towards the involvement of carers or other members of the multidisciplinary or multi-agency team in the care of the client?

Intentional use of self in developmentally needed or reparative relationships

It has been recognised for many years that one of the helping, healing roles that nurses play in their relationships with clients is that of surrogate parent. As Peplau (1988) puts it, 'permitting the patient to experience older feelings in new situations of helplessness, but with the acceptance and attention that encourages personality development, requires a relationship in which the nurse recognises her surrogate role' (p. 57). Clarkson (1995) sees the developmentally needed relationship as one that, 'provides a reparative or replenishing relationship where original parenting was deficient, abusive or overprotective'.

The theoretical underpinning for a surrogate role has come mainly from the psychoanalytic stream of ideas on human development and the therapeutic process. In the UK, the ubiquitous influence of the medical model has limited the impact of these ideas on psychiatric nursing practice mainly to therapeutic communities. A notable example is a model of psychosocial nursing that has evolved at the Cassel Hospital (Griffiths & Leach 1998). Here not only nurse/patient relationships but the whole social matrix of the community has developed as a 'culture of enquiry'. The client's difficulties in living are revealed, contained and explored in the daily life of the community and a newly emergent self nurtured.

Development can be seen as a lifelong progressive unfolding of our potential both as human beings and as unique individuals. The emergent self grows and flourishes in a loving, nurturing, encouraging environment, in a way that expresses itself in a sense of wellbeing. In an unfavourable environment, where the emergent self is not prized and nourished, development will be restricted, weakened or distorted in a way that expresses itself in increased vulnerability and dysfunction.

One of the most significant research-based theories of human development is attachment theory (Bowlby 1969, 1973, 1980, 1988). Attachments can be said to lie at the heart of family life. They create bonds that can provide care and security across the life cycle. They can evoke the most intense feelings of joy in the making or of anguish in the breaking and can lead to problems if they become insecure (Byng-Hall 1995). Attachment behaviour reflects the human need to be close to significant others on whom, in early life, our physical survival depends. For the majority of children, between 57% and 73% (Byng-Hall 1995), attachment to one or more caregivers provides a secure base from which to explore the world with a degree of trust and confidence and for the self and self-esteem to flourish. For others, those who do not receive 'good enough' parenting, insecure attachment patterns may develop and future relationships be undermined as the result of the replication of these early 'scripts'. The need for attachment and a secure base continues throughout life (Ainsworth 1991). The knowledge that someone is concerned for you and has you in mind supports autonomous, resourceful behaviour, even when an attachment figure is not immediately available. This has significant implications for mental health professionals who, in the context of a caring relationship, often become a temporary attachment figure for their clients. If this dynamic can be worked with in an aware way, then the opportunity exists to do reparative work with the client.

Self-enquiry box

Gather some small objects together. Objects you have in your pockets or a bag will do. Choose objects to represent yourself and members of your family. Arrange them in the form of a family 'sculpt', that is, a placement pattern that says something about your family system. Try not to deliberate too much at this stage – go with what intuitively feels right.

You might like to try a family 'sculpt' representing:

- your family of origin, when you were a pre-school child
- your family during your school years
- your family when you were an adolescent/young adult
- your family as it is now
- your family as you would like it to be.

Ask yourself:

- How have the 'sculpts' changed over time?
- What have been the important transitional points?
- How have I and others in my family been affected by these transitions?
- What do the 'sculpts' have to tell me about my attachment relationships and patterns?
- What needs to happen for my family system to change in the way I would like it to?

Many situations may undermine the capacity of a family to provide a secure base.

Fear of losing or the actual loss of an attachment figure This may be the result of the death of a parent or parental separation and divorce. It may be in the form of threats to abandon the child or the use of conditional love to control the child.

The attachment figure is unavailable Long-term illness in a parent, either physical or psychological, may mean the parent is unavailable or only intermittently available as an attachment figure. In this situation some children will take on a 'parentified' role, becoming caregivers and attachment figures for their parent.

While this role reversal may be appropriate later in the life cycle of the family, in childhood and adolescence it can restrict a young person's growth towards independence, making it difficult to separate. In other circumstances a child may feel excluded by another child or the other parent, who has 'captured' the attachment figure.

Scapegoating and misidentification by attachment figures In some families a child will become the focus of blame for the family's ills and may come to act out that role. In other circumstances a child becomes identified with someone else in the family, the 'black sheep' or someone with whom the parent has or had a difficult relationship, which is then re-enacted in their relationship with the child.

Abusive relationships with an attachment figure The most damaging example of a situation that undermines attachment is where a child is emotionally, physically or sexually abused by someone they would naturally turn to for security. They may feel unable to turn to the other parent for protection for fear of the consequences or because the other parent is unwilling to hear.

Many of these early experiences can be re-enacted in helping relationships, which prompt a replication of 'old scripts'. It is not uncommon for clients to have anxieties about being abandoned or not to feel cared for, despite the attention they receive from their nurse, and of course this can never be enough to make good what was missing from the parenting they received. It is not uncommon for adult survivors of childhood sexual abuse to feel that they have not been heard or believed by professional helpers whom they share this experience with. There is, unfortunately, sometimes a basis in the here and now for this conception. Hearing the client's story can be painful and difficult and the response to it can be muted or incredulous. The client may then begin to feel unheard and unprotected by the nurse just as they were unprotected by significant adults as a child. The currents of powerful feelings – hate, anger, anxiety – that may surface can create in staff both a strong need to care, but also at times, a sense that they themselves are being abusive.

There is an important issue here about the importance of believing clients' stories, even though occasionally they may be fabricated. Early experience may be 'known' at some level and have a profound influence on the behaviour of the client in the here and now, without them necessarily being able to recover the memories of formative experiences or the thoughts and feelings they gave rise to. There can be a number of reasons for this. Firstly, some experiences can be too painful and disturbing to remain in awareness and are shut out of consciousness. Secondly, parents will often disconfirm or discount a child's experience so that the child is no longer sure what to believe or whether what they are experiencing has validity. Bowlby (1988) gives a number of examples of psychologically distressed adults who as children witnessed a parent's suicide but were told that they had died from other, more 'natural', causes. Children may be repeatedly told 'to be grateful', 'to think yourself lucky' or 'you've got nothing to be unhappy about', by parents who find their children's hurt, anger or sadness an uncomfortable echo of their own unacknowledged pain. The consequence of this is that children will begin to disown their discounted thoughts and feelings. Finally, we want to believe that our parents are good parents. We want to believe they love us and are protective towards us. Not to believe so, even when a child's experience is of frequent neglect or rejection, is too threatening.

It can be seen from this brief comment on what is a complex process that there are implications for mental health professionals. It would be easy to disconfirm or discount key events in the client's history if we are not able to stay open and be a validating witness to their unfolding story. If we cannot hear what happened and contain the distress for the client, then it is unlikely they will be able to face that experience. They will not be able to begin the task of re-evaluating it, so that it is no longer such a powerful source of distress, and no longer has such a limiting and disruptive impact on their life.

Attachment theory conceptualises a process by which we internalise models of our attachment figures and of ourselves in relation to them, which then become part of self. What we experience as self is a reflection of the way significant others have behaved towards us. Thus if we have been cared for in a way that was predominantly loving and sensitively responsive to our needs, we are likely to have internalised an image of ourselves as both a loving and lovable person. If the reverse was true and the care we received was predominantly insensitive, an overly adapted self is likely to develop, which is lacking a sense of self-worth, and we will be demanding and insecure in our relationships with others.

While the 'psychological mechanics' of the process differ, there seems little difference in the significance given to attachment figures in the development of the self, between the psychoanalytically oriented views of D.W. Winnicott (see Phillips 1988) and Alice Miller (Miller 1990) and ideas of humanistically oriented writers. Rogers saw the unconditional positive regard of others as being a core condition for the development of what he called the organismic or true self. In other words, if our emergent self is accepted and prized, it is likely to flourish. On the other hand, if we experience rejection, disapproval, or conditional positive regard, the expression of our selfhood is likely to be overlaid by a false self. The false self may enable us to survive and gain some attention and positive regard but at the cost of a growing alienation from our authentic being. It is not just positive regard from others that we need. We need to feel good about ourselves and if this need is not met it is difficult to function in the world. As Thorne (1992) puts it, 'Our capacity to feel positive about ourselves is dependent on the quality and consistency of the positive regard shown to us by others, and where it is selective (as to some degree it must be for all of us), we are victims of conditions of worth' (p. 31). Positive regard from others is internalised and becomes a sustaining sense of self-worth that enables us to recover from the wounding life experiences of disappointment, failure, rejection and loss that inevitably come along. If our inner core of self-esteem is low, then we are vulnerable to the misfortunes of everyday life and they may overwhelm us with feelings of worthlessness. The alienation from our true self is maintained by our negative self, which continues to censor any expression of the true self that does not meet our internalised conditions of worth. It may, for example, be very difficult for some people to acknowledge certain feelings or needs, because to do so would seem to undermine their sense of self. The negative self can for many people be punitive, critical and impossible to live with. They frequently feel a sense of not being good enough in various dimensions of their lives as their organismic self seeks expression.

Self-enquiry box

You might find it useful to explore aspects of your own negative self. One way of doing this is to consider the many shoulds, oughts and musts we all carry around that can have restricting and limiting effects on our personal growth and undermine our self-esteem.

Write 12 open-ended statements:

I should.......................

I ought..........................

I must..........................

Now complete the statement with whatever comes to mind. Don't deliberate, go with whatever comes up.

Example

I should know.

I ought to be happy.

I must do better.

Now examine your statements. Ask yourself:

* Which ones am I most drawn to?
* Is this a value that I can own and try to hold to in my life?
* Is this a value that I continue to subscribe to but no longer accept as being relevant to my life now?
* Where does it come from?
* How does it affect the way I feel, think and act?
* Do I want to discard it altogether or change it so that it is less prohibitive?

Bowlby sees development proceeding along a number of possible paths, some leading to adaptive behaviour, others leading to increased vulnerability and maladaptive behaviour. Whether a child is securely or insecurely attached in their relationship with significant caregivers is seen as a key factor in determining which pathway an individual takes. Patterns of attachment established during the early years of life tend to persist and will be replicated in other attachment relationships a person makes as they journey through life. While there is some persistence, the developmental pathway is not seen as unchanging, since secure bases provided by other attachment figures in childhood, adolescence and adult life can provide an emotionally corrective experience that enables people to move from an insecure to a secure pathway.

In talking about the therapeutic stance in developmentally needed relationships, Bowlby identifies a number of 'therapeutic tasks'. First and foremost is the need to create a secure base from which the client can begin to explore their inner and outer worlds and share thoughts and feelings. The mental health worker will therefore need to be with a client in a way that is accepting, respectful, attentive and reliable and will also need, as far as possible, to see and feel the world through the client's eyes. Important to the experience of a secure base is the ability of the professional helper to contain a client's anxiety and distress. This psychological holding takes place when the mental health professional is experienced as an accessible and supportive presence in the client's life and as someone who communicates a genuine concern and care, who is not critical or rejecting, but stays with the client in their distress, does not react against it by, for example, giving extra medication, but reflects on it and tries to understand it. This is analogous with the way young children are held and comforted when frightened or distressed. When this happens, anxieties begin to subside and the client is less likely to act out their distress in disturbed, problematic ways. Gradually the client learns that intense feelings, fears and fantasies can be contained, reflected on and made sense of, with the expression of disturbing thoughts and feelings in disturbed behaviour being correspondingly reduced.

The secure base may be difficult to achieve and maintain. Insecure attachment patterns express themselves in the therapeutic relationship along with transferential feelings and fantasies. For example, a client may withdraw if he feels the nurse is getting too close for comfort. This happens not because the client wishes to end the relationship, in fact the very opposite. Instead it will be an attempt to maintain the relationship at a distance the client feels able to bear. Another example might be a client who senses the nurse's emotional reserves are low and that she or he is unable to provide the emotional nourishment needed. Their relational pattern might be to become more demanding in response to anxiety about being 'pushed away'.

 Geoff's story

Theme: reparative relationships

Geoff is a 27-year-old who has had frequent contact with the psychiatric services since the age of 18. He has been diagnosed as having a personality disorder and is usually referred in a depressed and suicidal state. His threats of suicide are often of a dramatic and alarming nature, including dousing himself with petrol and threatening to set himself alight, or on another occasion threatening to jump off a motorway road bridge. He drinks heavily and sometimes takes street drugs.

Central to Geoff's early history was, at the age of 8, finding his mother dead, having committed suicide by cutting her wrists. His father, a morose man, who showed little interest in him, began drinking heavily after his wife's death. Geoff was subsequently brought up by an aunt, his mother's sister, who cared for him in a dutiful way but with very little emotional warmth. He left her care at 16 and lived on the streets in London for a while, where he found some sense of belonging to a 'family' group. The traumatic loss of his mother and the insecure attachments to his father and his aunt left Geoff feeling abandoned, unlovable and 'a jinx'. This latter image of himself, which became embedded in his psyche, originated from his aunt who often told him he was 'a jinx on all our lives' and seemed to scapegoat him for things that went wrong in her own family. There was very little family discussion of his mother or her death and he can only talk in a very vague, flat way about his early relationships.

Geoff's relationships with girlfriends have usually ended as a consequence of his demanding and possessive attitude and an excessive need to please the object of his affections. Any distancing or disapproval in the relationship he reacts to with prolonged, withdrawn, angry, grief-stricken silences. He is currently unemployed and lack of work is a major preoccupation. It is difficult for Geoff to attribute this to the insecurity of many jobs these days and the ebb and flow of economic circumstances, rather than to his own lack of worth and personal rejection. Crises have often followed the breakdown of a relationship or the loss of a job.

Geoff is currently living in a hostel for young adults with severe emotional problems and attends an outpatient therapy group. The hostel community and the group have provided a secure base for Geoff to begin to recognise and explore the patterns of behaviour that replicate themselves in such a disruptive, distressing way in his current life and relationships. It is difficult at times for both the group and the community to contain his unresponsiveness and his brooding, threatening anger and there is concern when these episodes occur about the risk of self-harm behaviour. Despite these anxieties, the group, the hostel community and Geoff's key worker have been able to maintain a matrix of caring relationships that is allowing Geoff to begin his developmental tasks. There are careful and sensitive limits set in relation to drinking and drug taking, violence and being present, but beyond these conditions of care there is a prevailing sense of unconditional positive regard towards Geoff which is helping him to acknowledge his own worth and value and appreciate himself more. Geoff has surprised himself by discovering a sense of humour. This allows him to laugh at certain frustrations and disappointments, for example not getting a cleaning job at a local supermarket, a let-down that previously would have undermined his sense of self and precipitated feelings of hopelessness and desolation.

Once a secure base has been established, the client may feel safe enough to begin to explore some of the difficulties that arise from their patterns of relating and reacting. I do not see this as 'doing therapy' in the formal sense, although it is a form of 'social therapy': being with the client in different settings, participating with them in the activities of everyday life and using opportunities to engage in purposeful conversation with a client about the issues that create problems of living. Issues arise in the context of living with others, working with others, taking recreation with others and managing the responsibilities of everyday life. The more involved the nurse is in the social matrix of the client's life, the more attuned they can be to the social transactions that take place. These everyday transactions (and sometimes the transactions between the nurse and client) provide 'here and now' examples of old scripts – the past in the present. If these patterns can be recognised, people can be supported in improvising new ways of relating and reacting that are not influenced so strongly by past experience. In the light of the experiential learning that comes out of an ongoing reflection on the 'here and now', old scripts are updated.

In applying attachment theory to the therapeutic process, a particular reference is made to the significance of the client reconnecting with and expressing feelings associated with their experience of attachment relationships (Bowlby 1988). Often stories of neglect or abuse will be told in a flat, impassive way that gives little hint of how the child in the story felt. Miller (1990) emphasises how children adapt to parental needs and conditions for love and approval to such an extent that feelings such as anger, hate, jealousy, anxiety and unhappiness are disowned. This leads to the development of a false self in which our emotional being remains largely unacknowledged and unexpressed. In an empathic, accepting, containing relationship it becomes possible to re-own that lost part of self. Bowlby suggests filling in the 'emotionally blank' story by empathetically engaging with the hurt, angry, sad, frightened child and articulating those feelings. Doing so can give clients a powerful sense of being heard and of it being safe to own and discharge these painful feelings.

 Angela's story

Theme: reparative relationships

I suppose I'd always known it, but never really faced it. I'd been very depressed for about 5 years and had several admissions to hospital. There were other problems as well. I used to get panic attacks and I was very thin, anorexic really. In some ways I didn't mind going into hospital. I always had this feeling that I would be safe there and that this time they would help me. I didn't talk much about my childhood to the doctors or nurses – nobody asked really.

I began talking about it with my CPN. She was a bit older than me, someone I trusted and felt comfortable with. I was telling her about the last time I was in hospital and this male patient came into the female dormitory one night and tried to get into bed with a young girl. I remembered lying there feeling very frightened and not being able to go and get the night nurse. Then I began to talk about how I'd felt like that when I was a child and not being able to tell my mother that my two stepbrothers were sexually abusing me. I couldn't believe it was me saying it, in fact I couldn't believe that what I was saying was true. But Kate (CPN) listened and took what I said seriously. I think she said something like, 'You must have felt very frightened and very alone'. It seemed like she had really heard me and was concerned for me in a way my mother never was.

After I'd told her I felt very quite panicky but stifled it, holding it inside, not able to show it. That was the first time. Since then we've talked about it often and it's been very painful emotionally. There were times when I had this fear that she would forget to come and I remember feeling resentful about all the other patients she had to see. I suppose I just had this great need to feel protected at that time. I remember feeling quite angry with her and feeling let down in a way that I can see now I was never able to feel towards my mother. I suppose I'd begun to idealise Kate a bit and it was good for me to recognise that she wasn't perfect, just as parents are not perfect. It helped me to feel a little more forgiving towards my mother and to understand how difficult it was for her.

As well as talking, she asked me to write letters, from myself as a 10-year-old girl to myself as an adult and then to reply. It sounded daft but I found it helpful. I was able to express a lot of thoughts and feelings that were quite difficult to talk about. It also helped me to care for myself and to say to my 10-year-old self – 'You were not responsible'.

I've started attending a group for adult survivors who have been abused as children. I'm learning that it wasn't my fault, that I didn't deserve it and that I'm not a bad person. I'm also beginning to learn to trust people and to be a bit more confident and assertive. Looking back I now see my depression as that 10-year-old girl feeling abandoned and frightened, reminding me that she was there and needed to be taken care of.

174

Bowlby describes the role of the therapeutic helper as being a companion to the client in their exploration. The client is seen as the 'expert' on their own experience, who with support and occasional guidance can discover for themselves the true nature of the models that underlie thoughts, feelings and actions and begin the process of restructuring them. Growth and recovery are seen as a naturally occurring process. 'Fortunately the human psyche is like human bones, in its inclination towards self-healing' (Bowlby 1988).

The job of the therapeutic helper is to provide the healing conditions. Similarly Winnicott was more concerned with care in the service of personal development than cure. He saw the therapeutic process as holding the client's conflicts and distress while development and resolution took place. For Winnicott the significant moments in therapy were when the client 'surprised himself'. Perhaps it is this capacity of clients to 'surprise themselves' that mental health professionals attempt to facilitate through their helping relationships.

Any theory can become dogma and impose itself on an attempt to understand the client's experience. While attachment theory as a basis for practice has arisen from the experience of clinical practice and has been rigorously tested by research studies, like all theories it still does not capture the lived experience of the individual client. As Moore (1996) puts it, 'Each person is a mystery never to be completely understood'. No theory will explain the mystery of being that person. What is much more important is being with people and allowing the mystery that is both our lives to be enacted and better understood.

Person-to-person relationships

18

The person-to-person relationship is a more human, de-professionalised approach to working with people struggling with mental adversity. It is a helping relationship in which there is more mutuality and equality. A person-to-person relationship requires us to be 'real' in our interactions, which means being more open and genuine, bringing more of ourselves into the social encounter. It is potentially the most liberating and growthful of all the helping relationships, for both the client and the practitioner, but also one of the most difficult to achieve and manage. It requires a significant shift in attitudes – from seeing people as psychiatric patients who are suffering from pathological syndromes and in need of treatment, to seeing people as people who at this moment in their lives are experiencing a state of psychological overwhelm, from which they can emerge and grow.

If this stance is to be more than mere tokenism, then it requires us to relate in a different way to people using the mental health services. It means recognising that the problems of living people present with, while they may be more urgent and sometimes desperate, are not qualitatively different from our own. It means recognising that the person seeking help is an expert by experience on their own life and carries within them the potential for self-healing and recovery. It means working within more diffuse boundaries than is the norm in therapeutic relationships, replacing a quasi-parental role with a more fraternal one. Person-centredness is essentially a non-directive way of helping and healing. The task is not to authoritatively prescribe the way to recovery but to be an enabling presence for the person in their quest to find within themselves the resources and the wisdom to grow through an experience of disabling distress. Joseph & Worsley (2005) neatly encapsulate the person-centred view, arguing that given the right social environment, human beings have an 'inherent tendency to grow towards their potential for optimal functioning, a guiding principle that applies even when working with people who are deeply distressed'.

The person-to-person relationship is much more about being than doing. It is a basic philosophy, rather than a technique, which involves being with people in a way that creates the conditions for growth and change. Carl Rogers, the originator of person-centred counselling, described this way of being as relating to others in a way that is genuine, accepting, and characterised by an empathic attunement to the other's inner world. When this way of being is lived out in our personal lives, it connects us with our core selves and frees more of our potential for living. When lived out in our professional relationships, it facilitates others to engage in self-exploration, self-discovery and constructive change. This remained a central theme in Rogers' practice, writing and research for over forty years (Thorne 1992).

Person-centred therapy has been exposed to a lot of criticism over the years, much of it centring on Rogers' claim that the core conditions were the necessary and sufficient conditions for change. The opposing view has been that, while the core conditions are necessary, they are not sufficient to facilitate growth and change and that the judicious use of techniques such as the re-attribution techniques of cognitive behavioural therapy produces better outcomes. Thus the core conditions have come to be seen as the relational background against which 'real therapy' takes place. This claim has been strongly refuted in a recent review of psychotherapeutic outcome research, which concludes that in all therapies 30% of the positive outcome is related to the client–therapist relationship and 40% to the client's own inner resources (Bozarth & Motomasa 2005). This suggests that specificity – that is specific psychotherapeutic techniques for specific disorders – has a relatively small contribution to make to recovery and, as Rogers consistently affirmed, it is the compassionate presence of the practitioner that awakens the client's capacity to live a more fulfilled life – to live well. In person-centred practice the relationship is the therapy – it is the relational depth which provides the secure base for people to face their dysfunctional way of being and surviving, a way of being that has caused such suffering, and for healing and growth to take place (Mearns & Thorne 2000).

But we are not concerned here with formal psychotherapy per se, but with the therapeutic use of self which lies at the heart of the work of many mental health professionals who would not consider their practice as encompassing formal psychotherapy. It is my contention and experience that if a person in extremis is able to perceive the practitioner's warm acceptance, genuineness and empathy, then over time they will liberate themselves from their *mind made manacles* and begin to develop in the direction of becoming a fully functioning person. The therapeutic use of self has been the central focus of my own action research over several years (see Chapter 21). Action research starts from a pertinent question – my question has been: 'Is it possible for me to work in a non-directive way within the mental health system, to trust the actualising potential of people to grow in the direction of resourceful living given the presence of enabling and empowering relationships?'. Much of the content of this book has been distilled out of that experience.

Over the past 30 years, person-centredness has entered the realms of psychiatry through the back door and been adopted by many mental health professionals of all disciplines as the philosophical and practical basis for their work, without them necessarily recognising humanistic psychology as its theoretical source. It resonates strongly with their desire for a more human approach to care. To hold person-centred attitudes and to live them in your personal life and professional practice can be challenging. Psychiatry, as a tradition that confers on practitioners a powerful expert status and the political function of custodians of the mad, and with its pathological orientation and obsessive concern with evidence-based practice, is not a milieu in which person-centredness is likely to flourish. That it can and does stems from the experiential and intuitive knowledge of healing and growth of individual practitioners in both their professional and personal lives. Once you have experienced the creative nature of person-centred relationships, out of which emerges a flow of possibilities leading to self-directed change and growth, then you know this way of being in relationship to others creates the necessary and sufficient conditions for growth, recovery and sustained mental health.

I want to emphasise here that this is no easy thing to achieve. As suggested above, the traditional culture of the psychiatric system is in many ways the antithesis of person-centredness, although it has in the past decade taken some genuine steps in that direction, in response to the voice of service consumers and survivors. Also the education, supervision and management of mental health professionals does not, on the whole, provide a social milieu in which these personal qualities can flourish. There is a tendency to feel that we have come to our chosen profession with these attributes already well developed and that professional training simply awakens us to their potential for facilitating others' growth and change. Of course there are people who acquire these attributes in good measure in their early life, people who are transparently real, who communicate a warm acceptance and who are able to sensitively attune themselves to the inner experience of others – but they are the exception. Most of us have to work hard at being more open to the flow of our inner experience, to become more congruent and authentic in the way we live our lives. Most of us have to learn to accept and affirm ourselves as worthwhile human beings. Most of us have to discover a way of being that is more empathic and compassionate towards ourselves. We cannot relate in this way towards others in our professional lives if we do not live it, if this way of being does not permeate our lives. It will not be deep enough to enable people wounded by the lacerations of life to begin their healing journey. This unity of personal and professional growth can take place if practitioners are committed to reflective practice, have supervision that has the practitioner's congruence as its focus, and through participating in personal development groups and in personal therapy. If we are serious about making person-centred philosophy the cornerstone of our practice, then we should seek out these developmental opportunities.

Box 18.1

A broad hypothesis of therapeutic human relationships

If I can create a relationship characterised on my part by:

* a genuineness and transparency, in which I am in touch with my real feelings
* a warm acceptance and prizing of the other as a separate individual
* a sensitive ability to see the world and himself as he sees them

then the other individual in the relationship will:

* become more integrated and more effective and show fewer characteristics normally termed neurotic or psychotic
* have a more realistic view of himself and become more like the person he wishes to be
* value himself more highly and become more self-confident
* become more understanding and accepting of others
* become more open to his experience and deny and repress less
* cope more resourcefully and creatively with the stresses and problems of living.

Source: Rogers (1967), pp. 35–37.

Genuineness as a way of being

Genuineness, or congruence, refers to the capacity of the helper to be with the client in an authentic way, not hiding behind any pretence or defence. This degree of 'realness' is hard won. It develops gradually as the result of a commitment to self-awareness, through which the practitioner becomes more in touch with their true self. This parallels the therapeutic process, which is also concerned with reclaiming and integrating disowned parts of the self, facilitating the individual's growth towards becoming a fully functioning person. The helper and the client can therefore be seen to be on the same journey. It can be argued with good reason that practitioners will be unable to take a client further in their personal growth than they have been prepared to go themselves, with any degree of acceptance and empathy. There can be no openness to the experience of others unless we are open to our own experience. Congruence is not something that is turned on and off, but is a way of being in the world, a way of relating to others in both our personal and professional lives. It is only possible to live our lives with real integrity when our outer and inner being are in harmony.

Being aware of the feelings, images and thoughts that flow within us when we are working with a client does not mean that we have to disclose everything we experience. In fact it would not be helpful to do so. What we can helpfully disclose are those feelings, thoughts or images that surface in the here and now as we work with a client and may help them in facing and overcoming the issues that confront them. The key question is, 'What is likely to be the therapeutic benefit of my disclosure to the client?'. For example, we may be working with someone who is quite withdrawn and isolated and have a strong sense of hopelessness resonating within us. If this is not our hopelessness, it must belong to the client and can help us connect empathetically with his world.

It can be useful to respond in an authentic way to the client's story and how they present themselves by providing a mirror through which they may reframe troubling life issues or a negative self-concept. This might involve valuing and validating some aspect of the client's behaviour. For example, when working with a client who has been sexually abused as a child, it might be helpful to disclose how angry we feel for that child, that they were not protected and that they should feel to blame. Such openness can allow clients to connect with their own anger and re-evaluate the sense of blame and shame they feel.

Mearns & Thorne (1999) identify a number of reasons why genuineness is important in helping relationships. Firstly, it contributes to the degree of trust a client feels in the practitioner. Some level of trust can be gained through role expectation and the knowledge and expertise of the helper, but a deeper sense of trust emerges from a practitioner's honesty and openness. Secondly, a helper who is willing to be judiciously open about their failings, uncertainties and vulnerabilities, creates a greater sense of equality in the relationship, is more approachable and increases the client's confidence in their ability to understand. Thirdly, the practitioner's congruence models a way of healing that the client is being encouraged to take. A practitioner's acceptance of themselves, their feelings, weaknesses and rough spots, enables clients to own feelings and failings and articulate that experience in a less defensive manner. Finally, genuineness is important because the helper's responses are then an honest reflection of the effect on another person of what the client shares of themselves and their lives. Mearns and Thorne see this as a powerful therapeutic phenomenon that provides the challenge and support which facilitates growth and change.

It is worth keeping in mind that many people referred to the mental health services will have experienced emotional hurt and abuse in significant relationships in the past and may find it difficult to enter into a person-to-person relationship and it may be hard for them to accept the helper's expression of interest and care as genuine. While the person-to-person relationship can be of great benefit, some people need time to work through these issues in a transferential relationship before they can begin to relate in a more person-to-person way.

Self-enquiry box

Being more fully ourselves in helping relationships

It is worth giving some thought to which aspects of yourself you express openly in your relationships with service users you work with. What are some of the issues raised by normalising relationships in this way?

My feelings of love	My humour
My feelings of anxiety	My spirituality
My feelings of anger	My sexuality
My feelings of joy	My interests
My feelings of sadness	My values
My feelings of disappointment	My creativity
My feelings of regret	My knowledge
My warmth	My vulnerabilities
My appreciation	My fallibilities
My needs	My lifestyle
My tactile self	My personal circumstances
My playful self	My caring self

The ethics of practitioners' self-disclosure

Linked to congruence is the question of what is appropriate self-disclosure for mental health workers in their helping relationships. We first of all need to recognise that reciprocal self-disclosure is a necessary condition for forming and deepening social relationships. It is a social skill without which our relationships would be very superficial and dissatisfying. In professional helping relationships, clients are expected to disclose a great deal about themselves and their lives, while helpers disclose very little. When helpers do step out from behind a façade of invulnerability and communicate something of their own experience, it is often appreciated by service users. This reciprocity gives the relationship more equality. It is no longer so one-sided, the client gives something back. The fact is that while the dominant discourses in psychiatry created a chasm between those who are diagnosed mentally ill and those who are not, there is in reality no such delineation. What is falsely portrayed as a chasm is in reality a small step for any one of us, particularly at those times when our vulnerability is exposed by the challenges and demands of life. The 'us and them' perspective is maintained, partly because we see ourselves reflected in the suffering of others and in our discomfort seek to distance ourselves from what is – however labelled and however extreme – an expression of the human condition. As the psychoanalyst Harry Stack Sullivan (1953) famously and succinctly remarked, referring to people suffering from psychosis, 'We are all more alike than different'.

The concept of the wounded healer has recently found some expression in psychiatric literature with more practitioners being prepared to come out about their own psychiatric histories (Redfield Jamison 1995, Perkins 1999, May 2001). Mental health professionals have tended to be guarded about their psychological vulnerabilities, often with good reason, since to be open about mental health problems was to risk having doubts cast about their fitness to practise. The key issue should not be whether mental health professionals suffer emotional problems, some severe enough to be diagnosed as a mental disorder, but what they do with that vulnerability. If it is ignored and denied, then there is the danger of this distress adversely influencing the helping relationship. If it can be faced, understood and healed, then it can be a source of compassionate, empathic practice. Understanding the experience and meaning of a client's distress is likely to be enhanced by an appreciation of the nature of our own wounds and our own healing process. The concept of the wounded healer has its origins in the shamanistic traditions and beliefs of most ancient cultures. Healers were often people who had suffered, who had visited the spirit world and encountered the spirits responsible for human suffering and returned with the sacred knowledge of healing. There is for me some echo of these ancient traditions in the experience of the mental health professional who is able to discover and make judicious use of the healing from his or her own 'long day's journey into night'.

A few years ago I suffered the loss of my eldest son through suicide. He was a beautiful beanpole of a boy – intelligent, a fine artist, blessed with a wonderful sense of humour. That he came to feel so humiliated by life, drifted out of reach of the love and support of his family and friends, and in that isolation chose to end his life remains a source of great anguish. It was a desperate, grief-stricken time for myself and my family and I wondered at times how I would survive the overwhelming desolation and guilt; how I would live with the painful reality of his death; how I could continue my vocation. It is a personal tragedy that has taught me a great deal about survival, healing and recovery. For a long time after his death, I existed in that dark realm of self-loathing, recrimination and despair; preoccupied with the question of why it had happened. Healing came through the love and understanding of those family, friends and colleagues closest to me who, like Orpheus, entered my personal Hades bringing a life-affirming song. Gradually their loving support and affirmation reawoke my own compassion, acceptance and forgiveness and enabled me to reconnect with the spirit of life. It has left me, I think, with more humility about what therapeutic influence I might have; more respect for the resourcefulness and self-healing qualities that people have; and more certain that in our confusion and suffering, the empathic, affirming, transparently real presence of others 'calls to you like the wild geese, harsh and exciting – over and over announcing your place in the family of things' (from *Wild Geese* by Mary Oliver).

Acceptance as a way of being

Many people who are referred to the psychiatric services have chronically low self-esteem. This may have arisen out of an early experience of neglect, rejection or abuse. It may have its origins in the experience of conditional love in early life. This may be compounded by social impoverishment and the experience of becoming a mental patient, which reinforces doubts about self-worth and can eclipse an individual's personhood. As Barham & Hayward (1995) show in their absorbing study of the lives of people who have suffered a serious mental illness, a person's social identity can become defined by their psychiatric histories. Whatever the origins of low self-esteem, a person may seek to protect their vulnerable self in defensive behaviour.

Given a history of oppressive relationships, it is not surprising that some people may find it difficult to trust the helper and seek to maintain a distance in the relationship or to sabotage the relationship through defensive strategies. They may be withdrawn and guarded with the helper, behave unreliably, question the helper's motives, put the helper down, put themselves down as not being worth helping, behave in aggressive ways, deny, minimise or seal over their problems. When clients present in these ways, we need to try and stay aware of the hidden agenda – 'Can I really trust this person?'. Being with people in an accepting way, if it is consistent, serves the function of helping to create trust and a safe base from which they can begin to explore and make known their inner selves which relate to the world in distressed and disturbed ways. Being with people in an accepting way offers a mirror for them to begin to re-evaluate their worth.

A number of other terms have been used to describe acceptance: a non-judgemental attitude; unconditional positive regard; non-possessive warmth; respect; valuing; affirming; prizing. It is not an easy attitude to hold to. To accept some clients can feel difficult – feelings of dislike, disapproval or irritation may be around in the helper's consciousness or just below the level of awareness. This may be based on limited knowledge of the client and if we can focus on understanding the meaning of their behaviour, then any antipathy is usually dispelled and we are able to relate in a more accepting way. Where our feelings persist, it is worth asking ourselves questions such as: 'Who does this person remind me of? Does this attribute that I find so irritating also belong to me? How am I stereotyping this person? How is it that I become impatient/bored/critical/distant when I'm with this client?'. Listening openly to ourselves for an answer to these questions can bring into awareness our projections, prejudices and unacknowledged needs and fears.

Mearns and Thorne draw attention to the possibility that the institution within which helping takes place may operate as a conditional culture. The person referred to the psychiatric services may, for example, be expected to be compliant in the helping process, to accept explanations of their problem, to gratefully go along with their care programme and then be discharged. Where people do not conform to this passive role, they may get labelled non-compliant, disengaged, manipulative, over-dependent or resistant. It can be very easy in these circumstances to bend to the pressure of the institutions and become a conditional helper rather than face being seen by colleagues as naïve.

Learning to be with others in an accepting way requires us to be accepting towards ourselves. We must be willing to look at our own needs, vulnerabilities, inadequacies, failings and strengths. This can take place in a number of different learning structures that offer a safe and supportive opportunity for self-enquiry. Personal development groups, staff support groups, co-counselling, supervision or personal therapy are in my view essential elements in the training and professional development of mental health workers. This commitment to self-exploration, self-acceptance and personal growth is not narcissistic or self-indulgent. It springs from the recognition that working in a person-to-person way requires us to show the same respect for ourselves that we wish to show to clients. If we can value and appreciate ourselves, if we can acknowledge our failings and fallibilities, then we can be freer in the way we engage with others.

Empathy as a way of being

Empathic listening and responding is a core condition that contributes centrally to the therapeutic use of self. It means being able to enter the landscape of another's world, to see it, as it were, through his or her eyes. It means being sensitive to the flow of feeling we find there, to the meanings that make up this person's perception of the world. It means being able to communicate that understanding accurately.

Empathy is much more than a communication skill, although it is often taught as if it were simply that. It is a process in which we are able to put aside our own frame of reference and experience the other person's world as if it were our own. Empathy is an essential ingredient in human relations. It is the social cement that holds families, communities and societies together. To enjoy good relationships is to be empathic with others. Where individuals have discordant relationships with friends, colleagues, within their family, or with social groups, then invariably that quality of empathy is missing from their social transactions. We develop this interpersonal quality as we grow up and grow older. The toddler becomes sensitive to the moods of its parents, we identify with our friends in their joyfulness and miseries, we immerse ourselves in another's world in our most intimate relationships and as parents we become attuned to the feelings and needs of our children. The images in art, in film, in literature and music also draw from us an empathic response. At times, however, this human quality remains blocked in our interactions with others. In a professional context, it can feel safer to stay within our own frame of reference than to become involved with the client's meanings and feelings. This leads to helping that comes too much from the head and not enough from the heart – we need both.

How do we become more empathic? A useful place to start is to pay attention to the quality of our listening. Am I listening with my attention free enough to really hear, to hear not just the words but the meanings and feelings that may lie beneath them? Am I open enough with those with whom I have a working alliance to communicate what I experience as I hear their story? If I can be more in touch with my own experiences of joy and despair, anxiety and security, attachment and loss, hope and despondency, self-worth and doubt, then, paradoxically, I am likely to be more receptive to this experience in others.

We are all engaged in the same struggle of being human with all the joys and sorrows of the human condition. As Carl Rogers reminds us, the deeper we go, the more universal human experience is. This is not to say that my experience of, say, the loss of a parent, will be the same as yours. It is important to guard against the tendency to project our own experience onto others and mistake it for empathic insight. But having experienced the emotional pain of loss does give me a reference point to help me find you where you are. As Kierkegaard observed, 'If you really want to help somebody, first of all you must find him where he is and start there. This is the secret of caring' (cited in Davis & Fallowfield 1991).

Rogers considered empathy often to be an intuitive response to the experience of another person. 'There are times when I am listening to people that ideas or images surface as if from nowhere into my consciousness. I find that it is usually worth trusting your intuition enough to share these thoughts with the client.' This can be done in a tentative way: 'The thought occurred to me ...' or 'I have this picture, I'm not sure whether it will mean anything to you or throw any light on what's going on in your life at the moment'. There seem to me to be different types of knowing; cognitive knowing – a logical, analytical knowing – is the dominant form in our culture. Other forms of knowing – emotional, imaginative, intuitive knowing, which are a function of the right brain – are undervalued in Western society. Cultivating our intuitive, imaginative potential can, I believe, prove a valuable asset in the therapeutic use of self with clients.

Why is empathy so important in skilled helping? Firstly, an empathic response promotes the flow of conversation, helping people articulate what is often difficult to put into words. Secondly, it is very reassuring to be understood and accepted. People often feel isolated with their worries and concerns. There is an awful sense of alienation in the belief that nobody will understand. This leads on to the gathering sense of hopelessness and despair which underlie many acts of self-harm and suicide. Being understood gives a person a sense of having an ally. From that position they are more likely to examine honestly some of the problematic situations that confront them and work at re-evaluating themselves and aspects of their lives. When someone begins to understand and accept my experience of myself and my life, which may seem to me frightening, weak, foolish, bad, bizarre, and can communicate that understanding and acceptance to me, then I can begin to understand and accept myself. I can begin to claim some of the 'disowned' parts of myself. As Carl Rogers puts it, at its deepest level an empathic response works on the edge of the client's awareness.

As we enter the client's world and sense some of the confusion, anxiety, anger, helplessness, sadness etc. we might find there, we must try and stay aware that this feeling is theirs and not ours. It is all too easy to over-identify and take on the client's feelings. In the busy work schedule of mental health practitioners we often do not take the time to free our attention from the client's distress and may carry it into our next contact or into our off duty time. Debriefing with a colleague after an intense session, using this as an opportunity for reflective processing; writing up an account of the session, as it were capturing the feelings in words and transferring them to the page; and of course regular supervision; all play a part in giving us temporary closure in our work with a client and help us manage the emotional burden of the work. Of course sometimes the client's experiences may touch the raw edge of an unhealed personal wound and remind us that we have our own healing journey to complete.

Breggin (1997) puts empathy at the heart of creating a healing presence:

> To create healing presence, we fine tune our inner experience to the inner state of the other person. We transform ourselves in response to the basic needs of the person we are trying to help. Ultimately we find within ourselves the psychological and spiritual resources required to nourish and empower the other human being. (p. 5)

An intuitive way of being

In a fascinating study of intuition in psychotherapeutic practice, Rachel Charles describes how the ascendancy of logic and reason has left intuition in a subordinate position to the extent that it has been largely disregarded by psychologists and psychotherapists. This seems extraordinary, given that intuition 'can be pivotal in understanding human dilemmas and in helping solve life's problems' (Charles 2004).

The mental health professions, in pursuit of professional credibility in an age of evidence-based practice, have largely turned their backs on intuitive care. Reflecting on my own work, I recollect many occasions when I now wish I had trusted my intuition rather than cognitive appraisal as a basis for my response. I recall with lingering sadness and regret a talented man who hanged himself on a local heath, having spoken with me at length 2 days before. I knew subjectively that all was not well, but by all objective criteria he appeared to be progressing in his recovery from a severe depression. There was a mild euphoric sense to his manner that I interpreted as the joy of having come through, but which I see now as the gladness of a mind resolved to seek the ultimate end to his suffering.

What is it that creates within us this state of knowingness that seems to arrive unheralded and complete in our consciousness? The experience of not knowing how we know, we just know! Intuition is not the same as empathy although they are related attributes. Empathy is an attunement to the experience of another person, often although not exclusively at an emotional level. There is an element of resonance with the other person's experience and we get a palpable impression of what that lived experience is like. Empathic attunement is a vital element in social cohesion – we could not relate to each other with consideration and compassion were it not for our capacity to transpose ourselves into another's world. It is a facet of human relating that allows us to feel deeply connected to each other and is an antidote to alienation. Often empathic understanding has to be consciously worked at. We seek to understand an experience and its meaning through a reflective conversation, gradually finding our way into another's lived experience. At its deepest level it feels like a merging of one's consciousness with that of another, yet never losing that sense of separateness. By comparison, intuition seems to appear in our minds in the form of connections, thoughts, feelings, images or felt senses which are not the product of any conscious rational process.

Intuition has a valid place in the care process. We should not be shy of drawing on images, feelings, words, phrases, ideas and felt senses that surface unbidden in our consciousness in relation to people we are working with. Such intuition can provide helpful insights into a person's distress and problems in living. It can guide the flow and substance of the interaction and, used judiciously, can help deepen the relationship. Intuition seems to be a subliminal response to non-verbal cues, to the said and the unsaid, to the context of a person's life. It stirs our imagination and memory. It reverberates in our unconscious and offers up its wisdom. Sometimes we need to allow ourselves to be confused, to be content not to know what to say or do. If we wait expectantly, a way forward will usually emerge from the creative unconscious. Of course our intuition can be wrong and it is easy to overstate the case for the superiority of its insights and solutions. It seems wise to subject our intuitive inclinations to cognitive scrutiny, to check out the validity and appropriateness of our understanding and proposed actions. But being alive to our intuitive powers and cultivating them can lead to a more creative way of being and relating.

Not only should we be alive to this intuitive function within ourselves but we should seek to cultivate it in the people who seek our help on their recovery journeys. Many people recognise that still small voice inside which if we would only listen to it would act as a guide in life choices. Over the past few years I have worked with a gifted young man recovering from what one might describe as extraordinary, sometimes overwhelming, states of consciousness that have had a disruptive impact on his life. A significant part of the healing process for him has been to intuitively seek an inner source of wisdom for an understanding of his perplexing experiences and as a guide to his recovery. The source has become personified in his mind as a beneficent entity that he is able to contact at will through automatic writing. Reading some of this remarkable script, I have been struck by the loving-kindness, insightfulness and pragmatism of this inner voice – a voice that he has now come to trust and value. I suspect this phenomenon is a manifestation of the archetype of great wisdom and of great love that resides in us all and his breakdown has enabled him to receive a great gift that could be an inspiring and sustaining facet of his life.

So how do we begin to develop our intuition? Firstly we need to challenge the prevailing belief that intuition is anathema to the rational mind. We should not mystify it, but recognise it for what it is: a coalescence of impressions, thoughts, images, feelings and felt senses, mostly perceived subliminally, stirred in our imagination and memory and synthesised into a meaningful whole, in which form it reaches consciousness. It is a valid source of knowledge about ourselves and our world and is the wellspring of creative living. We must free ourselves from the dogma that abounds in psychiatry to create sufficient space for intuition to flourish. If we cling to an established view, we are unlikely to be open to intuitive insights which challenge an 'existing truth'. Although it takes courage in the scientifically oriented culture of psychiatric medicine, I believe we should bring more of our intuitive self into client work, clinical reviews and supervision. Often when I meet with clients, we will start with a 5-minute meditation. I find that this helps clear the mind, allows us to become more attuned to each other and to be open to any intuitive thoughts, feelings, images that present themselves to be worked with.

The neglected core conditions

In his seminal work Carl Rogers described six core conditions necessary for growth and change. The relational qualities we have described above – genuineness, acceptance and empathy – have been the subject of a vast amount of exposition, while the other three conditions have been somewhat neglected. These are:

- the incongruence and anxiety of the client
- psychological contact or engagement
- the client's perception, at least to a minimal degree, of the practitioner's genuineness, acceptance and empathy.

These are vitally important aspects of therapeutic work in the arena of mental health care. Many people find it hard to engage with psychiatric services or, more pertinently, psychiatric services with them. The reasons are not difficult to understand. Firstly, many people have had negative experiences of mental health services. They may have experienced traumatic admissions, been over-medicated, subject to physical restraint and/or seclusion, detained compulsorily, been exposed to dehumanising, disempowering psychiatric interviews and mystifying, stigmatising diagnoses – why wouldn't they want to disengage from services and maintain a physical and psychological distance from mental health workers?

Secondly, many people find their turbulent inner worlds too threatening and potentially overwhelming to encounter. They close down protectively and employ what has been described by Tait et al (2003) as a sealed-over way of coping. This guarded, enclosed way of being can make it difficult to feel that any real psychological contact has been made; conversation may be kept to a minimum and diverted away from any discussion of their inner process. So much of a person's energy and attention goes into maintaining this survival strategy. To engage more fully in life and to be more open to relationships is to risk exposing and facing distress-filled experiences from the dark corners of the psyche. In one client I have come to know this guardedness and reticence about the emotional traumas that have shaped her life were reflected in the content of her abusive, defamatory voices which repeatedly warned her against talking to anybody about them.

Another client, a young man I have worked with for some time, seems to exemplify this sealed-off way of being. It is difficult to move beyond superficial, emotionally neutral conversation and any attempt to engage at a deeper level is met with evasion. His most poignant and revealing communications are through his body language – deep sighs, alarmed looks, displaced tension, moments of distraction, hurriedness, overdressing – all of which speak of anxiety leaking from his sealed-off inner world. Beyond all this fearfulness and the psychological sanctuary/prison he has created for himself I have an intuitive image of a warm, funny, artistic, intelligent young man. I think his breakdown cast him into a bleak and paranoid landscape which was so frightening that to risk returning there to learn and grow from that experience is daunting. Yet I feel he will make that journey. Reflecting back to him some of his bodily expressions takes us on short excursions into that inner world. It is a beginning!

Thirdly, it seems to me that a lack of psychological contact can simply derive from interaction between a client and mental health practitioners becoming routinised and from the client's viewpoint just not worth the effort. There is the same focus on the presentation of symptoms, the same preoccupation with medication compliance. Little attempt is made to attune to the individual's personal world and to understand the survival meaning in their presentation of self in everyday life. Miller (2000) argues strongly for *personal consciousness integration* to be at the hub of therapeutic conversations. She argues that non-ordinary states of consciousness are widely experienced and potentially growth-enhancing. They become problematic and labelled psychotic when externalised, projected and acted on indiscriminately, precipitating a state of confusion and conflict between the person's inner world and consensual reality. As Miller says:

> Most recipients of psychiatric rehabilitation services cease to discuss their non ordinary experiences with professionals; they have learned that the most profound and challenging experiences of their lives are ignored and labelled psychopathology by the mental health system. When they express anxiety about these experiences typically their medication is increased. (Miller 2000, p. 346)

Instead of seeking to provide emotional containment to clients in their troubled, dissonant states of mind; instead of trying to help them make sense of their unquiet mind, we suppress emotional discomfort with powerful drugs which further disconnect people from the source of their distress. It is this incongruence – the unawareness of the flow of experience within – that leads to distress leaking out or exploding out in discordant, dysfunctional behaviour. After a while people seek more medication or different medication in response to an increase in their emotional discomfort and are driven to seek refuge in a life circumscribed by their fearfulness.

In such circumstances it can be enormously difficult to enter this defended, drug-suffused world, yet I find that if I can accept it as an affectively charged part of a person's phenomenal world, an experience that has significant meaning for them, without disregarding, devaluing or pathologising the experience, then a window of opportunity will often present itself for a reflective dialogue on those experiences. Such *islands of clarity* may be brief initially but to be in real, empathic, non-judgemental contact with another person helps anchor the client in consensual reality and shines the light of rationality on what may be frightening and confusing experiences. One person with whom I have had some involvement typically engages in delightful reality-based conversation which will then quite suddenly, as the result of some internal stimulus, enter another dimension of thought resulting in the dialogue becoming distinctly surreal. Stories of seduction and rape by celebrities who seem to populate her world are disclosed and the conversation usually ends with an angry tirade displaced onto whoever happens to be present. It is like being cast in a psychodrama.

Mae's story

Theme: realness, warm regard and empathy in helping relationships

Mae is a 47-year-old woman who has been a service user since her mid-twenties, when she was diagnosed as suffering from a manic-depressive disorder. It is her lows that are most disabling and distressing and she has made three suicide attempts to end what she describes as the 'numbing misery' of her episodes of depression. Although there is no clear cyclical pattern to Mae's disorder, the worst episodes have tended to occur during the spring. She has always resisted a diagnostic label and has been a reluctant though mostly compliant self-medicator.

Mae recognises two selves: her 'dull grey self', which seems dominant and recurrent, and her 'coloured vibrant self', which emerges briefly and usually as a prelude to a depressive swing. She does not understand why her dull grey self should have such a grip on her life. It seems to Mae that if these two parts of herself could merge, her personality would have more balance.

Mae's personal and family history is that she is the daughter of a white English mother and a black Afro-American father. Her parents never married and she was adopted shortly after her birth. She grew up in a white middle class family with her two brothers by adoption. She remembers her childhood as unremarkable yet one in which she always felt her parents' love and approval was conditional on her meeting their expectations and standards; as she grew older, this led to frequent arguments and a gradual distancing in their relationship. This was compounded when at 16 she became pregnant and her parents arranged for her to have an abortion. Mae believes that this confirmed for her parents that they had 'taken on a wild child' who 'wasn't the daughter they had in mind'. Mae carries an emotional legacy from that period in her life which hasn't been fully resolved and seems to trouble her increasingly as she moves through her middle years, childless and not in a permanent relationship.

Mae's CPN, Gloria, has been involved with her and her care for the last 3 years. Their relationship began with the development of a working alliance in which the goals included helping Mae to recognise and manage her depressive thoughts, feelings and behaviour more effectively and to contract with her some strategies for maintaining her safety when suicidal ideas became too intrusive. The relationship now seems to have deepened in a way that seems helpful and respectful to Mae and more involving and satisfying to Gloria. She feels her relationship with Mae is more like a friendship, though both recognise that they are meeting in a professional context and that it is Mae's issues, feelings and needs that are the focus of their interaction. Recently they have talked a lot about what it means to be childless and the emptiness and loss Mae has expressed resonated for Gloria with her own experience of being a surviving twin, an only and lonely child. Drawing on this emotional experience she is able to relate in an empathic way to Mae's story.

Gloria's experience as a black British Afro-Caribbean woman raised Mae's consciousness of her own black identity and helped her identify with the richness of black American culture. There seemed to be an important association, for Mae, between this largely unacknowledged part of her identity and the 'coloured vibrant self' that emerged during her 'highs'. Mae talked about a deeply held but seldom expressed fear that she had been 'given up' because she was black. She talked about her unknown father in idealised terms and reconnected with painful feelings of hurt and anger towards her birth mother which had been intensified by having to 'give up' her own child.

The warm regard and realness of Gloria's relationship with Mae is helping her gradually to 'feel at home with herself'.

The ethics of involvement

The person-to-person relationship requires involvement. This raises some interesting and important questions. How can I have an authentic relationship with someone that I am paid to engage with and perhaps would not choose to spend time with socially if the context were different? How is it possible to draw boundaries between this type of relationship and a friendship? What constitutes over-involvement? What if clients become attached to me? What if I become attracted to the client sexually and what if they become attracted to me? How can I end a person-to-person relationship?

Perhaps the key to all these questions is honesty and openness. Yes, I am paid to engage with the person in my care but that doesn't mean that my interest and care has to be any less genuine. Yes, it is a role but it is a role that is infused with myself to the extent that it becomes the role of no role. I want to be with a person in need in a real or authentic way that earns their trust. If I reveal so little of myself in my helping relationships that people do not experience me as a person, there is little on which to build a trusting relationship. To engage in a way that is emotionally distant seems to me to dehumanise the relationship, and care then becomes a mechanical act.

I want to relate to people in a fully human way and that means bringing along my feelings. It means that I will like and feel a great deal of affection for some people and at the other end of the continuum, will at times feel antipathy towards others. It means that I will often be deeply affected by the painful struggles and adversities that people face. It means that I will at times feel angry at the behaviour people exhibit or at the social injustice and oppression that they experience. It means that I will at times feel anxious when faced with the distress and disturbance the client brings and experience a sense of powerlessness when faced with the complexity of a client's problem. It means that at times I will feel sexually attracted to the clients that I work with.

It does not mean that we have to express or act on the feelings that surface in our consciousness. Often there are good reasons why we should not. Firstly, clients do not want the burden of our feelings, the responsibility for meeting our needs. They need to feel that we will be able to contain their distress and that the problems and needs they bring are paramount. Secondly, people who seek help from the psychiatric services are often very vulnerable, both emotionally and socially, to insensitivity and exploitation. There is a power imbalance in helping relationships that creates opportunities for unethical practitioners to exploit people using the service, materially, emotionally and sexually.

All professions working in the mental health arena have codes of professional conduct that offer clear guidelines for working with vulnerable clients. All underline that sexual relationships between practitioners and clients will almost certainly be a breach of the code of professional conduct, be subject to disciplinary action and may constitute a legal offence under the Mental Health Act. They caution practitioners against using their power and influence with clients to meet their own needs or to benefit financially or materially and question 'whether it is ever appropriate to have anything other than a purely professional relationship with the client' (UKCC 1998, 1999).

These rules governing the conduct of professional relationships which are by nature intimate are sensible. Boundaries must be set for the protection of both clients and practitioners. But in a caring culture that aims to normalise and 'de-professionalise' helping, the line between what is justified therapeutically and what is ethically questionable is thinly drawn. Is all affectionate physical contact taboo? Is socialising with a client outside working hours always unacceptable? Is a client's attachment to a helper necessarily undesirable? Should a client's sexual attraction to a key worker or a practitioner's sexual attraction to a client be seen as impropriety? Is friendship never permissible? Many clients appreciate a practitioner's willingness to engage in a relationship that has the qualities of friendship. What is valued is the ordinariness of these relationships in which the client is not exhausted by the helper's desire to help but are anchored in reality and normality by ordinary companionship. As Ram Dass & Gorman (1989) put it, 'The more you think of yourself as a therapist, the more pressure there is on someone to be a patient'. In my view it is possible and often desirable in long-term contact to bring the qualities of friendship to the helping relationship without losing our discipline and integrity. What turns a committed helping relationship into an 'over-involved' and potentially unethical relationship is the intrusion of the helper's needs and feelings, in a way that skews the relationship towards dealing more with these needs and feelings than with those of the client.

Overall the problem is more one of under-involvement than over-involvement. Often mental health professionals – lacking an emotionally sustaining work environment – relate in routine, institutionalised ways with clients, ways which lack the humanity, vibrancy and spirit of a person-centred approach. Knowing as I do the compassionate nature of most people who enter the mental health professions, this detachment from clients can only be seen as a defensive strategy against the anxiety of bringing one's self into the work with all our fallibilities and vulnerabilities, recognising that the distance between ourselves and our clients is but a small step. We function professionally in an incongruent way, unaware or only dimly aware of the flow of feeling and thought within us. Such a detached interpersonal style leads only to superficial relating which is unlikely to facilitate growth and healing for either the client or practitioner.

The ethics of sexuality

As Gallop (1998) observes, sexuality in the context of helping relationships can be particularly difficult if it is not dealt with openly. If it is ignored or denied, either at an individual or at a team level, and not acknowledged as a commonly occurring dynamic in helping relationships, it increases the risk of practitioners being exposed to compromising situations and of clients being sexually exploited and their trust betrayed. If a client's sexual attraction to a practitioner is treated in a censorious way, they can feel humiliated and guilty. If the practitioner reacts by becoming more distant, the client can feel rejected. These issues need to be brought to supervision and other appropriate staff forums and discussed openly and respectfully, acknowledging the anxiety and uncertainty they can create. This is unlikely to happen if there is gender stereotyping in which male staff are exposed to accusations of predatory sexual behaviour with little recognition that female clients sometimes use their sexuality to seduce and entrap staff. Female staff too may be given little support in dealing with the sexual attentions of a client, the implication being that they are to blame for getting over-involved with clients and leading them on.

Gallop observes that over-involvement may sometimes reflect both the practitioner's and the client's unmet need to feel 'special', which creates a dynamic for symbiotic relationships that are potentially exploitative. Staff may harbour rescuing fantasies believing that they, through their special relationship with the client, can save them from destructive behaviour patterns. Clients may respond to this attention by feeding the practitioner's fantasy that they alone have made a difference. Relationships in which this dynamic is active run a great risk of transgressing professional boundaries as the client's emotional demands on the practitioner increase. Occasionally staff may use power coercively to exploit clients sexually, sometimes seeing this as a legitimate development of their therapeutic work. Others may use power in a more paternalistic but nonetheless damaging way that fosters an emotional attachment leading to a sexual involvement.

Sexuality is part of normal human interaction. Attraction and playful flirtation is an enjoyable element in many social transactions. For some clients, the owning and expression of their sexuality is part of the recovery process and it would be surprising if professional carers were not at times a focus for that sexual interest, given the intimate and caring nature of the relationship. But social signals can easily be misinterpreted, particularly where a client is socially isolated or has a pressing unmet need to feel special and for a loving, sexually consummated relationship. In such a scenario the warmth of a helper's interest and care may be taken as a cue that they are willing to enter into such a relationship. Unfortunately this often ends with advances being rejected and the hurt and angry client making formal complaints of sexual harassment or abuse against the mental health worker. There is a need for us as helpers to be more aware and proactive in reasserting our boundaries and to work through the resulting issues and feelings in an open and supportive way with the client before this degree of emotional investment and sexual interest takes hold.

There can, as we have seen in the previous chapter, be a transferential element to feelings of love and attraction to a professional helper, who becomes the nurturing, protective parent or attentive lover, with whom the client seeks to satisfy unmet attachment needs. However, it would be unhelpful to interpret all transactions between staff and clients in which an emotional and sexual attachment develops as the past in the present. In ongoing caring relationships in which there is often a social as well as a therapeutic dimension Eros is bound to enter the interplay sometimes. Where this attraction is reciprocal, it can be impossible for a practitioner to ensure professional boundaries are not transgressed and it is unrealistic to expect them to continue working with the client.

Rebecca's story

Theme: over-involvement in practitioner–client relationships

Rebecca is a recently qualified staff nurse working in an acute admission assessment unit. She is a primary nurse for a group of six clients. She has found herself thinking more and more about Liam, a 27-year-old man with a history of depression and alcoholism, who is in her client group. She has had a lot of therapeutic contact with Liam over the past few weeks and enjoys his mildly flirtatious, humorous conversation and his appreciation of her as a nurse. They have met a few times in the hospital cafeteria for a coffee after Rebecca's shift has ended and she has occasionally been shopping for him, things she would not normally agree to do. Gradually their conversations have become more reciprocal, with Rebecca sharing personal information and talking about a recently ended relationship.

A friend and colleague, recognising Rebecca's over-involvement, mentioned it to her, only to be met with resentful annoyance at her intrusion and Rebecca's insistence that she was quite capable of managing her relationships with clients. The matter was not reported to a senior member of the team and neither did Rebecca bring the issue up in supervision. She felt that Liam was benefiting therapeutically from their relationship and that she could help him transcend his depressive personality and destructive drinking. During one of their conversations Liam asks her if it would be all right for him to contact her socially when he is discharged. He tells her that he feels considerably stronger emotionally as a consequence of her help but worries how he will cope when he leaves the unit and no longer has her support.

Following his discharge they meet socially and soon begin dating. After 3 months they move into a flat together. It is not long before Liam is drinking again and their relationship is in crisis. There are frequent angry exchanges in which he accuses Rebecca of never being off duty, of analysing him and trying to run his life for him. Rebecca decides the relationship is over after he accuses her of seeing other men and attempts to rape her. Three weeks later Liam is readmitted following an overdose taken after several weeks of heavy drinking. Rebecca has no alternative but to report her relationship with Liam to her clinical team leader who arranges for Rebecca to be transferred to another unit. She is required to attend a disciplinary interview at which she agrees to seek counselling and to make the management of boundaries a focus of her supervision.

The spiritual dimension of therapeutic care

19

The meaning of spirituality and the nature of spiritual care are probably two of the most important yet largely ignored themes to emerge in the context of mental health care as we move into the 21st century. Nolan & Crawford (1997) argue that, in the quest for empirical respectability and a scientific knowledge base, we have become disconnected from mental health care's deepest roots: the spiritual care of those experiencing disabling distress.

Mental health professions claim to take a holistic view of patient care, yet training and practice rarely go beyond the physical and psychosocial to include the spiritual (Dyson et al 1997). There is a hesitancy and discomfort about engaging people in a consideration of their spiritual needs. This is not surprising as there is a widespread assumption that spirituality and religion are the same and that spirituality is therefore the domain of the chaplain or leaders of the patient's faith community. We need to recognise that organised religion provides just one (albeit important) way of connecting with and expressing spirituality.

The spiritual realm of experience may be difficult for service users to talk about precisely because they are unsure of how it will be received. There is a fear that it will be disregarded or worse pathologised. As one respondent to a survey put it, 'To invalidate a person's spirituality no matter how distorted it is, is to invalidate the real core sense of self and I think you then risk doing untold damage to somebody' (Mental Health Foundation 2002). Many people have extraordinary experiences of consciousness that they interpret in a spiritual way, whether occurring in the context of a psychological crisis or not. These deeply felt experiences may take the form of voices guiding or calming; thought insertion of a benign nature; the sense of a benevolent presence; 'showings' of a revelatory nature; or affective experiences in which a person feels enveloping moments of security and peace, of joy, of new strength, of love, of hope and optimism. Such experiences may be transitory but they remain vividly in the memory and can have a transformative effect on an individual's life. Romme & Escher (1993, 2000), in their groundbreaking work on voice hearing, point to many examples of individuals both with and without psychiatric histories who experience their voices in a mystical or spiritual way and for whom orthodox psychiatric interpretations just do not ring true. What is important in relation to these psycho-spiritual experiences is how they are understood, coped with and integrated into an individual's life, a process that is aided by being able to confide openly with others who are accepting and appropriately responsive. Research by Macmin & Foskett (2004) into the spiritual and religious experience of mental health service users concluded that when people are fully heard and their spiritual life acknowledged:

> Their own spiritual resources began to emerge and their breakdowns were more likely to become breakthroughs. They encountered parts of themselves which they did not know existed and which helped them make sense of their crisis. They spoke of the power of humour, healing, blessing, inspiration, prayer, compassion, salvation, faith, inner change and the value of sacred places and spaces in their recovery.

Spiritual care

What is spiritual care? In a review of the literature Dyson et al (1997) identify a strong relational theme in spirituality: how I relate to myself; how I relate to others and the animate world; how I relate to God; and the interconnectedness of those three elements.

Relationship to self

The first of these, how I relate to myself, is concerned with the question of loving myself. Can I have regard for myself, care for myself? Can I recognise my essential goodness, despite all my flaws and failings? The dogma of Christianity, like psychiatry, has tended to have an unhelpful bias towards a view of humankind as essentially flawed and sinful. In the case of the Church people are seen as having fallen from grace, and in psychiatry, which embraces a psychoanalytic perspective, people are seen as driven by the promptings of the id to behave, in fantasy or reality, in self-gratifying ways. In both cases the basic conception of humankind is one of moral weakness, which requires on the one hand absolution and on the other treatment. What is so badly missing in the mainstream Christian Church and in psychiatry is a belief in the essential goodness of people. Self-denigration and a pervasive sense of unworthiness occur frequently in the stories of people in distress and it is as much through an experience of loving kindness as through psychological interventions that people come to prize themselves more.

Relationship to others

If we reflect a little on the second of Dyson's observations about the relational nature of spirituality – how I relate to others – there can be no doubt that some people, both high profile figures and many, many ordinary individuals, relate to others in their work and everyday lives in a way that is infused with spirituality. They engage with people in a way that transcends the potential barriers of mental illness, disability, culture, ethnicity, class, education and poverty, and communicate understanding, a warm acceptance and compassion. There is a similarity here to the unconditional positive regard that Carl Rogers describes as one of the core conditions for facilitating growth and change. Although Rogers spoke out against institutional religion, towards the end of his life he made reference to a spiritual dimension in helping relationships. He describes moments in his therapeutic work when 'my own inner spirit has reached out and touched the inner spirit of other. Our relationship transcends itself and becomes part of something larger' (Rogers 1986a).

In his account of Rogers' life and work, Thorne (1992) refers to a spiritual awakening that for some people seems to occur in person-centred therapy. He concludes that in the process of self-actualisation we may discover at our deepest centre the human spirit which is open and transcendent, a discovery that launches us on a spiritual journey and changes our way of being in the world.

The experience of severe mental health problems can cut a person loose from their moorings. They feel adrift in unfamiliar oceans, in search of landmarks, alienated from others. It can seem, at times, as if the person is lost in chaotic seas of madness. To care well for someone suffering from a troubled mind and disabling distress is in some way to share their experience, to enter their chaotic world as if it was our own, but without losing the capacity to return to our own moorings. Relating empathetically, Rogers contends, is one of the most powerful elements in the healing process because 'it brings even the most frightened, [disturbed and chaotic] client back into the human race. If a person can be understood, he or she belongs' (Rogers 1986a). Such compassionate understanding and acceptance is at the heart of spiritual care.

Similarly Breggin (1996), writing about the psycho-spiritual care of deeply disturbed people, emphasises the importance of the principles of love and liberty in the caring relationship. He argues that healing is facilitated through loving relationships, in which there is a 'treasuring of others that is reverent, caring and empathic', and by nurturing and respecting self-determination. If we can find within ourselves the psychological and spiritual resources to nourish and empower others, essentially an attitude of loving kindness, we are able to create a healing presence (Breggin 1997). He goes further in suggesting that at times people, like places, can seem enveloped in an aura that nourishes, heals and inspires. If we were to ascribe a Christian interpretation to such phenomena we might attribute it to God's presence, seeing it perhaps as a manifestation of Christ's message 'where two or more are gathered together in my name, there I am'. But it does not require a belief in mystical realities to recognise that at times we connect with people at a relational depth in which what is strengthening and healing evolves in a place beyond words at a transpersonal level.

Inglesby (1998) suggests that the use of a spiritual/religious lens can help make sense of madness. Religious imagery can be seen as a metaphor that bridges the chasm between ordinary experience and the unintelligible world of experiences we term psychotic. She argues that mental anguish can be seen as part of a journey of redemption and renewal. For many people, the experience of becoming deeply depressed or lost in the chaos of a psychotic experience can be like a descent into a personal hell. Yet it is a place from which renewal is possible. The hope is in the energy and movement that is locked into anguish and turmoil; as Nietzsche said, 'Only out of chaos may there be born a dancing star'(cited in Inglesby 1998). The hope is also in the willingness of mental health workers, family and friends to witness and validate the experience of suffering and to provide companionship to that person on their journey in search of 'the truth that heals'. It is difficult to return alone and alienation can lead to despair and annihilation of the self. The return to a way of being in the world that is different from before, that suffuses life with meaning and a deep sense that 'all will be well', is a recovery pathway. What is recovered is a stronger sense of identity and a more authentic and soulful way of being. This is in contrast to a rehabilitation pathway which aims to return people as near as possible to the point from which their descent into turmoil began. As Inglesby puts it, 'the descent may have been necessary to find a path out into the light'.

We need also to consider here our relationship with nature, with the animate earth that sustains us. Traditional Western Christian teaching supports the notion of the supremacy of humankind over nature and as a result we have become dislocated from the natural world, losing our sense of respect and reverence for this biosphere, the earth. In denial about the perilous circumstances of our species we adopt an attitude of blind faith in the innovation of science to find solutions to the damage we continue to inflict on our world to satisfy our rapacious, materialistic, hedonistic lifestyles. Eco-psychology draws our attention to the relationship between our estrangement from nature and the level of dis-ease we experience, reflected in the increasing incidence of mental health problems (Roszak et al 1995). In damaging the world we are damaging ourselves. Man did not weave the web of life, he is merely a strand in it. We have to reconnect with the benevolence and beauty of nature – it is only through a reunion and communion with nature that we will heal the world and ourselves.

As the 19th century nature poet John Clare wrote during his long incarceration in Northampton Asylum:

> Poets love nature like the calm of heaven
> Her gifts like heaven's love spread far and wide
> In all her works there are no signs of leaven
> Sorrow abases from her simple pride
> Her flowers like pleasures have their season's birth
> And bloom through regions here below
> They are the very scriptures upon the earth
> And teach us simple mirth where'er we go
> Even in prison they can solace me
> For where they bloom God is and I am free.

Relationship to God

The third theme to be considered is our relationship with God. While many people will seek God and express their spirituality through one of the world religions, others seek spiritual nourishment and begin their journey to their spiritual centre through psycho-spiritual counselling, through the practice of meditation or yoga, through art, music and poetry, or through a reverence of nature. Perhaps what it means to be in communion with God is to be in touch with a benign power that exists within us all, that allows us to see more clearly, feel more deeply and know more surely. For many this power signifies a divine presence in our lives; for some it is experienced as a life-affirming force, a universal pulse of nature that connects us deeply to the animate world; for others it is enough simply to accept that our lives relate in some unfathomable way to a universal mystery.

The person struggling with psychological disabilities is often dispirited and demoralised. We intuitively know, though this is seldom acknowledged in the professionalised arena of mental health care, that the recovery of the spirit is necessary to the recovery of wellbeing. The power of the arts and nature to restore the spirit and aid the recovery process has long been recognised. The enlightened care provided for the mentally ill at The Retreat, York, in the late 1700s included gardening, art and music. Yet in modern times these important sources of psycho-spiritual healing are available to the few rather than the many. There have been several imaginative schemes to bring the arts into places of healing which are so often soulless buildings (Senior & Croal 1993). The use of poems in public settings such as *Poems on the Underground* is an example of the way in which spiritual nourishment can be brought into everyday lives. *Start*, an inspiring creative arts programme for mental health service users in Manchester, offers courses in painting, ceramics, textiles, photography and horticulture that have proved central to the recovery of many people (Teall 2003, Teall et al 2005). In Ipswich *Inside Out* run a programme of arts workshops for people with severe and enduring psychological problems that has as its central philosophy a 'belief in the creative process to strengthen the spirit'. The programme includes a wide spectrum of the arts – singing, painting, sculpture, photography, creative writing, drama, dance and drumming – led by local artists (www.insideoutcommunity.com). The creative process engages people at all levels – cognitively, emotionally, physically, spiritually, imaginatively and intuitively. It energises, awakens, and enables people to live their lives more vibrantly, creatively and spiritually.

Throughout history people have sought solitude and silence as a source of healing, to commune with nature, to know themselves, to paint or write, or to come closer to God. Some of the most inspiring spiritual vision has come from people who have chosen a life of solitude. As Thomas Merton said, 'It is in silence, not in commotion, in solitude and not in crowds that God best likes to reveal Himself most intimately to men' (cited in Lane 2006). In the noise-infested frenetic nature of contemporary life we seem to have lost sight of the value of stillness, quietude, solitude and have come to fear it and avoid it. There is a fear of boredom; our capacity to open our senses, intuition and imagination to unfilled moments has become dull. We find it hard to tolerate the personal demons and the essential aloneness of our existence that may surface into consciousness in the space created by silence. Yet we know in the depths of our being that the presence of quiet spaces in our lives allows the soul to breathe so that we may replenish our energy and restore our spirit.

Storr (1988), in discussing the value and significance of solitude, argues that the capacity to be alone is linked with a sense of a personal life; with self-realisation, with becoming aware of our deepest needs, feelings and impulses. He goes further in suggesting that these moments of inviolate solitude are sacred; they are encapsulated moments of communion with God whether we pray or not, whether we believe or not. For most people a monastic way of being is not desirable or possible. We need the stimulus and joy of interpersonal living, but there can be little doubt that opportunities for solitude and silence need to punctuate our lives in order for us to sustain wellbeing; just as punctuation brings meaning to the written page so silence brings meaning to the experience of our unfolding lives.

The troubled and turbulent mind craves peace and order but there is little chance of finding this in our acute wards which are often places of bedlam, or populated by dull-eyed individuals in a state of drug-induced tranquillity. There is a great need for sanctuaries of silence and stillness within our healing environments where people can contemplate, rest and restore themselves. Even in the therapeutic conversation we are often too quick to interrupt a silence with some interjection when a person is deep within a profound and healing silence. It is in the companionable silence of a therapeutic space that people encounter themselves and begin their recovery journey. In my own practice, with the client's agreement, I like to begin each therapeutic conversation with a few minutes of meditative silence. It is time which allows us both to be fully present, to gather ourselves for the task, to attune to each other. I sometimes find that in those few silent moments I connect to a flow of loving kindness that infuses the ensuing interaction. I cannot pretend that this is always present in my professional life, though I strive through spiritual practice to open myself more freely to its presence.

The term asylum means refuge, a place where a person can escape the problems of living that threaten their sanity and survival and find a haven of peace and safety in which to recover. The parkland in which mental hospitals were once set provided nourishment for the soul. Some years ago a man I came to know, who from time to time became lost in a psychotic world, was allowed to camp in the woods on the hospital estate during his periods of hospitalisation. The solitude and closeness to nature seemed to soothe his turbulent persecuted mind, rooting him in reality and restoring his equilibrium far more effectively than antipsychotic medication. He claimed that it was 'communion with the spirit of nature' that cured him. His strong attunement to the natural world made him responsive to its moods – the new vibrancy of spring, the glory of summer, the mellowness of autumn, the still inwardness of winter – to such an extent that he was forced to abandon his urban life and seek sanctuary and sanity in a remote, self-sufficient rural life, where he could live in harmony with the cycles of nature.

There is often an unnamed absence in people's life that cannot be made good by a materialistic, hedonistic lifestyle. Erich Fromm (1993), in his analysis of Western culture in the 20th century, describes a society dominated by the acquisitive motive: we must have success, status, money, qualifications, a bigger house, a better car, material possessions, a husband/wife, children, sources of entertainment. These have become the benchmarks of our worth, from which our sense of self-esteem and the esteem of others is largely derived, with the result that we look for fulfilment from what we have. They may give us some transitory pleasure but they do little to nourish the spirit and maintain our sense of wellbeing. Fromm argues that there is a moral imperative for turning from this 'having mode' and embracing a lifestyle that places more value on what he refers to as the 'being mode', which is concerned with finding ways of being at peace with oneself, with others, and with the world. It is about caring compassionately for others, for the world and for ourselves.

When we are being truly human, we are able to recognise the divine in others and in the world and have a greater awareness of the interconnectedness of all things.

In many large urban areas, faith communities – be they Muslim, Sikh, Hindu, Buddhist, or the many denominations of the Christian Church – provide a stronger sense of community and personal identity than any other neighbourhood groups (Copsey 1997). Religious and spiritual beliefs are profoundly important to many people with mental health problems (Mental Health Foundation 2000, 2002). They provide a source of support and comfort and add a powerful sense of meaning to people's lives. Copsey argues that there is a need for mental health professionals to engage in a dialogue with local faith communities in multi-faith areas in an open way without expecting them to take a Western world view of mental health problems, which largely excludes the spiritual dimension of people's lives. Rationalistic, secular beliefs about health and wellbeing may be difficult to reconcile with the teaching of world religions that put living an ethical life as a central theme in the avoidance of suffering. There is a need for mental health professionals to develop a greater sensitivity to the beliefs and practices of clients. The problems of living that people present with, the confused and painful experience they are troubled by, must be seen in the context of cultural and religious beliefs.

If care in the community is to mean more than professionalised care, faith communities that are central to the lives of many service users must be encouraged to become involved in providing help and support and to develop a more informed understanding of mental health problems. For while religion and membership of a faith community is a nourishing experience for most people, for some it can be damaging. Religious doctrine and the attitude of some faith communities have at times left people feeling a sense of blame and failure for having psychiatric problems. Others have felt rejected by their faith communities at a time when inclusion, warmth and support were most needed.

If we are going to work in an authentically holistic way, to include the spiritual, we must recognise our own need and take steps along the path of our own spiritual development. In postmodern Britain there is a growing recognition that all kinds of dogmatism are flawed. Science, whether physical, biological or behavioural, does not offer absolute truths about the meaning and experience of being human and in a largely secular society neither does organised religion. Yet the need for one's life to have meaning and purpose remains as strong as ever. Finding answers to the question of what invests our lives with those qualities is part of the quest for a more spiritual life. Often that need surfaces and becomes more compelling at times of crisis. For others a spiritual journey is prompted by a nagging sense of dissatisfaction and incompleteness.

Self-enquiry box

There are a number of guided visualisations and meditation exercises that are that are helpful in developing a spiritual awareness. You might like to try the following:

Exercise 1

Sit comfortably on a straight-backed chair with your feet flat on the floor. Give a little more of your body weight to the chair. Allow it to support you. Take a few deep breaths down into your abdomen. Allow yourself to settle, to become quiet and still.

Now imagine yourself walking along a path through some fields – the path is gently rising and ahead of you is a hill. The sun is shining and there is a light refreshing breeze. Be aware as you walk of the birdsong. Be aware of the flowers amongst the meadow grasses and the breeze stirring the leaves of nearby trees. Imagine yourself crossing a footbridge over a busy stream and following the footpath up through some deep cool woods. You emerge from the wood and follow the path winding round the hill towards the summit. As you walk you stop from time to time to enjoy the changing vista of the countryside stretched out below and to bathe in the peace and solitude of the place. As you approach the summit you become aware that you are about to meet someone, your inner guide – a wise person, connected with the evolution of your life. A person whose eyes express a great deal of love and care for you. Allow yourself to visualise this person. Allow a clear image to form. Now imagine yourself talking with your wise person. Ask about any issue, problem, choice, opportunity that you currently have in your life. Be open to the answers to your questions, allow them to surface in your consciousness. At the end of your conversation your wise person gives you a gift of symbolic significance to you. Something you need at this moment in your life. Receive what you are given. Thank your inner guide. Now imagine yourself walking back down the winding path carrying with you the answers to your questions and the gift. Picture yourself walking down through the wood and crossing the stream. Walk back across the meadows to the start of your walk.

When you are ready, bring your attention back to the here and now. Consider what you have learned and how you can incorporate this learning into your life.

Self-enquiry box

Exercise 2

Sit quietly for a minute or so.

Become aware of the experience of your body. Become aware of your thoughts without getting caught up in them. Notice your feelings, however faint, without being drawn into them. Now allow yourself to scan your life in the present and the past. Allow your recollections to settle where they will. As you do this, be aware of the effect on your body, your thoughts, your emotions. Experience whatever is there. Now give your attention to developing an attitude of loving kindness towards yourself. If it helps, repeat to yourself 'May I be peaceful and happy'. Try and maintain this compassionate focus towards yourself for a minute or two. If you find your attention wandering, gently bring it back to an expression of care for yourself.

Concentrate your attention on a friend. Bring them to mind. Be aware of your feelings. Now give attention to developing an attitude of loving kindness towards your friend. Try and maintain this compassionate focus for a minute or two.

Concentrate your attention on a person whom you dislike or who dislikes you. Bring them to mind. Be aware of your feelings. Now give attention to developing an attitude of loving kindness towards this person. Try and maintain this compassionate focus for a minute or two.

Concentrate your attention on a group of people, a community, or a nation, particularly those who are experiencing oppression and adversity. Bring a representative image to mind. Be aware of your feeling. Now give attention to developing an attitude of loving kindness towards them. Try and maintain this compassionate focus for a minute or two.

Concentrate attention on the earth, on its sustaining beauty and its abuse. Bring a representative image to mind. Be aware of your feeling. Now give attention to developing an attitude of loving care towards the earth. Try and maintain this compassionate focus for a minute or two.

NB: Initially you may find it difficult to locate your feelings or they may be very faint. Reconnecting with feelings comes with practice. It comes from sitting quietly and becoming mindful of your bodily sensations and from there to the emergent feeling. Giving your attention to a feeling allows it to surface more fully into consciousness. Sometimes you may be surprised by negative feelings. These should be acknowledged without becoming drawn into them. They can be helpful moments of learning about yourself and your relationships and lead to changes in how you relate. It may be difficult to access your feelings of loving kindness. Recollecting a moment in time when you felt that way or experienced loving kindness from others may be a way into that feeling state. Above all, this exercise requires patience. Once your flow of feeling is freer you are able to bring it into your everyday life.

The shadow side of helping

20

We would like to think that what draws us into the mental health professions is the motivation to be of service to others, to respond in a skilled and selfless way to the needs of people coming to the service for help.

This saintly viewpoint is rightly questioned in that it is often our own unmet needs and unresolved issues that prompt us to engage in such work. I am not suggesting that the mental health professions should have in place some ultra-sensitive selection process that screens out all but those with the highest motives – who would be left to do the work! What is important is that professionals become sufficiently self-aware as to acknowledge some of their own issues and needs that may intrude unhelpfully into their work with clients. Acknowledged needs can find expression and satisfaction in our personal relationships; unacknowledged needs may unconsciously intrude into our working relationships. This view is shared by Brandon (1976), who argues that helping others is for some a way of concealing 'desperate personal needs'. We may give care and advice to people which we are unable to give ourselves. We may prop up our own sense of adequacy against the inadequacy of others.

John Heron also takes up this theme strongly in arguing for what he calls 'emotional competence' in helpers (Heron 2001). By this he means that our own anxieties and distress, accumulated from past experience, should not drive and distort our attempts to help others. He describes three levels of competence:

Level 1 At this level a person's helping is always contaminated by hidden agendas and has an oppressive, hindering, intrusive or impersonal quality of which the practitioner is unaware.
Level 2 At this second level the helper acts in emotionally clean ways most of the time but sometimes slips into compulsive, distorted helping without realising it.
Level 3 At this third level the helper slips much less often and, more importantly, recognises when it happens and can take steps to correct it. People who work at this level will usually have done some psychological work on past distresses which gives them more awareness and the ability to act intentionally more of the time.

The second level is widespread amongst both professional and lay helpers and often leads to 'contaminated helping'. Specific examples of 'contaminated interventions' are legion and can be outlined in relation to the six categories of helping interventions originated by Heron (Box 20.1).

Box 20.1

Contaminated interventions in helping relationships

Prescriptive interventions

Giving advice when it is not needed; 'taking over', overriding the client's autonomy and responsibility; being coercive and imposing in giving advice; giving moralistic prescriptions – 'you should'; being controlling; not allowing clients the dignity of risk and the right to fail; not allowing clients to say what they need or choose; not being assertive in giving advice and prescriptive care when it is needed; giving advice the helper needs to hear themself; use of threats or force.

Informative interventions

Not giving information about diagnosis, drugs, resources or legal rights that is wanted and needed; imposing 'mystifying' explanations and interpretations; labelling and stigmatising clients; not listening to or respecting the client's frame of reference; giving false information; making unrealisable promises of help or promising overly optimistic outcomes.

Catalytic interventions

Asking too many questions; using blocking tactics to control the agenda; attention not free for the client; staying in safe territory, avoiding difficult issues; manipulating the client into being over-disclosing; engaging in a compulsive search for 'answers'; focusing on the helper's issues in the client's story or avoiding them; maintaining a distant professional stance, not fostering any sense of mutuality or equality; sexual or emotional exploitation of a client's transference.

Cathartic interventions

Not reaching out to clients in distress; not 'giving permission' to be upset; discounting or placating distress; talking over a client's distress; missing or ignoring cues to distress just below the surface; pushing people into catharsis inappropriately or too soon; giving 'conditional care'; being overwhelmed by the client's catharsis that finds an echo in the helper's own unacknowledged distress; being controlling rather than containing when clients become distressed.

Challenging interventions

Avoiding or talking around issues because of the helper's anxiety about raising it directly; not raising issues because of the helper's fear of retaliation, of hurting the client, or of spoiling the relationship; being apologetic and defensive in raising issues; not being assertive in raising issues so that challenges can easily be dismissed or ignored; challenging clients aggressively or judgementally; swings from evasiveness to 'hard truths' and back again to evasiveness because of the helper's anxieties; the helper 'overtalks', denying the client the space to assimilate and question what has been said; avoids or anxiously raises agendas that would be difficult for the helper only to find the client accepts them without undue concern; abusive verbal assaults on clients.

Supportive interventions

Support is given in a patronising or insincere way; support is given intrusively, rescuing the client, showering them with help and care when they are struggling resourcefully with their problems; not recognising and reaching out supportively when help is asked for overtly or covertly, not allowing the expression of dependency needs; holding clients in a dependent relationship, blocking the clients in their efforts to support themselves or draw on other sources of support.

Source: Heron (2001).

Self-enquiry box

- You may find it helpful to reflect on these examples of 'contaminated interventions' in relation to your own practice. Challenge yourself! We can all recognise ourselves in some of the outlined interventions. Your attention may also be drawn to patterns in your way of relating to clients of which you are not so aware.
- Ask your clients what they have found helpful and not so helpful about the way you have worked with them.
- You may find it valuable to explore the outcomes of your self-enquiry in supervision.

Egan (2006) takes a broader view of the shadow side of helping, suggesting that alongside the helper's shadow side and the client's shadow side is also the shadow side of the helping process, which can be contaminated by all of these.

Not everyone wants to be helped or can be helped. The client may seem to engage in a relationship and the helping process with serious intent but does nothing to tackle their problems or seize opportunities offered. This passivity or reluctance has to be acknowledged and explored before there can be any change. Sometimes this centres around dependency needs. A client may have a need 'to be held', to feel cared for to a greater degree and for a longer period than the helper or the multidisciplinary team realises. They need time to feel that the relationship will provide them with a safe base from which to begin to assert their autonomy and become more effective in meeting the demands and challenges of everyday life. The helper may strongly value independence and self-reliance in their own life and may have personal anxieties around dependency, all of which can have an unnoticed influence on their attitude towards the client. This may express itself in feelings of impatience and blame towards the client for their lack of progress, to which the client may react by retreating further into passivity and dependency.

Clients sometimes manipulate helpers in order to meet their hidden agendas. They may seek to arouse the helper's concern by threats of self-harm or actual harm – one client I have come to know carried a noosed rope around with him for several years as a constant reminder to us of his at-risk status. Other clients may stop taking medication, or not turn up for an appointment, ruminate on the likelihood of impulse behaviour of a threatening nature or leave the ward without telling anyone – behaviours which have a powerful impact on professional helpers. Clients may sometimes retreat into symptom behaviour and helplessness and, by clinging to a sick role, avoid the discontinuation of care. Clients may emotionally, and sometimes sexually, seduce helpers in order to meet a need to feel special, to feel loved, appreciated and valued. Clients may be non-engaging and non-compliant with helpers or the service as an expression of their resentment at the way they have been treated by mental health and social services in the past. All these issues can be considered part of the client's shadow side that can hinder the development of helping relationships and therapeutic work.

207

The process of helping also has its shadow side. The history of psychiatry is chequered with examples of abuse. The stigmatising, disempowering, excluding attitudes and practices of the institutional era of psychiatry still exist in community-oriented services of today. Many long-term users of the services have little choice or say in their care plans and are subjected to under-stimulating programmes of day care that do little to meet their needs for socially valued work and leisure activity. Many users feel hindered rather than helped by excessive doses of neuroleptic medication which often add to their disabilities. In reviewing the evidence for drug-induced disability, Breggin (1993) estimates that 10–20% of people treated with the phenothiazine group of drugs will develop tardive dyskinesia.

The professionalisation of caring and what Brandon (1997) calls the 'therapeutic egos' of many helpers create a culture of disparagement where people whose behaviour is distressed and disturbed enough to become the objects of 'expert' attention are pathologised and treated. Personhood becomes submerged beneath the mantle of mental patient and the individual excluded to the margins of society from where it is very difficult to reclaim citizenship. The tendency to pathologise behaviour that deviates from the arbitrary social norm seems to be increasing. The current Diagnostic and Statistical Manual of Mental Disorders (DSM-IV) contains 390 categories of mental illness, whereas DSM-III had 205. It is argued (Coleman 1998) that rather than representing the advancement of scientific knowledge it reflects psychiatry's encroachment into normal human responses. Life inevitably involves suffering. Happiness is not a divine right. There are no easy answers to the adversities and the pain of living. Yet our culture seems to promote a utopian view that there is a solution to all the problems of being human. This is often reflected in the unrealistic expectations of professional help, held by both clients and helpers, who look for the 'big fix', instead of a small but definite change that results in a problem being managed better rather than resolved.

Like many helping professionals, I have been slow to recognise my own feelings and needs, which have at times intruded in a way that has hindered clients in their journey of recovery. I have at times not been proactive in getting the help and supervision I needed. This is in part the result of cultural conditioning, reinforced by a work culture that places a high value on independence, self-reliance, stoicism and selflessness. As James Hillman observes, 'We have been brought up to deny our needs. To need is to be dependent and weak; needing implies submission to another' (cited in Hawkins & Shohet 2000).

 Ruth's story

Theme: contaminated helping

Harry is a man of 37 who has suffered from a manic-depressive disorder and alcoholism for some years. His key worker, Ruth, visits him weekly, providing a supportive alliance within which early relapse signs can be monitored and coping strategies implemented. There is some evidence that Harry is drinking again and he has not been at home on two occasions when his key worker had called. Ruth is aware of feeling quite angry towards Harry for what she sees as his 'deceptive' and 'irresponsible behaviour'. She feels let down by him after all the 'hard work' she's put in. On her next visit she aggressively confronts Harry and threatens to discharge him if he is unwilling to follow the agreed care plan. She leaves feeling unhappy, guilty and compromised professionally.

In supervision Ruth is able to discuss this incident with a senior colleague. She recognises that an 'over-investment' in problem resolution in her work with clients is a pattern that often leads to her blaming herself or blaming clients for a lack of therapeutic endeavour. She traces this to her own experience of a much-loved alcoholic father, whom both her mother and herself were never able to 'help enough'.

 Martin's story

Theme: contaminated helping

Martin is a mental health worker at a supported housing project. He has been Jeannie's support worker since she moved to the project 2 months ago, after a lengthy period in hospital. Jeannie had been admitted in a disturbed, distressed state of mind, complaining of hallucinations and delusions. She has made a good recovery but is a vulnerable young woman with a pressing need for a secure supportive relationship. She is in her twenties, single and grew up in foster care and various children's homes, following parental desertion. Jeannie tends to search Martin out on the slightest pretext and has clearly become attached to him. Martin feels flattered by her regard for him and plays along with the flirtation that has crept into their conversations, at one level seeing it as a normal expression of sexuality and entirely appropriate in a caring culture that seeks to normalise professional helping relationships. Gradually social excursions become opportunities for discreet intimate exchanges and Martin finds himself increasingly attracted to her. It is not long before Jeannie tells Martin that she is in love with him and clearly signals her willingness to enter into a sexual relationship.

Martin feels confused. He is currently unattached, as is Jeannie. There is mutual attraction that in other circumstances would lead to an emotional and sexual relationship. Yet he is aware of having crossed a professional boundary in allowing a mutual attraction and emotional involvement to develop as it has. He is aware that in the past he has knowingly drawn clients both male and female into enmeshed relationships with his personable attention, only to withdraw defensively when demands began to be made which ethically he could not fulfil. In supervision he is able to acknowledge the feeling of power he experiences when people idealise him and need him in the way Jeannie does now. His supervisor recognises that Martin's unmet narcissistic needs are intruding in a potentially damaging way into his work with clients.

Part

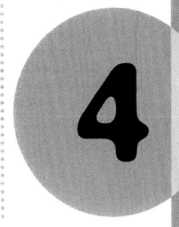

Personal management

4

Introduction

A recurring theme throughout this book has been the importance of practitioners being committed to their own growth and development. There is a need to avoid the potentially damaging split that so often occurs in professional caring, in which the practitioner's vulnerabilities, needs and problems of living are denied and only the client's vulnerabilities and neediness are seen.

We cannot be effective as practitioners if we live an unexamined life. Knowing ourselves allows us to relate more sensitively and empathetically to others, for as Carl Rogers argued, what is most personal is also most universal. To be more intentional and authentic in the way we relate to people is to be less influenced by the unconscious motivations of our own unacknowledged needs and unresolved distress. This final part of the book sets out three ways in which personal management as a vital, integral part of professional development can enhance practice.

Chapter 21 considers the place of personal development within professional education. The first step in this process is developing self-awareness. It is argued that if we remain blind to our own defensive communication patterns, our oppressive attitudes and prejudices, our own needs and feelings, our personal wounds and undealt-with distress, then it is unlikely that we will be able to engage with service users in ways that will be experienced as helpful and healing.

Chapter 22 explores ways in which work-related stress can be creatively managed. The energy and resourcefulness we are able to bring to the helping relationship will depend greatly on our ability to take care of ourselves. The high rates of sickness, absenteeism and burnout amongst mental health professionals suggest we are not very good at doing this.

Chapter 23 examines the importance of regular, planned opportunities for guided reflection on practice. There are times when our work as mental health practitioners seems hardly worthwhile; when it seems to achieve little; when clients seem lost in their distress. There are times when the experience and problems of living that people bring seem crushing and insurmountable. There are times when we feel impotent, inadequate and drained, with little left to give. It is because helping relationships can be so challenging and depleting that good supervision plays such a vital part in replenishing practitioners and in developing and sustaining competent, creative practice.

Personal development in professional education

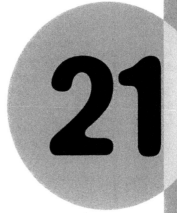

21

Relationship skills are the key attribute that mental health professionals bring to their work. Such skills are not easy to acquire and training programmes at pre- and post-registration level need to find creative ways of helping students and practitioners to develop depth as well as breadth in their skills repertoire. This depth, I would argue, comes from personal development work and should be seen as a prerequisite for effective psychological helping.

Practitioners in mental health seek to engage with people, often very vulnerable and troubled people, in a way that helps them move towards a more effective way of being. At its best it is an empowering, enabling process that is rooted in a belief in the potential of people to recover themselves and their circumscribed lives from enduring and disabling distress. To fill out this role, practitioners need a thorough psychosocial training that goes beyond communication skills, beyond psychological strategies and techniques, and brings the self more fully into the role. This chapter looks at how personal education, concerned with the 'art of being', can coexist in the academic context alongside a curriculum concerned with 'knowledgeable doing'.

A great deal of professional education is characterised by what Knowles (1991) defines as didactic, pedagogic teaching and learning and is principally concerned with cognitive knowing. Clearly this is not an appropriate way to meet the need for personal development. An experiential, student-centred approach offers a more fruitful teaching and learning style. By experiential learning I mean the active and interactive involvement of people in structures that engage them holistically. The educational process needs to engage people at a feeling, intuitive and sensory level, as well as the cognitive, if they are to become skilled in the intentional and therapeutic use of self. Experiential structures are designed to create opportunities for gaining self-knowledge, for learning how to relate to others in more authentic ways. They are concerned with knowing how to be present with people in ways that are enabling and healing. Learning takes place within collaborative relationships with teachers and fellow students, in which responsibility for the learning process is shared. The underlying philosophy is that of student-centred teaching (Rogers & Freiberg 1994).

Student-centred, adult-oriented approach to teaching helpfully parallels the collaborative relationship between practitioner and client and mirrors the person-centred philosophy of care programmes. Relationships of empowerment need to permeate the culture of caring organisations and the supporting educational culture, involving students and teachers, practitioners, clinical team leaders and service managers, if service users are going to experience the help they receive as enabling and empowering. Power differences need to be acknowledged as a dynamic in all human relationships and managed awarely, in ways that are anti-oppressive. In a supportive and empowering educational culture, students can take responsibility for determining their learning needs and become resourceful in getting those needs met.

Much of the experiential learning methodology has come from the field of humanistic psychology and from the arts. When used imaginatively and facilitated well, these structures can contribute in an exciting, relevant and effective way to professional development. There is a rich seam of structures to draw on, some examples of which you will have already experienced in this book:

- co-counselling structures
- guided visualisation
- expressive writing
- journal keeping
- encounter-style personal development groups
- intrapersonal and interpersonal awareness exercises
- expressive art
- role play
- improvisation
- mask work
- story-making
- sculpting
- psychodrama
- movement exercises
- meditation
- action research.

My own experience of facilitating drama-based experiential groups suggests that personal development that has significance for professional practice can take place in an educational context (Box 21.1). An approach to experiential design drawn from drama therapy seems to offer a challenging but safe structure in which students are less likely to become overexposed to the point of vulnerability and shut down protectively. Students find the self-discovery talk and openness to feeling in a cohesive group to be a strengthening and enlivening experience. Such groups can create a context in which inner empathy can develop so that the help offered to clients is less likely to be contaminated by the mental health worker's own needs and feelings. Another interesting outcome from this type of educational work is the increase in awareness of the non-verbal channel of communication. The process of helping normally depends heavily on words and we become blinkered to the subtle yet significant messages conveyed by body language. Drama exercises that focus on bodily communication can reawaken us to the dance of life. Finally, students often observe that they are able to relate in more spontaneous ways as a consequence of participation in drama-based experiential groups. Gersie (1991) suggests that many of us have internalised

---

Box 21.1

Key learning experiences reported by students in a drama-based experiential learning group

- Giving and receiving support
- Increase in knowledge of self
- Increased awareness of group processes
- Increase in openness/self-disclosure
- Affective learning/being more in touch with feelings
- Increased interpersonal awareness
- Increased spontaneity and confidence
- Raised awareness of bodily communication
- Strengthened ability to reflectively process experience

Source: Watkins (1995).

---

critical judgements about our capacity to be creative which have blocked our imagination and creative energy. Finding the freedom to be creative in such a group can increase the vitality and spontaneity available for everyday life and relationships.

Self-awareness

Increasing self-awareness is the first stage of learning how to use ourselves as therapeutic agents. If we remain blind to our defensive communication patterns, to our oppressive attitudes and prejudices, to our own needs and feelings, to our emotional wounds and undealt-with distress, then it is unlikely that our engagement with people using the service will be experienced as helpful and healing. This unknown side of ourselves – the shadow side – will appear like an uninvited guest in our interactions with clients. It is difficult to stop ourselves reacting in a hurt, angry way to rejection or criticism from clients if we are blind to our need to feel 'special' in our relationships with them. It can be difficult to accept non-compliance if our need for control, and the anxieties that surface if control is lost, have not been examined. It can be difficult to see past the vulnerabilities and neediness of clients if we do not recognise our own needs and fallibilities. It is unlikely that we will be effective in nurturing the self-esteem of others if we have a fragile sense of our own self-worth. We cannot expect to work helpfully with people of a different gender, sexual orientation or ethnicity to our own, if we have not considered the biases we have inherited from our culture and how they influence our interactions. We cannot create a helping dialogue if we are not aware of the inner distractions that prevent us from having our attention free for people. These kinds of statements about the art of helping seem to me to represent the case for self-awareness and personal development work to be an essential core running through the initial training and continuing professional development of all mental health staff.

Heron (2001) argues that it is important that helpers free themselves from past hurts and develop emotional competence if needs and feelings that have their origins in past relationships are not to spill over into our helping relationships. By emotional competence he means that we will be in touch with our feelings and can both appropriately control and discharge our distress. It means that we have choice – we are in charge of our feelings rather than them being in charge of us. Traditionally the helping professions, particularly nursing, have sustained a culture which overvalued the control of feelings. To acknowledge feeling upset or, worse, to show that upset, could have resulted in practitioners being thought inadequate and unsuitable. Stress-related problems and burnout follow in the wake of a failure to recognise the emotional labour of professional caring and to create a culture in which practitioners' feelings are respected (Smith 1992). We cannot care empathetically for people, recognise and respond to their feelings, if we are not in touch with our own. It can be difficult to allow and respond appropriately to a person's distress if we cannot face and deal with our own emotional pain. We may not see the signs of distress in others or, if we do, we may fail to reach out. Alternatively we may smother others' distress in comforting words and actions, when the safe discharge of distress and the gathering of insight into the context for the distressed reaction would be a more therapeutic response.

Self-esteem

Many people suffer from low self-esteem. Their experiences of life, particularly early developmental and educational experiences, have not allowed them to internalise sufficient self-regard to weather the winds of fortune that blow through life. Their self-esteem is either too externally regulated or internally sensitised. In the former, self-esteem may be frequently punctured by minor experiences of disappointment, let-down and failure that are part of everyday human experience. In the latter, self-esteem is sensitised to particular events, so that an individual crumples when exposed, for example, to criticism or to not being centre stage. Self-esteem is not derived from seeing only our positive qualities and talents and defensively ignoring our flaws and failings. It involves being able to acknowledge our imperfections, changing what we can change and accepting what we can't. Self-esteem comes from living a life that contains and expresses what we value for ourselves. Sometimes when we feel bad about ourselves it is because we perceive ourselves as falling short of certain standards or values which, if we took the trouble to examine them, we would not wish to own. They are values that we have picked up from our parents or teachers or they may have been imposed by our culture.

For the mental health practitioner, low self-esteem may make it difficult to find the confidence to engage with some clients and sustain a relationship. Doubts and uncertainties will frequently surface about being good enough to do the work. Things that clients may do or say will be experienced as hurtful. Relating to people in an honest way becomes difficult. Some practitioners may feel they have nothing worthwhile to say or feel that they won't be listened to. Others may find it difficult to be open to the appreciation and regard of others.

Personal development work in the context of professional education should sustain and enhance the self-esteem of practitioners. It should develop relation-

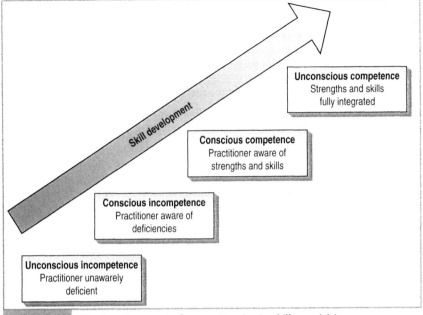

Figure 21.1 ● The development of competencies in skill acquisition.

ships and educational structures within which a person can become known and feel valued and validated. It should create a forum in which the conscious incompetence of a practitioner can be safely disclosed as a starting place for development (Fig. 21.1). Clearly, if insufficient trust exists then practitioners are more likely to defensively adopt a position of unconscious incompetence and practise in unaware ways which are potentially harmful. Educational groups that have personal development as a desired outcome, support groups and supervision offer the opportunities to work on and strengthen self-esteem. An important step in building and sustaining self-esteem is being able to obtain feedback from others (see Self-enquiry box below).

Self-enquiry box

Being able to obtain good feedback is an important skill. The following proactive strategies can be helpful in getting feedback in a way that is experienced as enhancing rather than diminishing. Try them out in your conversations with colleagues and clients.

Negative assertion involves making a negative statement about some aspect of yourself or your practice that you are dissatisfied with. It invites a supportive response from others.

Positive assertion or positive enquiry involves making a positive statement about some aspect of yourself or your practice that you are pleased about. It invites validation and appreciation.

Continued

Self-enquiry box—cont'd

Negative enquiry involves inviting negative feedback about some aspect of your practice that you perceive others to be unhappy with. It allows you to maintain some control over the timing and focus of the feedback.

Open enquiry involves asking open questions that invite general feedback about yourself and your practice.

Receiving negative feedback – be aware when the observations of others seem valid and when they seem invalid. Ask for more information if you need it. Try to be open to feedback without becoming defensive. Be aware of how certain criticisms puncture your self-esteem or are particularly hurtful to receive. Try and identify your associations with them. Acknowledge the feelings negative feedback has left you with.

Receiving positive feedback – be open to the feedback. Be aware of any tendency to diminish or dismiss it. Consider whether this is a familiar pattern. What do you feel when someone gives you positive feedback? What associations can you make with those feelings?

Self-enquiry box

You may find it useful to reflect on Johari's window (Fig. 21.2) as a structure for developing self-awareness. Each panel of the window represents a way in which our 'self' expresses itself in our everyday lives.

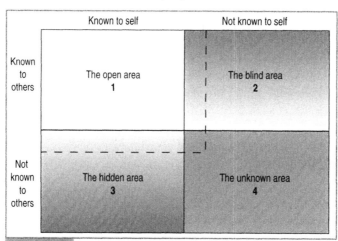

Figure 21.2 ● Johari's window.

Panel 1 is the part of ourselves that we know best and that is known to others – our persona, the self that we commonly present to the world. Panel 2 is that part of ourselves that is seen by others but which we deny or are unaware of. Panel 3 is the part of ourselves that we know of, a familiar companion, but one that we keep hidden from others. Panel 4 is that part of ourselves which is largely unconscious but which expresses itself in our actions and reactions.

Since drawing and painting are effective non-verbal ways of exploring the self, I suggest now that you take a large sheet of paper. Select some colours and draw or paint an image to represent the self that you present to the world most of the time. Try to allow yourself to paint/draw in a spontaneous way. Don't think too much about it, just do it and see what emerges. There are no prizes for artistic achievement! Take about 10 minutes to do this and then put it aside, out of sight. Take a second sheet and draw or paint an image to represent yourself at times in your life when you have felt most fully alive. You may find it helps to spend a few minutes quietly scanning back on some of those moments in your life. Now select some colours and begin to draw/paint again, allowing yourself to be as free as possible about this. Again, take about 10 minutes. Now compare the two. One way to do this is to brainstorm a list of adjectives that come to mind when you look at each drawing. You might like to consider what prevents you being in touch with the self expressed in the second picture more of the time.

Research

As indicated above, to become an emotionally competent, interpersonally skilled practitioner able to work with people at relational depth requires a commitment to personal development. This is achieved through holistic learning and good supervision. Research offers a third and important possibility. Research in the humanistic tradition is very different from empirical research – research on people. In humanistic research the researchers are also the researched upon, hence it is research with people rather than research on people. In a cooperative enquiry for example, two or more people with a common research interest decide the focus of the enquiry and the methodology by which data can be elicited and subjected to critical evaluation (Heron & Reason 2000). Essentially it involves 'going several times round an experiential learning cycle in a formal structured way with full awareness and intent in order to enquire systematically into some facet of experience' (Heron 2001, p. 128). The growth of knowledge that accrues from such enquiries is firmly rooted in experiential knowing. This living–learning experience is not a process exclusive to mental health professionals in pursuit of an evidence base for practice but one which could also be used by groups of clients to learn more functional and satisfying ways of being. Heron makes the even more challenging and exciting suggestion that a client and a practitioner could set up a cooperative enquiry into some aspect of their relationship.

One group of practitioners I have been associated with, concerned about their own levels of work-related stress, the absenteeism and high attrition rate in the service as a whole, decided to research the determinants of wellbeing in the workplace. They started with a shared list of influences, positive and negative, and a self-assessed wellbeing score on a 10-point scale. Participants also brought to consciousness and shared with each other an image that represented their state of wellbeing at that moment in time. It was decided early in the discussion that the research question would reflect an empowered sense of personhood, i.e. that each of us, at least potentially, holds the personal power necessary to enhance or diminish our own sense of wellbeing. This resulted in considerable discussion about the impact of socio-political events and organisational decisions on our lives over which we have little control. A convincing case was made for the nobility of the individual in adversity, holding that even in the direst of circumstances qualities such as courage, fortitude, hopefulness, acceptance, spirit, love, self-belief had a sustaining influence on wellbeing.

Eventually the research question was framed as 'In which ways can I/we sustain and enhance my/our own wellbeing in work environments where stress is a ubiquitous presence?'. The group agreed to monitor and rate their wellbeing weekly over a 3-month period and to keep a time-line of events that impacted on it. The six members met as co-counselling partners weekly, supporting each other through the experiential cycle (Fig. 21.3) and met fortnightly as a group to critique each other's feedback on personal learning. At the end of 3 months the participants produced individual reports which were subjected to a process of cut and paste whereby common learning themes were transposed into a single report that captured the collective truth of the experience.

The outcomes of this enquiry, an abstract of which is offered below, had an influence not only on the six practitioners involved but also on the wider clinical team whose curiosity was stimulated to the extent that they became peripherally involved in the enquiry. There was a perception, backed up by some evidence, that working in an organisational culture which was very focused on the task of meeting targets and improving audit ratings, that the wellbeing of the workforce was low on its agenda. The prevailing credo seemed to be 'If you can't stand the heat get out of the kitchen'. Alongside this was an acknowledgement that we as professionals need to be more assertive in securing what support we need to practise effectively and reduce the sense of burden that can accrue from the emotional labour inherent in the work.

Abstract: *One key piece of learning was that a great deal of anxiety in the workplace comes from unprocessed experience that sits in the psyche emitting distress signals. There must be opportunities, informal and formal, individual and collective, to reflect systematically on the work. Unsurprisingly perhaps, the enquiry group found the co-counselling structure and the group feedback experience itself had a significant effect on their sense of wellbeing. The enquiry, and in particular those two structures, gave them permission to be more 'holistically present' in their work, more transparent in their interactions with clients and colleagues. Another significant theme was the importance of being true to deeply held values in the arena of work: not acting in accordance with personal values, such as being non-judgemental or from a place of loving kindness or from a place of realistic hopefulness, creates waves of dissatisfaction that undermine happiness and wellbeing. At the end of the enquiry participants visualised second wellbeing images, comparing these with the ones produced earlier. The images had changed from a pot plant withered and limp from lack of care to an unfurled leaf new in its greenness; from a featureless silhouette to a fully seen, vibrant figure.*

Action research

Another example of research that can play a significant part in practitioners' personal and interpersonal development is 'action research', which originated in the work of social scientist Kurt Lewin in the 1940s and which is now recognised worldwide as a credible research model. It has been widely used in education, management and in social and health care work as an approach to professional/ personal development and the enhancement of practice. Action research is empowering to practitioners; it entrusts them with the responsibility for the development of practice and for contributing to the knowledge base that underpins it. Knowledge is not a static entity: the leading edge of knowledge is always growing and changing. Traditionally the creation of new theory has been seen as the preserve of academics and researchers and because this confers considerable power and status there has been an investment in keeping it that way. That view has been challenged by the process of action research, enabling practitioners to make a valid contribution not only to evolving practice but also to new theory or the reconfiguration of old theory (McNiff & Whitehead 2006).

Action research is often one-person research, although as we have seen above a research question can be a basis for a collaborative enquiry and can have a much wider sphere of influence on practitioners and practice through the interest it creates and through the dissemination of learning. It is based on the experiential learning cycle or action–reflection cycle (Fig. 21.3) in which the systematic reflection on some aspect of practice leads to new learning and the change or enhancement of practice. The term 'the reflective practitioner' became a watchword in the brave new world of nurse education in the 1990s and offered a credible basis for student-centred learning and self-appraisal. But this is no easy process to engage with, relying as it does on the holistic awareness of the practitioner, the ability to be open to the flow of their inner experience and judiciously congruent with that experience in the way they behave. This requires a healthy degree of self-acceptance. If I cannot accept my fallibilities and weaknesses along with my strengths and qualities, I will not be able to reflect authentically on my experience. Tuning into an experience, exploring it reflectively, understanding it and teasing out the learning from it requires a sophisticated degree of self-enquiry skills.

Action research begins with a question pertinent to improving practice:

- How do I relate to clients in a way that is effective in encouraging and strengthening their engagement with services?

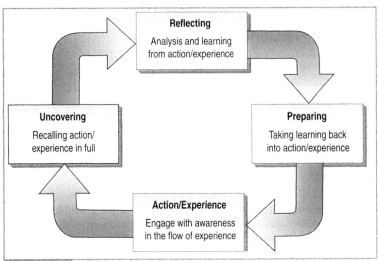

Figure 21.3 ● The action–reflection cycle.

- How do I improve my ability to enable clients to make informed choices about whether to take medication?
- How can I be more effective in identifying and responding to clients' spiritual needs?
- How can I relate to clients in a way that emphasises their strengths rather than fallibilities and deficiencies?
- How can I become more effective at working with risk without infringing the person's freedom and autonomy?

Such research questions usually spring from values that are deeply held by practitioners, the expression of which is in some way restricted in their current work. So, for example, implicit in the last question could be a strongly held belief in the rights of people to be at risk and the necessity of risk for growth, maturation and autonomous living.

Action research is a rigorous methodical process that aims to generate and validate new learning of value to the practitioner and the wider practitioner community. McNiff & Whitehead (2006), in their inspiring text on action research, identify the steps of this process in the form of questions.

- What is my concern?
- Why am I concerned?
- What kind of experiences can I describe to show why I'm concerned?
- What can I do about it?
- What will I do about it?
- What kind of data can I gather to show how the situation unfolds?
- How will I evaluate the potential influence of my learning?
- How will I ensure that any conclusions are reasonably fair and accurate?
- How will I test the validity of the evidence-based account of my learning?
- How will I modify my concerns, ideas and practice in the light of my evaluation?

Box 21.2 provides an example, in outline, of a proposal for an action enquiry.

Box 21.2

Outline proposal for an action enquiry

What is my concern?
How do I stay true to non-directive ways of working with people referred to mental health services?

Why am I concerned?
I am concerned because I hold values that respect the sovereignty of a person over their own life; the right of people to decide for themselves what they need to regain internal and external harmony and wellbeing. This assumes the universal desire of all humans to avoid suffering and seek wellbeing. Within the mental health system these rights are often disregarded by the imposition of authoritative or prescriptive

care. I concede from the outset that autonomy as an inviolate right would not be possible in mental health care as by its very nature, serious mental dysfunction can diminish a person's capacity to act with good judgement in the interest of personal wellbeing. The research does not aim to promote such a utopian ideal but is concerned with endorsing non-directivity as the value base for practice and towards which all practice gravitates.

What kind of experience can I describe to show why I'm concerned?

I am aware that a dichotomy exists within me, and within many colleagues, between a non-directive attitude held cognitively and my/our actions which are often strongly directive. Often I am seduced by a person's apparent passivity or helplessness into taking a prescriptive stance; or pander to my own ego needs to be seen as an authoritative, knowledgeable, professional. Sometimes I lapse into authoritative mode when anxious about the person's capacity to stay safe or act with reasonable judgement and control. On occasions I allow myself to be persuaded by the anxiety of families or colleagues to act in ways contrary to a client's wishes. I'm conscious of practising within a system that coercively and legally exercises the power to take away a person's freedom and to treat them without their free and informed consent. It is a system which pathologises troubled or unusual states of mind, creating a situation where knowledge resides with the expert setting the scene for benevolent authoritative care which is either accepted passively, reluctantly, resentfully, or is rejected. None of these outcomes are satisfactory as they do nothing to enhance a client's sense of personal power and resourcefulness in the face of their suffering.

What can I do about it?

I can maintain a level of conscious competence/conscious incompetence in relation to non-directivity in my practice. I can reflectively examine all instances where I deviate from this position towards more prescriptive ways of relating. I can reflectively examine all instances where a non-directive stance is challenged by the presenting mental state of clients, but is maintained. I can seek to promote non-directivity in forums where practice and issues are discussed.

What will I do about it?

All of the above; plus make the non-directivity of my practice open to collegial scrutiny in team meetings and make it a focus of managerial and clinical supervision.

What data can I gather to show how the change in practice unfolds?

I can use Six Category Intervention Analysis (Heron 2001) as a structure for reflecting on my interactions with clients and rating myself on a directive–non-directive scale. So, for example, in the catalytic category I am interested in who sets the agenda for our contact and conversation, to what extent do I attune to the client's world rather than impose my own perspectives. Similarly in the prescriptive category, how consultative or collaborative am I; to what extent do I enable clients to make their own decisions. In the supportive category, can I be supportive in a way that is not withholding yet avoids rescuing. Further, I can seek feedback from clients on their experience of the collaborativeness of care, the extent to which they feel their care is self-directed and the extent to which this results in a shift in self-perception toward a more empowered, resourceful self-concept.

How can I evaluate the potential influence of any learning?

While the research is oriented towards changing my personal practice, there is the potential for authenticated claims as to the efficacy of non-directivity in the arena of mental health care to influence colleagues to shift the value base for their practice. In living out non-directivity in my work and promoting this as a value base I am inviting other practitioners to question and reflect on their own practice from that standpoint.

Continued

Box 21.2

Outline proposal for an action enquiry—cont'd

How can I show my conclusions are reasonably fair and accurate?

I can subject the data and learning as it emerges to a review and critique by a research supervisor and to a validation group who would be made up of a clinician, an academic, my supervisor and a service user meeting at regular intervals through the project. Their task will be to help me determine whether I am able to provide reasonable evidence that non-directive ways of working are compatible with an acceptable standard of care, that people are mostly capable of deciding what they need to recover harmony in their lives and that non-directivity leads to a more empowered and resourceful sense of self and as a consequence reduced vulnerability. Similarly but less formally I would anticipate and welcome continuing questioning from colleagues about my congruity – do I walk the talk – and about the ethics of non-directivity and about any claims for the efficacy of this style of working.

How can I evaluate the validity of the evidence-based account of my learning?

My validation group act as guardians of the rigour of my methodology and will draw my attention to any deficiency in this process and any learning claimed that is unsubstantiated. The issue here is transparency; transparency on my part in the reflective cycles and in the deductive process. I would expect my supervisor and validation group to challenge me if my openness about the process was in question.

How will I modify my practice in the light of new learning?

It is of course difficult to say at this stage – I will know when I get there! But there are some hunches I have about how my practice or at least my conceptions of practice may change. One of these is that I am not as important as I sometimes think I am in the lives of clients; I am not this omniscient presence on which they rely. People are much more resourceful than we give them credit for. Recently a client, who had been a cause of considerable concern because of the persecutory world he seemed often drawn into, took himself off on an unplanned impromptu trip to India in search of healing and resolution. He lived for several months in cheap hotels surviving on his benefit entitlement accessed from global cashpoints, a course of action that would test the courage and resourcefulness of most of us. I anticipate trusting people more; trusting them to find their way out of the chaos, the troubled state of mind, the dysfunctional way of being, and the distress that has surfaced in their lives. Any expertise I bring is concerned with supporting them in that process.

I believe action research has an enormously valuable role to play within the multidisciplinary community of mental health practitioners, particularly in the evolution of practice that has at its heart humanistic values. While we each have a unique individuality, we are not a separate 'I', we are part of an open system made up of others by whom we are influenced and in turn influence. We live in a pool of ideas and values that inevitably pass through that 'semi-permeable membrane' that gives us an illusory sense of the integrity of the psyche. Some of these ideas we incorporate into our value base, our way of thinking about the world and our way of being. Sometimes when our established values are challenged by big or radical ideas, our ways of thinking and acting get shaken up, which can have a profound effect in all sorts of ways. For me, one idea on practice and philosophy of such profundity was the idea of *the living learning experience*, which lies at the heart of therapeutic communities. It was an idea not just encountered intellectually through reading but witnessed being lived out by colleagues in their practice and residents in their care. And it was through a dialectical reflection on this experience that most influence on me occurred. It may be that the value base and the ideas on practice that I have explored in this book may strike a chord with you and your practice aspirations and influence you to become more humanistic and congruent in your work. They may become the basis for your own action enquiry.

Action research takes place from this ontological perspective. It is social action research – it engages interest and involvement; it influences people. While you, the 'I', may be engaged in a one-person research enquiry it is never in isolation. The value base you start from will be shared or differed from by others and the ideas about practice that flow from your enquiry will be viewed with sympathetic interest by some and antipathy by others, which will provide the spark for many dialogues. Building an evidence base in the course of and at the conclusion of your research that living and working according to certain values has significant implications for good practice will impact on the therapeutic environment and will not be research that sits neglected in a library archive.

Taking care of
ourselves

Taking care of others, particularly people with severe psychological disabilities, can be demanding and stressful. The energy and resourcefulness that we are able to bring to the helping relationship will depend greatly on our ability to take care of ourselves. Professional helpers are generally not good at this, not good at identifying and meeting their own needs. The high rates of sickness, absenteeism and attrition are an indicator of the presence of stress and burnout amongst mental health staff (Thomas 1997). There are several reasons why mental health professionals are not very good at self-care; often the culture of caring occupations carries an unspoken belief that, come what may, staff cope, so that to acknowledge being stressed or upset is to risk being thought neurotic or unsuitable. The wider culture too imposes expectations in the form of gender-linked values and beliefs, such as, 'women are expected to put others' needs before their own', or 'men are expected to be tough-minded and strong'. Onyett (1998) observes how 'macho cultures' develop in community mental health teams and contribute to staff stress. There is what he describes as an 'addiction to accomplishment' in which nurses take on more and more work and boundaries around hours worked begin to slip. In this kind of work environment, interaction with colleagues becomes exclusively work-oriented with little time for the kind of informal social contact which can be experienced as depressurising. At a deeper, more personal level, we are sometimes drawn into helping or caring occupations as a covert way of meeting our own neglected and denied needs. In other words, we give to others what we ourselves need. We recognise in others the vulnerable part of ourselves which is difficult for us to own, and that becomes the hook for projecting our own vulnerability and neediness. Taking care of ourselves starts with owning that vulnerability and neediness and recognising it as part of the condition of being human.

The challenge in our work can be stimulating. People often say they work better under pressure and it certainly seems to be the case that up to a certain point stress does improve performance. Beyond that point, however, our performance begins to deteriorate. If we are subjected to sustained stress, either at work or in our personal life and do not adequately de-stress, then we run the risk not only of becoming inefficient and ineffective in our work but also of burnout and ill-health (Fig. 22.1). We can become so accustomed to living on the down slope, that we become unaware that we are stressed until stress symptoms become so intrusive that we can no longer ignore them.

Figure 22.1 ● The human function curve.

Hawkins & Shohet (2000) suggest that burnout is a process which begins quite early in the careers of helpers. It arises principally out of an over-attachment or an over-investment in helping clients. Most of us struggle with the issue of non-attachment. We often lurch between the poles of impotence and omnipotence, feeling a sense of inadequacy and failure at one moment and infallibility the next. Non-attachment does not mean not caring, it means 'I care but I don't mind'. I care for clients compassionately in their struggles to manage the problems of living more effectively. But if they are motivated to escape from that struggle into symptom behaviour, or for a time seek refuge in a more dependent way of being, or seek relief in street drugs or self-harm behaviour, then I don't mind. If I did I would soon become disillusioned, demoralised and exhausted. Nurses suffering from burnout show less empathy towards clients, adopt a depersonalising, cynical approach to care, and minimise contact, seeking refuge in administrative and routine tasks (Santa Maria 1998).

Self-enquiry box

This exercise will help you become aware of how stress affects you.

Reflect back on a recent stressful period in your life. Focus on the way in which you were affected. You may find it helpful to categorise your list of personal reactions under the following four headings: *Physical, Emotional, Mental, Behavioural*. Stress tends to have a diverse effect on human functioning. If you find it difficult to identify effects in a particular category, you may be ignoring important signs of stress in your life. Now compare your list with Table 22.1.

Table 22.1 Examples of the effects of stress

Physical	Mental	Emotional	Behavioural
Headache	Forgetfulness	Discontent	Resisting change/
Indigestion	Poor	Anxiety/worry	inflexibility
Tense, tight	concentration	Apprehensive a lot	Cynicism
muscles,	Difficulties with	of the time	Absenteeism
backache,	decision-making	Tearful	Talking a lot
neckache	and thinking	Sense of	Overworking
Sleeplessness	things through	hopelessness	Losing interest
Menstrual	Putting oneself	Irritable, annoyed	easily
problems	down	Angry more of the	Apathy, inertia
Diarrhoea	Beating oneself	time	Withdrawn
Tiredness,	up	Easily exasperated	Destructiveness
exhaustion	Imagining the	More despondent,	Drinking a lot
Restlessness	worst	sad, depressed	Insensitive,
Cold hands and	Changing one's	than usual	impatient with
feet	mind	Helplessness	others
Trembling	Confused,	Resentment	Avoiding people
Jumpiness	muddled	High, excitable	Taking less care
Frequency	Dreaming a lot	Doubt/Uncertainty	with appearance,
Sweating			diet, hygiene
Palpitations			Making mistakes
Tight breathing			Reduced
Pallor			commitment to
			work
			Complaining a lot
			Taking work
			home, 'busy'
			syndrome
			'Indispensable'
			syndrome

Stress, like beauty, is in the eye of the beholder. What we find difficult and stressful in our work, others may find less so. It is not so much that situations are stressful but how we perceive them. Take, for example, a person who despite having disabling problems resents the interventions of mental health staff, seeing them as intrusive and unwanted. Try as the staff may, all they get is abuse. Some helpers might find this behaviour very upsetting and stressful to deal with, perhaps seeing it as a personal rejection or a reflection on their adequacy as a nurse. Others may react differently, perhaps seeing the resistance and abuse in a less personalised way, interpreting it as the expression of the anger the client feels about his loss of control over his life or the oppressive care he has received in the past.

Looking after at-risk clients can be very anxiety provoking for some staff. It may be they are the sort of people who tend to anticipate 'the worst' – to catastrophise

– and as a result adopt a very controlling, directive approach to care. Others may be able to take a more balanced view and allow clients the dignity of risk in order to encourage self-responsibility and wise action. Here again we can see how stress can arise primarily from within.

Sometimes the stress we experience has more to do with some previous, perhaps distant, distressing experience, which is in some way mirrored by the current situation. In this case, we might find that feelings of anxiety, anger or sadness can be restimulated by the current event. If we find ourselves unreasonably upset by a particular person or situation, it is useful to ask ourselves, 'Who does he/she remind me of? When have I been in situations like this before?'. A client's abusive experience, or loss, may remind us of our own and if the issues and feelings around that experience have been incompletely dealt with, then we may find ourselves perturbed by the client's story.

Self-enquiry box

This exercise will help you identify key stressors in your work situation.

Look at this list of stressors and decide which apply to you. Add other stressors not on the list that apply in your own work experience.

- Having little say in what happens
- Frequency of organisational change/restructuring
- Having to deal with difficult behaviour, e.g. hostile behaviour, self-harm behaviour, non-compliant behaviour, high levels of neediness and dependence, high levels of distress
- Lack of appreciation/not being valued
- Cynicism and negative attitudes in others
- Lack of progress or slow pace of therapeutic change
- Increasing bureaucracy involved in delivering care
- High turnover of disturbed distressed clients in inpatient settings
- Heavy caseload of clients with complex problems
- Job responsibility unclear or unreasonable
- Duality of the role; custodian and carer
- Threat of litigation
- Threat of redundancy
- Poor appraisal process
- Not having appropriate skills/lack of opportunities for professional development
- Getting over-attached to clients; clients getting over-attached to you
- Lack of support/supervision within the service
- Target-driven nature of services
- 'Macho' management ethos
- Lack of resources to provide quality care
- Organisational culture and vision clashes with personal vision and values.

Now rate the items on your list with a high/average/low stress rating. Be aware of the number of high to average ratings present in your current work situation.

> Now ask yourself: What needs to change? The situation? The way I think about it? The way I react to it physically/emotionally? Perhaps all three?
>
> Now ask yourself: How am I going to do it? What resources do I have now that I could use? What new strategies could I adopt/learn that would be useful to me?
>
> You may find it helpful to read the rest of this chapter and Chapter 23 and then return to this task.

Most of us have a selection of strategies ranging from the ordinary to the exotic, which we use to manage the stress in our lives. I use the term 'manage' as opposed to 'cope with' or 'resolve' because the former implies treading water and the latter is often unrealistic – not all stress situations are resolvable. But what we can do is to manage the stressful situation and/or ourselves more effectively so that we are mostly on the up slope, making stress work for us rather than against us.

Managing stress more effectively involves answering three questions: What's the problem? What do I want to do about it? How am I going to do it? We have so far been considering the first of these three questions. The second question involves considering what needs to change for me to feel under less stress and pressure. I might decide that what needs to happen is to be able to stay more relaxed in busy, pressured situations or to leave work behind me when I'm off duty or that in amongst the demands of home and work I need some time and space for myself. Perhaps I need to increase the level of support available to me or to reward and nurture myself a bit more or to say what I think and feel about what frustrates me. We can think of these as desired outcomes which, if they were in place, would make a significant difference to our stress levels. Imagining how a situation might realistically change helps us to 'climb out' from under the stress in our lives – to take more charge of our lives.

The third question, 'How am I going to do it?' translates these ideas into action. Let's take 'Being able to stay more relaxed in busy pressured situations' as our desired outcome. We might decide that one helpful piece of action would be to join a yoga class to cultivate a more centred approach to life. We could also learn breathing techniques, which could be used at times when we felt under pressure. We might also try building three 5-minute relaxation periods into our working day – clearing the mind and letting the tension leave the body even for these short periods helps prevent over-stimulation. At home we could try an Alexander technique lie down which is a valuable way of releasing tension and restoring energy. (It involves lying on the floor with two or three paperback books under your head, having your knees bent and feet flat on the floor.) Another strategy we may decide to adopt is to ask for more support from others or to speak to our seniors about an unreasonable workload. These last two strategies may require cultivating some assertiveness skills.

We need to keep in mind when considering how we might take better care of ourselves how often intentions remain just that – intentions. It is helpful to ask ourselves, 'What is going to be my first move? When am I going to do it?'. Enlist the support of someone to help reinforce your commitment. Be aware of some of the things that might prevent you from getting started and from keeping it going. Ask yourself, 'How could I reduce these obstacles?'. Remind yourself of the gains. Reward yourself for your successes. Learn from your setbacks.

Self-enquiry box

This exercise will help you become more aware of your support system.

Take a large sheet of paper. Represent yourself in the centre. Map out all the people and groups that you experience as supportive. Put important sources of support close to you and less important ones further away. Draw in arrows to show whether support is one-way or mutual.

You may find in doing this exercise that you have a good, sustaining support system in your life right now. Conversely, you may find it is somewhat limited. Ask yourself, 'Do I give out a lot but don't receive? Am I open to support? Is the support that I get helpful, i.e. not rescuing, imposing or manipulative?'.

Now ask yourself:

- What are some of the things I could do to strengthen my support system?
- What else, apart from the people in my life, do I draw on for support?

Draw these into your support map. What else might you incorporate into your life that would be supportive?

One of the universal strategies that enable us to feel more comfortable in the reality of our lives is the presence of support: the people, or whatever there is in our lives that provides us with the comfort, encouragement, affirmation and advice that sustains and replenishes us. The extent to which we develop and use a support system is partly determined by our attitude to support. For some people it may have negative associations with weakness, inadequacy or being smothered, while for others support is seen as an enabling, strengthening presence. A supportive relationship is a great resource, but it is unreasonable to expect one person to meet all of our needs. The challenge is to develop and maintain a number of supportive relationships. We may, for example, unload a lot of our work frustrations onto a partner or a close friend when what we need is the support of a trusted colleague who knows our work and can stand with us non-judgementally in our frustrations and joys. Staff support groups can usefully meet this need. Of course, the best care teams *are* supportive to each other but it can be helpful to set aside a specific time each week for the team to review their work, share satisfactions and frustrations, learn from each other's experience and to team-build.

Clearly, it is not just from other people that support comes. We can support ourselves through valuing ourselves more, nurturing ourselves, through our spiritual beliefs, through the sanctuary of home and through replenishing contact with the natural world.

Some strategies for managing stress

- Develop your problem-solving skills. People tend to deny, ignore or muddle through problems with a consequent increase in stress. Confront the problem, explore the issues, decide on some ways forward, take the first step. (See Chapter 11.)

- Develop your assertiveness skills. Considerable stress can be caused by not being able to express your needs, put your point of view, make requests, say no. Be aware of your body/voice. Does it 'collapse' when you make requests or express your needs? Where do your eyes go? Stay relaxed. Get the person's attention. Be specific and concise. Be persistent. Stay in the same gear (don't get irritated or defeated). Give feedback ('Thank you for your time. This is important to me.'). Remember assertiveness is not aggressiveness: aggressiveness *denies* other people their rights and needs, while communicating assertively *respects* them.

- Be aware of how your thinking about stressful situations adds to your discomfort. Learn to use positive inner speech to challenge negative thoughts. For example, if you find yourself often worrying that you haven't done things right or well enough, ask yourself, 'Is there any evidence for thinking that?'. Remind yourself, 'I always do the best I can and my best *is* good enough'. Remind yourself, 'I don't have to be perfect to be valued and accepted'. Be aware of successes, accomplishments and positive outcomes in previous work. Be open to positive feedback from clients and colleagues.

- Notice your breathing. Hyperventilation is a common habit pattern that produces symptoms similar to the stress syndrome. Over-breathing in stress situations exacerbates the symptoms of stress. Slower abdominal breathing quietens and calms the mind and body.

- Learn the art of relaxation. We don't necessarily relax when we sit down to read a book or watch television. Doing a quick 'body check' at these times will raise your awareness of residual tension. Learning and practising mindfulness, meditation, yoga or tai chi can help. Learning the Alexander technique can help you use your body in a more efficient, less stressed way. Slow down the frenetic pace of your life. Spend time in quiet places.

- Nurture yourself: get enough sleep, take care of your nutritional needs, reduce caffeine/alcohol intake, treat yourself to a sauna or massage, take a weekend break, listen to some music, take a long bath, 'shower the day off'. Make yourself a favourite meal, put on your most comfortable clothes. Have some time to yourself. Make love. Enjoy your garden or the countryside. Be self-comforting. Be compassionate and forgiving towards yourself. Go on a retreat or a quiet day.

- Have plenty of distractors in your life – conversation, pastimes, interests, exercise.

- Regular exercise helps by releasing muscle tension and produces endorphins, providing a sense of wellbeing, supporting self-esteem.

- Unburden to a friend or colleague. Talking about a stressful situation helps us to see it more clearly or differently. Having a good shout/cry/swear/laugh helps unload distress and frees us for the next piece of living. Learning co-counselling and participating in a co-counselling network is a useful, more structured way of doing this.

233

- Artistic expression through art, music, dancing can replenish the mind, body and spirit.
- Developing a spiritual dimension to your life through one of the world religions or through a more personal spirituality can be a source of inspiration and strength.
- Develop and maintain a good support system, relationships which are a mutual source of help, advice, encouragement, affirmation.
- Create stability zones and rituals. Build routines and rituals into your day that are sanctuaries from the pressures of everyday life. Taking the dog for a walk, the drive home, pottering in the garden, taking short periods of meditative time out, allowing yourself to be enveloped by a favourite piece of music.
- Open yourself to the beauty of the natural world and the resolute pulse of nature.

 Self-enquiry box

The pleasure list

Think of 20 things that give you pleasure and list them. Now think about how often you allow yourself these pleasures – frequently, occasionally, rarely. Think about whether these pleasures are expensive, inexpensive or cost nothing. Finally think about whether you can enjoy these pleasures alone or whether they require company.

Reflect on your list and how you incorporate pleasure into your life.

 Self-enquiry box

Guided visualisation

Sit quietly for a few minutes. Now imagine yourself walking down a side street in a large city and up ahead you see a building that looks different from all the rest. As you approach, you see above the door a sign which reads 'This Building Is Dedicated to Silence. All Are Welcome.' Imagine yourself opening the door and stepping inside. There in front of you is a large octagonal room. The room is bathed in soft coloured light from stained glass windows. There are comfortable chairs placed around the room and you find one and sit down. As you sit there you become aware of an enveloping calm. You become aware of the peacefulness that surrounds you. Picture yourself sitting comfortably in this quiet peaceful space. Picture yourself relaxed, immersed in this oasis of calm. Imagine yourself refreshed by the silence that surrounds you. Imagine yourself restored by the soothing tranquillity that surrounds you.

When you are ready, imagine yourself unhurriedly getting up, walking out of the room, opening the door and stepping back into the street. Be aware of the calmness, the peacefulness that you are taking with you. Be aware that you can return to this place at any time.

Being a reflective practitioner

Why bother with supervision? Firstly, supervision is a significant source of support where we can focus on the difficulties, challenges and successes of our work and have our supervisor share some of the responsibility. Secondly, it forms part of our continuing learning as a professional. As Casement (1985) comments, 'As professionals we are in a process of becoming, that begins, continues, but never ends'. Douglas Winnicott, the paediatrician and psychoanalyst, famously spoke about the 'good enough mother', observing that it would be difficult for any mother to be 'good enough' in the face of the emotional and physical demands of the maternal role if she did not have the support of a husband or some other supportive adult. He referred to this triangular relationship as the 'nursing triad' and it offers a useful analogy for supervisory relationships. For practitioners to be effective – 'good enough' helpers – there is a need for a therapeutic triad within which the distress, disturbance and the psychodynamics that are played out in helping relationships can be safely held and explored. This is provided by supervision.

As we have seen in a previous chapter, the shadow side of helping needs to be an acknowledged presence if the care we provide is not to degenerate into an interaction in which meeting our own needs is the predominant, if unconscious, motivation. Whilst I believe it to be true that there is an altruistic trait and a capacity for genuine compassion that motivates many of us to spend our working lives in the helping professions, there are also undoubtedly other motives at play that draw us towards a caring vocation. The need for personal power is one obvious motivation that may manifest itself in the dynamics of the helping relationship, leading to authoritative, oppressive, disempowering care. Similarly we may not recognise our own dependency needs, projecting them onto clients and thus holding them in a state of passive helplessness. Also part of the shadow is our woundedness – the turbulence and trauma held in our own psyche – and it has long been recognised that it is the quest for healing that prompts many to become mental health practitioners (Barker et al 1998, Hawkins & Shohet 2000). None of this matters if we can raise our consciousness of these personal needs and wounds; if we can work awarely and congruently with clients and not do our personal healing work vicariously through them.

⭐ A personal story

A few years ago I found myself noticing that my feelings for a number of clients that I was working with at the time had seemingly intensified. Where there had once been a warm regard there was now a feeling that I recognised as love. This I found somewhat disturbing as love seems a misplaced emotion in the context of helping relationships – or at least according to the dispassionate psychiatric literature. I should add that one of the clients was a woman younger than me and although I felt some sexual attraction I had no desire to sexualise my relationship with her. Neither did I have any desire for exclusivity in my relationship with her – it did not feel a possessive kind of love. I felt very moved by her struggle to survive and to hold on to her sanity. I cared about her deeply but at the same time did not feel I was acting out some archetypal rescue fantasy or that I could release her from the storms of emotional pain that used to flood her psyche and plunge her into a despairing psychotic world. What I was conscious of was a deep need within her to feel loved – something she had not found in her abusive parental relationships or in her adult life. Love of course is best represented as an adjective because it is in acts of loving that it is communicated. There were many times when I wanted to express what I felt for her in physical contact, in affectionate words, yet I felt restrained from doing so, afraid of how that disclosure would be received.

As a much younger man my feelings of love had been rather muted and my expressions of love undemonstrative. This changed gradually as my children came along, but it has never been a feeling I have been comfortable with. There seemed such danger in that feeling somehow – bringing with it the risk of loss or rejection by the object of my affection or the fear that my own need for love was somehow too demanding, not legitimate. I should say that in my older adult life I have felt truly loved and I do not feel a pressing need to seek affection, love and regard through my working relationships.

I use this scenario to illustrate how emotionally unclear the interaction can be in therapeutic engagement with people in the psychiatric arena and how good supervision can be invaluable in reflecting on complex interpersonal issues in the therapeutic use of self. There were two outcomes from exploring this scenario in supervision. One was that I needed to be congruent in my contacts with her; it was important that she knew how I felt towards her, that I was not coming on to her and that I required nothing from her in return. It was simply the loving feeling of one human being for another. This was difficult for her to accept – there was distrust and some drawing back initially – she had been hurt too many times before, and I think felt happier with a more neutral professional relationship. Then she became more demanding and testing; if I was unable to respond to her immediate need she became quite angry, accusatory and dismissive. But gradually over time the disclosure of my feelings seemed to allow her to value herself more, to see herself as lovable and to comfort the hurt child within who had felt 'bad' and deserving of the mistreatment she experienced. The second outcome was a personal one – it felt to me as if I had been given a gift. Whatever it was in the dynamic of our relationship that penetrated my deepest defences, it drew out of me a profound feeling of love that somehow seemed unbounded, a slightly mystical experience which had hitherto been unavailable to me in my life.

The quest for a learning culture

For some time I have been puzzled by the fact that while the psychiatric professions have been talking about supervision for the past 30 years, promoting it as desirable, if not as a requirement for professional practice, it has still yet to become widely embedded within services. The reason for this is likely to be found in the prevailing culture of the organisation. Hawkins & Shohet (2000), in their excellent book on supervision for the helping professions, argue that it is the work culture that determines whether supervision is seen as having priority and value. They outline some examples of organisational dynamics that hinder the implementation of supervision throughout the service.

In some organisations the mindset about supervision is that it is indicative of problems. People say 'I don't need supervision this month I haven't got any particular problems'. Often it is reserved for students and junior staff and seen as unnecessary for more senior grades. Other organisations tend to give high priority to tasks and low priority to personnel. In strongly hierarchical cultures, where managerial supervision is given, there is often a defensive attitude. Staff may cover up difficulties, deny high stress levels or feelings of being overwhelmed by the demands of their caseload, fearing that they may jeopardise their prospects and professional standing.

Some organisations seem crisis prone. There is always some incipient crisis, or a very demanding work schedule to be met, that leads to supervision being squeezed out. Dealing with crises and managing a heavy caseload can seem like a badge of honour that meets staff needs to feel a valued and able professional. It is not only clients that create or perpetuate a crisis or a high level of need in order to feel worthy of care but staff too may collude in this process. There are also organisations that develop addictive cultures. Work becomes the predominant way in which employees give their life meaning, meet their emotional needs or resolve anxieties about being good enough; they work long hours, always have full diaries, take on more and more work, create dependency and an illusion of omniscience, losing the balance between work and leisure. Often others in the team will collude with this kind of addictive behaviour as co-dependants.

Such organisational dynamics are not uncommon and it would be difficult for supervision to become firmly rooted in these kinds of cultures. For supervision to flourish, the team or organisation needs to evolve in the direction of becoming a learning culture. In learning cultures:

- Supervision goes through the organisation and is seen as being as necessary for senior grades as for junior staff.
- Learning is not seen as something that takes place only in the classroom. All experience is seen as an opportunity for learning through engagement in cycles of reflection.
- Problems are seen as particularly important learning opportunities.
- Supervision is not seen simply as a context in which the supervisee and supervisor bring theoretical perspectives to bear on clinical issues but more as an opportunity for dialogical learning in which new knowledge may emerge from the collaborative enquiry that takes place.

- There are regular team development days.
- Space for informal reflection and discussion on the work.
- Encouragement to engage in action research.
- Self-appraisal refined and validated by feedback from managers and peers.
- It is a self-renewing culture in which the way things are done is continually being influenced by staff at all levels in the organisation.

Being a supervisee

It is all too easy to slide into a passive, aggrieved state of mind, feeling unsupported with little opportunity for change and development. There is, I believe, a case for mental health workers to be more proactive in getting more of what they need to function more effectively in their professional role. There are a number of options for getting supervision – from peer-group supervision to one-to-one supervision with a senior colleague from another part of the service (see Box 23.1).

Being proactive starts with what Casement calls 'self-supervision'. In recent years the term reflective practice has crept into the vocabulary of nursing as a valued criterion of professionalism. Learning from experience begins with the ability to notice and reflect awarely on what happens in our interactions with patients and clients. This is a skill that deepens with practice. Johns (1993) defines professional supervision as 'the milieu in which reflective practice is facilitated'. This process of self-supervision involves asking reflective questions: 'What did I do and say?' 'Why did I intervene as I did?' 'What did the client do and say?' 'What was I feeling?' 'How did the client feel?' 'What was the outcome?' 'What other choices did I have?' 'How do I feel now about the experience?' 'What have I learnt?'. This reflection on the process of care can be enhanced if supervisees write up significant interpersonal events in a log or journal.

Being proactive does not stop with setting up some form of supervision. We need to be active in taking our share of responsibility for ensuring we get the

238

Box 23.1

Supervision options

- Regular one-to-one supervision with a team leader/line manager
- Regular one-to-one supervision with an experienced colleague from another discipline or team
- Regular one-to-one supervision with a supervisor from outside the organisation
- Regular one-to-one supervision with a peer (sharing time equally in role of supervisor/supervisee)
- Peer-group supervision with clinical team leader or outside facilitator/supervisor or rotating facilitation responsibilities
- On-line supervision, here and now through the use of a web cam or retrospectively through written reflections

supervision we want. This involves negotiating and contracting. It is important that both supervisor and supervisee communicate with each other their view of the purpose of the sessions and explore how far their expectations match, including their initial hopes and fears. Boundaries need to be established by clarifying the frequency and duration of sessions, the sort of issues it is appropriate to bring, the question of confidentiality, managerial requirements and how supervision is to be evaluated.

Supervision for many mental health professionals represents a shift in practice habits and, as with any change, there can be blocks that prevent the desired outcome being realised. The blocks may be internal:

- Supervisees may feel themselves to be in an anxious, vulnerable position – the supervisory relationship, however benign and equal, is always likely to restimulate experiences of previous relationships with authority figures.
- Dependence/Independence issues surface, to which the supervisee may react by surrendering their autonomy or conversely by becoming resistant to feedback and guidance.
- There are likely to be anxieties about being judged. Supervision can evoke the 'inner critic', threatening to leave the supervisee feeling demoralised and de-skilled.
- Supervision commonly has false connotations of being told what to do, of having one's work overseen. Qualified professionals may also feel that their status and competence is detracted from rather than enhanced by having supervision.

The blocks may be external:

- The organisational culture of the psychiatric professions places a high value on emotional control and coping behaviour, which may not be conducive to supervision. This is understandable given the nature of the work, but if these attributes are over-emphasised, they detract from the humanity of staff. The essential fallibility and vulnerability of the person in the professional role can get masked and the 'real self' alienated. This can lead to professional detachment in which the person is hardly visible in the role, an engagement style not conducive to the development of therapeutic relationships.
- Mental health workers tend to collude in not recognising each other's stresses and problems. It seems that the profession whose business it is to care for others is notoriously bad at caring for its own workers.
- The dual role of line manager and supervisor may present problems and create blocks in the supervision process. There may be trust issues: 'How much of myself and my practice can I safely expose to someone whose managerial responsibilities include monitoring and appraising my work?'. Where the managerial task is seen essentially as enabling and the power held is based on relationship and expertise rather than position, then clinical supervision by line managers can be effective.

A further issue in managerial supervision is that the supervisee may experience a conflict between the organisational priorities and objectives for which the

239

manager has responsibility and their own. A consequence of this can be that the focus of the supervision dialogue becomes restricted or worse, degenerates into a 'checking ritual' of visits made, strategies implemented and outcomes recorded.

The role of supervisor

Many different grades of staff find themselves in a supervisory role. Senior practitioners, service managers, team leaders, academics are examples. Given the misconceptions that exist about the role of the supervisor, it is important that supervisors of clinical and casework practice are clear about the role a supervisor plays and are adequately prepared. Part of that preparation is to be aware of the underlying needs and issues that the supervisor may seek to meet through the supervisory relationship, with these possibly being detrimental to the process as a learning experience for the supervisee. For instance, the need for power or affirmation may be expressed in the supervisory relationship by the supervisor adopting a guru-like status. Vertical relationships in strongly hierarchical and patriarchal organisations such as hospitals and community health care services do not lend themselves to relationships in which collaboration on a basis of equality and mutual respect for the other's professional autonomy can easily flourish. As Johns identifies, there needs to be a shift in the emphasis of the manager's role from delegator and supervisor of work to enabler. A similar shift in emphasis would apply to the academic engaged in supervision – in this case from didactic teacher to facilitator of student-centred learning.

The key to good supervision is the relationship between supervisor and supervisee. In that sense it is analogous to the helper/client relationship and, just as in the psychotherapeutic alliance, the relationship is part of the therapy, so in a similar way the relationship in supervision is a key learning opportunity. The supervisee learns about enabling relationships through being in one. It needs to be stressed, however, that while the relationship may mirror the therapeutic alliance, the focus of the relationship is educational rather than therapeutic. Clearly, personal issues arising out of the supervisee's work experience which have a bearing on their professional effectiveness will quite legitimately be a focus for the supervision dialogue. A danger here is that the supervisee may be filling an unacknowledged need for counselling. Equally, the supervisor may be acting out a need to demonstrate their therapeutic skill or to prove their worth. In this scenario supervision would become more like therapy.

Butterworth & Faugier (1992) suggest the role and function of the supervisor is to encourage personal and educational growth and provide support for clinical autonomy. Hawkins & Shohet (2000) see the supervisor's role as a synthesis of education, support and management.

The educative function of supervision is concerned with developing the skills and understandings of the supervisee. This can be achieved through a process of guided reflection on their work with clients and patients. Through this exploration the supervisee gathers insights into the dynamics of their interaction with clients. They can explore the meaning of the client's behaviour and the meaning the client's behaviour has for them; how they intervened; the outcomes of that intervention and alternative ways of responding to this and similar client behaviour. This is not a process in which the task of supervisor is to be the all-knowing expert. While interpretation and guidance from the supervisor may be valued and helpful, the primary task of the supervisor is to facilitate critical thinking.

Didactic and prescriptive supervision may lead to what Schon (1991) refers to as a 'learning bind' in which both the educator and learner adopt stances which impede professional growth: 'an open dialogue, in which the learner's experience and intuitive knowing is valued fails to develop, and the learner feels in awe of the educator's mastery and expertise'. It can be helpful if supervisors are prepared to openly acknowledge their own puzzlement. As Lidmila (1992) comments, 'If the supervisor can accept his own puzzlement it will help practitioners accept their own limitations without feeling inadequate simply because they are confused about a client's behaviour or have made an intervention error'.

The supportive function of the supervisor is concerned with helping the supervisee to take care of themselves. Psychiatric practice is emotional work. Feelings arise through empathising with the clients, through encountering clients whose experience contains echoes of our own past or present, or simply through a direct experience of the anguish and suffering that is part of mental health care. While feelings often have to be put on one side in order to function effectively, not attending to those feelings leads to the development of defensive strategies for staying distant from patients, to the accumulation of stress and ultimately to burnout. Smith, in her study of the 'emotional labour of nursing', concludes that nurses are better able to care for patients when they felt cared for themselves by trained staff and teachers. Faugier (1992), in identifying some of the characteristics of the effective supervisor, comments on the need for the supervisor to be open to and able to stay with the feelings the supervisee brings.

The culture of the psychiatric professions has traditionally been non-cathartic, with emotional control and coping being excessively valued. Bringing personal feelings into the supervision dialogue can be threatening if a 'safe base' has not been established in the form of a relationship of trust; anxieties about being seen as over-emotional, over-involved, unable to cope or not tough-minded enough, may surface. It is important that supervisors are able to promote the view that an acknowledgement of feelings is both a strength and a constituent part of good practice in the human relations dimension of health care. We cannot treat people with sensitivity and compassion if we deny our own humanity.

The managerial function is concerned primarily with quality assurance. Many supervisors will have a responsibility to their organisation for the delivery of effective and ethical care and meet that responsibility through the supervision of practitioners' caseloads. This may involve looking at assessment data, care plans, strategies and progress notes. There is a responsibility to respond to unsafe and unethical practice and to temper therapeutic idealism with realistic optimism. However, the main task is to collaborate with the supervisee in reviewing their performance with the intention of enabling the practitioner to provide therapeutic care of a high standard. There may be some conflict of interest between the practitioner's ideas and aspirations and the organisation's vision of the service that can be provided. This conflict will need to be addressed and managed if the practitioner is to stay committed to the work and not become cynical and disillusioned.

As has been emphasised, it is the relationship that is the key to good supervision. Hawkins & Shohet (2000) have commented that the skills and characteristics that supervisors need are similar to those required for counselling. Many identify characteristics that are akin to the 'core conditions for effective helping' (empathy, congruence, openness, genuineness, respect, warmth, acceptance) originated by Carl Rogers in his extensive writing and in his therapeutic and educational work (Kirschenbaum & Henderson 1990). It would seem important that supervisors are able to communicate these qualities in their work with practitioners for the unfolding of personal and professional potential to take place.

Heron's interpersonal skills model, Six Category Intervention Analysis (2001), has value as a framework for developing a supervision dialogue. The model identifies a cluster of skills, which have a common intention and are accordingly grouped into one of six categories.

- Catalytic interventions, including active listening skills, questioning and reflective responses, are concerned with eliciting self-discovery talk.
- Challenging interventions, which may involve giving feedback, correcting or disagreeing, playing 'devil's advocate' and asking confronting questions. They are concerned with raising the supervisee's awareness of blind spots, such as unhelpful patterns of behaviour, thinking errors, deficiencies and strengths, unsafe or unwise practice and successes.
- Supportive interventions, which will have the intention to validate and affirm the supervisee and their work.
- Cathartic interventions, such as 'giving permission', empathic responding, literal description, re-enactment and the judicious use of touch and proximity, which are intended to assist the supervisee to verbalise and discharge feelings appropriately and safely. They may help the practitioner go into unacknowledged feelings being held on the edge of awareness which are relevant to the issues being discussed. Heron makes the important point that suppressed feelings act as a screen preventing us from seeing a situation as clearly as we might or from a different perspective. In addition they will trap energy which would otherwise be free for problem-solving. Hence new insights and understandings are likely to emerge from cathartic work.
- Informative interventions, which are concerned with providing information and interpretations relevant to the needs and interests of the supervisee. As has been noted earlier, when this is overdone it impedes the development of critical thinking and the growth of professional confidence and autonomy. On the other hand, if it is underdone, it can hold the supervisee in a disempowered state.
- Prescriptive interventions, which are ways of responding that assist the supervisee to find the way forward. The supervisor collaborates in a process of creative problem-solving, suggesting alternative ways of managing problems presented by the client or patient. As Heron points out, the style in which prescriptive interventions are made follows a continuum from consultative at one end to authoritative at the other. With this in mind, it is important that supervision does not perpetuate what Lidmila (1992) refers to as the infantile fantasy of 'omnipotent narcissism in the supervisor and idealisation in the supervisee'.

The narrative accounts of our work that we share in supervision are often problem laden. The problem is commonly located within ourselves as practitioners, rather than the relationship or the organisational context, and leads to conclusions of inadequacy or failure. According to White (1997), the narrative accounts that are shared are often 'thin' descriptions of practice and seldom represent the richness of a practitioner's work. He argues that the supervision can be seen as a re-authoring conversation in which 'negative truths' about practice can be deconstructed.

There are times when our work as mental health nurses seems hardly worthwhile; when it seems to achieve little; when the client seems 'lost' to their illness or retreats behind a wall of resistance and refuses to engage in the helping/healing process. There are times when the experiences of people seeking help seem crushing and insurmountable. There are times when we feel drained with seemingly nothing left to give. It is because the helping relationship can be so depleting that good supervision has such a vital role to play in replenishing practitioners and maintaining effective and innovative practice.

Self-enquiry box

Figure 23.1 outlines one way of thinking about the factors that influence our performance as practitioners. Consider which quadrant best reflects your experience. How might your supervision help change that experience?

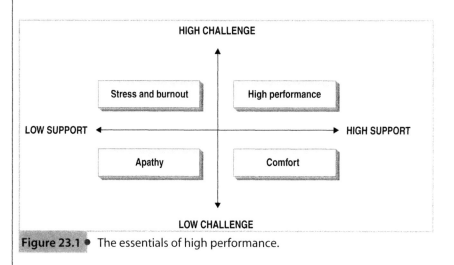

Figure 23.1 ● The essentials of high performance.

Appendix
A brief introduction to humanistic psychology

This book is largely rooted in humanistic psychology and it occurred to me that it might be helpful to include an outline of what humanistic psychology is and is not in this second edition, as many colleagues will not have encountered – a good humanistic word – this approach to understanding the nature of being human. It should be said that this is no easy task since the Human Potential Movement, as it was once known, is a broad church, including many different psychotherapeutic disciplines and many different theories of the emergent self and the dynamics of being human under its umbrella. Nevertheless we will not be too daunted by that fact and try to identify some common themes running through its constituent elements. For a more detailed overview, John Rowan's imaginative grasp of the breadth and depth of humanistic psychology is difficult to better (Rowan 2001).

Historical background

Most authorities would agree that the seeds of humanistic psychology germinated in the 1950s as a reaction by leading academic psychologists against a reductionist view of human behaviour as seen through the lens of psychoanalysis and behaviourism. There was a strong sense that these perspectives did not capture what it means to be fully human, did not recognise the innate capacity for socially constructive behaviour and potential for creative living. Leading figures in the inception of this new branch of psychology were Abraham Maslow, Rollo May and Carl Rogers – all greatly respected academics – and in the case of Rogers and May also pioneering figures in radical new approaches to psychotherapy. Their vision had been shaped by a fusion of Eastern ideas, where there is little distinction between spiritual, philosophical and psychological realms of thought and enquiry, and the challenging ideas of existential philosophy and phenomenology that captured the minds of many Western intellectuals in the second half of the 20th century.

Humanistic psychology emerged at a time when the austerity of the war years was beginning to recede and a spirit of freedom was in the air. Social convention and traditional values in many arenas of life were being joyously challenged. One way in which that freedom began to express itself was in an exploration of our potential as human beings, including extra-ordinary states of consciousness, which Maslow famously termed peak experiences. Personal development became a legitimate aspiration – not just educational attainment, socialisation and culturalisation, but a pursuit of cognitive, emotional, sexual, social and spiritual liberation and growth. While this has often been criticised as a having given rise to a narcissistically obsessed generation, at its core the Human Potential Movement had strong social values, sharing Carl Jung's belief that if you want to change the world you must first change yourself.

Because many humanistic ideas pose a radical challenge to the conservatism and hierarchy of the university systems, humanistic psychology has not become embedded in mainstream academia. Nevertheless it does have a respected and influential presence in some UK universities, mainly in faculties of education or management offering courses in counselling, human relations and in personal and organisational development – notably the University of East Anglia, Nottingham University and the University of Surrey.

The British Association for Humanistic Psychology in Britain and its practitioner branch, The Association for Humanistic Psychology Practitioners, provide a forum for the exploration and dissemination of humanistic ideas through the journal *Self and Society*, through networking and conferences, and seeks to enhance professional development and standards of practice through an accreditation system for humanistic practitioners (www.ahpb.org.uk).

Humanistic therapy

In the psychotherapeutic field, person-centred therapy, originated by Carl Rogers, one of the most influential psychologists of the 20th century (Thorne 1992), is still the most widely practised form of counselling in the UK but has remained largely outside the psychiatric system. There are two main reasons for this. Firstly, the concept of pathological distress and differentness is anathema to most humanistic practitioners, a theme taken up and explored in this book. Secondly, there remains an erroneous belief that person-centred approaches are ineffectual in helping people with severe and disabling distress. There is in fact substantial research supporting the efficacy of person-centred approaches to growth and healing (Bozarth & Motomasa 2005) and not just for those who succumb to the emotional backwash from the everyday problems of living but also for individuals experiencing more severe and enduring forms of psychological overwhelm (Sommerbeck 2005). Increasingly humanistic therapists and authors are arguing for humanistic practitioners to step more visibly into the arena of psychiatric care and to engage in a dialogue with the psychiatric professions about alternative conceptions of human distress and healing (Joseph & Worsley 2005, Watkins 2007).

Person-centred therapy, discussed in some depth in this book, is just one of many well-established approaches to psychotherapeutic helping that are strongly underpinned by humanistic values and beliefs. Gestalt therapy originated by Fritz Perls sees human development as a continuing process of creative, holistic adaptation. Habitual patterns of response to the challenges and opportunities of living, or fixed gestalts, diminish versatility and lead to dysfunctional ways of being. Immediacy – what a person is experiencing 'here and now' – and increasing awareness of that experience are the focus of gestalt therapy and the precursors of change (see Clarkson 2004). Focusing based on the work of Eugene Gendlin uses the concept of the *felt sense* experienced in the body/mind as a starting point for the resolution of problems of living and as a catalyst for personal growth and change (Gendlin 1981). Psychosynthesis, which developed from the work of Roberto Assagioli, infuses psychology of the person with a sense of soul and meaning. It is an approach to self-realisation which seeks to help people discover their spiritual nature and apply this discovery to everyday life (Whitmore 2004). Co-counselling, based on the work of Harvey Jackins, has a core belief that old hurts and accompanying distress get laid down in the body/mind and result in distorted ways of thinking, feeling and doing in a wide range of situations. They restrict a more flexible innovative response to changing circumstances as an adult. In the therapeutic process, which is mediated through reciprocal peer counselling, distress is released in catharsis allowing re-evaluation of past hurts to take place (see www.co-counselling.org.uk).

Humanistic groups

Group work remains an important facet of human potential work. The most widely practised humanistic groups are encounter groups – a term derived from existentialism meaning *a real meeting between people*. In *basic encounter* developed by Carl Rogers the core conditions for growth and change – empathy, congruence and acceptance – are created in the group, establishing a safe space within which members can interact in increasingly authentic ways (Rogers 1970). During a session individuals will work on issues that will have a resonance for several people in the group. The principle underlying this is that the deeper we go in an exploration of our humanness the more universal the experience is. Often – particularly early in the life of a group – the group dynamic will be a catalyst for an exploration of issues around trust, intimacy, alienation, acceptance which may be key themes in an individual's interpersonal life outside the group. It is not the leader's role to direct the group but rather to be authentically present and facilitate group interactions as they emerge in ways that enable members to encounter themselves and others more deeply. *Open encounter*, which has its origins in the work of Will Schultz, takes on a more interventionist style. Here the leader goes with the energy of the group; if a particular issue seems to generate energy within the individual and the group it becomes the focus for the work. The leader may suggest ways of working more deeply and fully on the issue, using techniques derived from different psychotherapeutic models such as gestalt, psychodrama and drama therapy (Schultz 1973, 1989). As with basic encounter, ground rules are established which permit and regulate the openness of the group interaction (see Rowan 2001 for a useful overview). A great deal of holistic learning goes on in well-facilitated encounter groups; members examine their presentation of self in everyday life and learn a more aware and authentic way of being. This may be a process that involves some pain but ultimately is joyful and liberating.

Psychotherapeutic approaches in the humanistic tradition trust the continuing capacity of human beings for creative adaptation; for growth and change; for constructive and resourceful living. They stress the responsibility of the individual to be self-directing in the change process. There is respect for an individual's personal reality, which is not interpreted according to the therapist's theoretical beliefs. Instead the therapeutic process enables the individual to distil meaning from their own lived experience – every person is seen as the author of their own lives. The presence of the psychotherapeutic helper is a facilitative one – a companion on a healing and growthful journey, rather than an authoritative expert offering solutions to human suffering. In the case of co-counselling and focusing, the role of therapist is dispensed with in favour of teaching people strategies for being their own (and others') agent for healing and change.

Education

Another arena in which humanistic psychology has been influential is in education and training. The humanistic approach to education, or affective education as it is sometimes called, posed a radical challenge to the traditional power structures in education and to teacher-centred learning in the 1970s and 1980s with the role of teachers growing more facilitative and student-centred. Classrooms then become not simply places where the intellect and cognitive skills develop but places where the uniqueness of the individual flourishes; where self-esteem and confidence are nurtured; where personal and social responsibility are fostered; and where imagination and creativity are encouraged. They are places where students learn the most important lesson, that of becoming resourceful learners, able to be increasingly self-directing in their quest for understanding, and in the process experience the joy of learning. The fact that this now sounds familiar and representative of many classrooms signifies the change that has taken place – 30 years ago classrooms were dominated by didactic, autocratic teaching styles and schools governed in a hierarchical way. There has perhaps been some drift back towards pedagogic teaching in our target-driven times but the culture of the classroom has been irrevocably changed by humanistic ideas (Rogers & Freiberg 1994).

Organisational development

Traditionally the culture of organisations was dominated by hierarchical structures in which power, from the top down, was often used oppressively. The concern for the task was high and the concern for people low. Research over the past forty years has consistently shown that hierarchical structures are damaging to people (Rowan 2001). Within such organisations people's sense of job fulfilment, of occupational wellbeing, of their value to the organisation, of their influence on the organisation's change and growth and their sense of commitment and motivation are all low. Not surprisingly, conflicts, anxieties, resentments and boredom in these cultures are high. The vision that came from humanistic psychology was that it didn't have to be like this, that organisations, just like individuals, could change in ways that released more of their potential. Essentially this flows from management styles that are more people-centred, from introducing consultative decision-making and recognising the human needs and aspirations of the workforce. One of the extraordinary things about organisations in which structures have developed which allow and encourage open communication and collaborative decision-making across the organisation is that energy increases synergistically and is available for creative problem-solving, implementing change and improving the effectiveness of services. Humanistic practitioners working as consultants in organisational development also bring some focus to the 'alignment' of the workforce with the vision and values of the organisation; the 'attunement' of people to each other which helps strengthen and harmonise relationships and enables the workplace to evolve towards becoming an 'empowerment' culture.

Research

Despite several decades of research in the field of psychology and sociology, relatively little of value has been contributed to the knowledge and practice of psychiatry since the 1960s when the inspired work of a group of contemporary psychiatrists coalesced into social psychiatry and revolutionised mental hospitals. Research has been dominated by biomedical studies oriented towards identifying the role of neurological deficits in psychosocial dysfunction and their drug treatment. Social science research has been scant and psychological research has been almost exclusively confined to refining and validating cognitive behavioural approaches to mental health problems. Part of the problem is that the research scene has maintained a certain exclusiveness, perpetuating the view that all *serious* research is done by academics and scientists based in universities, that blue ribbon research is empirical research and almost all other research designs should be viewed with incredulity.

So much qualitative psychosocial research lacks a human quality because it objectifies people. The researcher attempts in some way to capture and interpret some facet of human experience but ultimately fails because they are unable to uncover the fullness of the lived experience. Humanistic researchers would argue that what is required is research data that comes direct from the experience of the individual subject and is not filtered through a researcher. This has led to exciting new research paradigms that include cooperative enquiry (Heron & Reason 2000) and action research (McNiff & Whitehead 2006). These research methodologies have an enormous contribution to make to mental health care, creating opportunities for practitioners and service users to contribute to the development of practice and the advancement or reconfiguration of knowledge.

Humanistic ideas – a subversive paradigm

While some of the radicalism has disappeared from the Human Potential Movement it is still, in my view, positioned at the leading edge of human evolution, at both the individual and social level, and chronicles what is emergent in the condition of being human. It is subversive because its ideas challenge convention, orthodoxy, dogma – the 'immutable truths' that bind us to the status quo, limiting the vision and expansion of the psyche and our capacity to live creative and harmonious lives.

Personal power

Most of what is alluded to in the above paragraph centres on the way power is held and used. Our lives are lived out as an integral part of many systems in which the power dynamic has an enormous influence on our way of being. Power – political, social and personal – can be co-created and shared and is the wellspring of vital, resourceful living; but so often power is held and used in a way that diminishes and subjugates others. We see this in cabinet government into which the democratic voice of public representatives fails to penetrate, leaving citizens feeling politically marginalised, impotent and disillusioned; we see it in schools where pedagogic approaches to teaching are predominant, subduing the spirit of discovery and the emergence of self-directed, resourceful learning; we see it in health care where the power is held by authoritative experts in ever narrowing fields of expertise in which the whole person is never seen and the patient – as expert by experience of their own history of wellbeing – has no voice; we see it in the hierarchical power structures of organisations where macho management styles prevail and workers are slaves to targets, profit margins, dividends and executive bonuses; we see it in families where parents are unable to co-create sufficient parental power to provide a secure base for children to flourish or where one adult holds and uses power abusively.

Humanistic psychology upholds the power of the individual. Personal power is the source from which self-actualisation, self-efficacy and self-assertion flow into resourceful living. Carl Rogers, in a visionary book on personal power, a book that is as pertinent today as when it was first published, sees empowerment as the foundation for a *quiet revolution* in our institutions (Rogers 1978b). He points to a society in which inner strength is co-created and sustained in our families, schools and colleges, in the workplace and in our political institutions. Such a society would be one in which we assumed more responsibility for our own learning, became joyful seekers of understanding and creators of new knowledge; a society in which our voice was heard in the workplace and where we had some tangible influence on the growth and wellbeing of our organisation; a political system in which the power of the individual, enshrined in democratic principles, was not diminished by the remote centralisation of power and where the flow of public opinion informed political decisions. And in the mental health care system, which would be founded on an empowerment culture, people would recognise their inner strength and capacity for self-healing, transforming relationships with health professionals from passive recipients to active participants in care and recovery.

Holism

Holism is deeply embedded in the thinking of humanistic practitioners. Human beings are seen as open systems, a premise at the core of Eastern medicine that holds that mind, body and spirit are interrelated dimensions of the self and that the harmonious functioning of the whole is essential for health and wellbeing. The psychosomatic nature of many health problems is now widely accepted in conventional medicine, but the spiritual dimension of wellbeing less so, despite the fact that more and more people are now engaged in a search to find a spiritual core in a materialistic, hedonistic era offering only transient happiness and wellbeing. Our integral inner system is part of the larger social system and a larger still ecological system by which we are influenced and in turn have an influence. Much has been said in this book about the impact of the social and ecological conditions on our wellbeing. We cannot expect health and wellbeing if we become alienated from (as we have), or damage (as we are doing), the eco-systems of which we are a part and which sustain us. The *bad place we are in*, as James Hillman (1995) so rightly observed, does not refer to our state of mind so much as to the state of our world.

Holism has become identified with the 'New Age' culture that overlaps with and shares many of the ideas embedded in humanistic psychology. For some it is in the alternative 'New Age' culture that the radicalism of humanistic psychology now resides. Many who wholeheartedly embrace 'New Age' culture live out their values in a 'once removed' coexistence with the broad stream of convention. Others in the Human Potential Movement prefer to integrate into systems that provide structure to our society – the educational system, the health care system – and influence them from the inside. The politics of this can be seen in the twin concepts of alternative and complementary medicine. The alternative faction holds views that are often diametrically opposed to the ideas that inform science-based health practice and the conventions that regulate it. They regard anecdotal evidence of positive outcomes for clients as sufficient validation of their methods. Under this umbrella are found many esoteric therapies that work on the subtle energy systems of the body/mind. It is interesting that the metaphysical nature of ideas underlying these therapies is now beginning to have some cogency in the light of developments in quantum physics. This involves the concept of non-localised energy (Dossey 2001), that is energy fields not localised to the body but that radiate out and may be transmissible from one person to another. Transmissible energy may prove to be the therapeutic basis of many holistic healing practices. Other holistic therapists are more integrative and see the therapy they offer as complementary to evidence-based medical interventions. Many of these holistic practitioners are attempting to validate their approach to restoring health through rigorous methodological enquiry and seek to give their status credibility through a system of professional accreditation, registration and regulation.

An evidence base for the efficacy of holistic therapy does not seem so important to the many people who use it, if the growth of the alternative and complementary therapy sector is anything to go by. One cannot but think that people find in the presence of the therapist and in the total experience of the therapy session something that is vitally missing from most medical consultations. Quite apart from whether various techniques or interventions are effective, it is my contention that many therapists have a healing presence, a way of being with people that facilitates a release and relief from tensions held in the body/mind, allowing the natural healing processes to begin and a state of balance and wellbeing to be restored. Psychotherapy research seems to suggest that 40% of the positive outcome is attributable to a client's innate resources and 30% to the relationship with the therapist. The particular techniques or theoretical orientation of the therapist seem of little importance (Bozarth & Motomasa 2005).

Self-actualisation

Self-actualisation, one of the fundamental beliefs of humanistic psychology, is a belief in the innate capacity of humans to develop and grow in the direction of self-realisation. Maslow (1970) described this organismic growth as the actualising tendency in which our potential to become fully functioning individuals unfolds. This urge to become what we may become is a continuing force although it expresses itself most advantageously in a nurturing, facilitative social environment and can be impeded and distorted in unfavourable circumstances. Rogers talks about the conditions of worth imposed by significant others as a major factor in shaping and limiting the unfolding self (Mearns & Thorne 2000). Few of us ever express our full potential for living and being; few of us ever become fully functioning individuals, but humanistic psychologists take the view that this aspiration gives meaning and purpose to our lives as sentient human beings. Not only is each one of us charged with the responsibility for our own self-realisation but we hold a collective responsibility for the growth and flourishing of others. This facilitative process takes place in the intimate bonds of family relationships and in the wider social matrix of our lives.

Goodness and sinfulness

Ever since the well-documented difference of opinion between Rollo May and Carl Rogers about the potential for good and evil in the psyche of humankind (Kirschenbaum & Henderson 1990), the debate has continued within the canon of humanistic literature (Mearns & Thorne 2000, Worsley 2005). Psychology, like the Church, has tended to see humankind as afflicted by original sin, as having an innate tendency towards antisocial behaviour and in need of moral education enforced by the law. Despite the seemingly limitless capacity of humankind to inflict harm, Rogers took the view that there was 'no beast in man, there was only man in man' and that, given favourable and opportune conditions for growth, our innate tendency was towards socially constructive, harmonious living rather than harmful destructive behaviour. In addressing this question, Rogers did not deny 'that I and others have murderous and cruel impulses, desires to hurt, feelings of anger and rage, desires to impose our will on others, but that we also have the capacity to exercise judgement and choice in determining whether these impulses are acted on' (Thorne 1992). Over the years I have encountered many people who have acted in destructive ways towards others – women who have killed their children, men who have raped children, men and women who have inflicted extreme mental and physical harm on others. Sometimes true compassion and remorse has been evident in their stories, stories which inevitably contain a personal history of abuse and violence. But sometimes such contrition is not evident and in such circumstances what I have most noticed in my reaction to those individuals is a profound feeling of sadness. To feel such alienation from others and from one's own humanity that such harm can be perpetrated without remorse is a desperate condition. But I do not see this as evidence for evil at the heart of humankind, more that a person's essential goodness has been crushed. These individuals are people who have never acquired a sense of worth, never been able to experience and value themselves as sentient human beings and as a consequence are devoid of fellow feeling.

The real self

In humanistic psychology a key concept is the 'real self'. This is the authentic centre of our being, the 'I', the core elements that make us uniquely who we are. To talk of the true self is to talk of the emergent self, the self revealed in the continuing process of actualisation. In becoming a person we develop a number of sub-personalities (Rowan 2001) or configurations of the self (Mearns & Thorne 2000), personas which we adopt as a way of dealing with the complexity of life. Many of these configurations of the self are growthful and functional, are ways of being through which the realisation and enhancement of self occurs. Other configurations of the self can be limiting and block the actualising process. It is not difficult to relate to that sense of stuckness and the accompanying emotional discomfort that occurs when our true self or the self we have the potential to become is blocked. Many people who seek help from the psychiatric services are disabled by the dominance of dysfunctional configurations of the self – the 'victim self', the 'persecuted self', the 'inadequate self', the 'dependent self', the 'fearful self', configurations which block self-actualisation and the unfolding of their potential to live well. Therapy in this context is concerned with creating the conditions for growth in which the dysfunctional self is transcended by the emergence of a more vital and resourceful persona which is an expression of the authentic self.

While it is difficult to define the experience of the real self, we all have some sense of who we are behind our masks as we seek to live more transparently and authentically. Rowan (2001), drawing on and adding to Maslow's seminal work, describes the characteristics of a self-actualised person (see Box A1) which I have respectfully adapted in the interest of greater accessibility. Even a cursory glance at these human attributes brings recognition of our own personal quest to express such qualities and values more fully in our lives. They are the very hallmarks of humanity and the prerequisites for harmonious joyful living.

Authenticity

All of us will have experienced what it's like to be with someone who relates in an authentic way. There is a strong sense of their genuineness, their realness. To use a contemporary slogan they 'talk the talk *and* walk the walk'. There is often a comfortableness and confidence about them; they are at peace with themselves and are able to live in a more transparent way. Such individuals are more open, more in touch with how they feel and what they think, and behave in a congruent way. Their personal values are lived out, with these providing an ethical backbone to their everyday lives.

Most of us value authenticity and aspire to be genuine, but to some degree engage in a deception in the way we present ourselves in everyday life; we don our mask to face the world. It is the mask we know best, enabling us to function most effectively within our personal reality, but it is still a mask, and while it may express something of our authentic self it is also a disguise. Sometimes we become so identified with our mask, our false self, that we forget how to be real. Rogers spoke a great deal about congruence in human relations. It was his view that many people, as they grow through childhood and into adulthood, become shallower and lose touch with their 'deeper experiencing'. He argues that in order

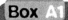

Box A1

Characteristics of the self-actualised person

* Acceptance of self and others
* Autonomy: empowered, resourceful living; being responsible for one's life
* Spontaneity: the freedom to express thought, feeling and action
* Ethical way of being: living congruently with one's deeply held values
* Creativity: evolving creative ways of living and being
* Humility and respect for others as sentient human beings
* Kinship: a deep sense of connection with others and with the ecology of life and a desire to live in harmony with the natural world
* Relationships: capable of relating to others in loving, growth-enhancing ways
* Solitude: a desire for aloneness in which to know oneself and for some to come closer to God is balanced with a desire for communion with others
* Peak experience: a capacity for mystical experience, extra-ordinary states of consciousness
* Humour: a capacity to recognise and laugh at the absurd in the human condition
* Outward looking: energies focused on external projects, often social or humanitarian, not self-absorbed
* Resistance to cultural norms when they are in conflict with being true to oneself
* Life appreciation: a capacity to experience and experience again the joy of living in the everyday elements of life
* Perception of reality: open to the fullness of reality rather than a taking a myopic view
* Resolution of dichotomies: there is a synergy and harmony between thought and feeling; intuition and reason; the feminine and the masculine
* Authenticity: living according to Polonius's edict to Hamlet, 'to thine own self be true'
* Attach importance to means not ends: see life as a journey, or series of journeys, not a destination
* Core values guide a person's walk through life and are a source of authentic happiness; becoming the person they are is a high order value
* Imperfections: perfection belongs only to the gods. Even self-actualised, fully functioning humans have faults and failings

Source Rowan (2001).

to 'receive approval and be loved we suppress those feelings and experiences of ourselves that are deemed unacceptable ... impairing our ability to be congruent, whole and genuine'. All of his work was concerned with the process of 'becoming a person, with discovering, accepting and when appropriate expressing and living the deeper fuller levels of one's being' (Kirschenbaum & Henderson 1990, p. 155).

The congruity of the helper is one of the core conditions for therapeutic growth and change. Without the realness it is difficult for a client to trust the compassionate presence of the practitioner; to believe the positive regard and the empathic reflections are genuine. The congruity of the humanistic practitioner is therefore a prerequisite for therapeutic engagement (Mearns & Thorne 2000).

To become more authentic in the way we practise and live our lives requires a certain fearlessness. It takes courage to face and acknowledge our real self:

> It requires a commitment to ensuring that we do not run away from thoughts, feelings or physical sensations which arouse confusion, excitement, anxiety, or the fear of stumbling on unwelcome discoveries about one's way of being in the world. (Mearns & Thorne, p. 97)

We must know our own minds if we are to become a harmonious whole. This is not a process that occurs automatically, it requires us to be intentional and seek out ways of knowing ourselves more fully. This quest may seem to many readers like self-obsession, but it is in this deep knowing that we find our compassionate selves. I would contend that we all experience and frequently deny those promptings to be something more; to live out our potential. In the Human Potential Movement the quest for authenticity is seen as the right and responsibility of all human beings, a quest that gives meaning to our existence.

Awareness

Of course we cannot help but be aware – it is a condition of being alive. Even in lower levels of consciousness such as sleep there is some awareness of inner and outer stimuli. What we are concerned with here is what happens to our awareness or attention in the process of living. Humanistic psychologists would say that to have our attention free is a condition necessary for authentic living. Often in everyday life our awareness is scattered, held perhaps by some past experience, or perhaps focused on some forthcoming event, with the consequence that awareness of the present is limited. To be fully in the moment, to be aware of what is happening within and around us now, moment to moment, is to be fully alive to the world; fully alive to others; fully alive to ourselves.

The frenetic nature of contemporary life makes it increasingly difficult to live awarely; so much seduces us; so much competes for our attention; we have become slaves to time. As the 'tramp poet' W.H. Davies put it, 'What is this life if, full of care/There is no time to stand and stare'. How then do we live more awarely? Awareness has been central to Buddhist teachings over the centuries and has been taught through meditation practice. Mindfulness is an approach to living popularised in the West by the Vietnamese Buddhist monk Thich Nhat Hanh. In his writings he offers a way to wellbeing through the practice of 'mindful living' (Thich Nhat Hanh 1975). The practice is rooted in the mindfulness of breathing, which with practice expands out into mindfulness of mental functions, of bodily sensations, of other people, of the task we are engaged in and of the world we are living in. He suggests a daily meditation practice of *following the breath* or *counting the breath* and a weekly day of mindfulness. This involves living mindfully from the time we wake and rise in the morning until we retire in the evening. It means that bathing, eating, cleaning, gardening, reading, talking, is carried out unhurriedly, mindfully, with our attention held enraptured by that moment of living. When potentially distracting or disturbing thoughts or feelings come to mind, they are noticed, acknowledged and allowed to pass, which they will if we choose not engage with them. Sustained practice leads to mindfulness as a way of being, enabling us to live more awarely and peacefully in the here and now. It is of interest that psychologists and psychotherapists in the West have in recent years begun to research mindfulness as an approach to treating recurrent depression (Williams et al 2007).

The transpersonal

If humanistic psychology is concerned with the study of human potential, then of course that must include the extra-ordinary, mystic, ecstatic, transcendent states of consciousness that human beings frequently experience. An interest in transcendent states dates back to the beginnings of humanistic psychology and the work of Maslow (1973) on peak experiences. These are moments of intensity triggered by some event in which we become so absorbed that the boundaried self seems to dissolve away and we lose ourselves in the moment. We joyfully become the music; we reverently merge with the landscape; we are blissfully absorbed in a sunset; we are spellbound by a text; we are enraptured by love. Sometimes these egoless moments of intensity can have a spiritual overtone as we sense the presence of the Divine in all things. Other types of transpersonal experience may take the form of voices, visions, a sense of being touched, of being guided, or of being bathed in light, or of an 'angelic presence'. Many people report experiencing unaccountably intense feelings of peace, joy, strength, reverence or wellbeing, often though not always at times of crisis (Hardy 1979, Hay 1990). While these moments may be singular in a person's life they can leave a strong and lasting impression, deepening their connection with the transcendent potential of their own being and opening a window, if only briefly, to another dimension of reality.

It is not difficult to see how these kinds of experiences – what in psychosynthesis counselling would be regarded as the promptings of the 'higher self' – can have a profound effect on how we live our lives and on our sense of wellbeing. It is not difficult to see either how many such experiences get pathologised and labelled psychotic. There is a pressing need for transpersonal psychology to be embraced by psychiatry. Sometimes 'soul work' can be disturbing! Some people are 'called' by unusual states of consciousness, sometimes by persistent and troubling states of depression or anxiety, to make a pilgrimage within in search of a spiritual core to their lives. We do them a profound disservice if we are unable to accompany them gladly on their journey (Barker & Buchanan-Barker 2004).

Humanistic psychology is a positive psychology of being human. It is a liberation psychology, liberation from what Maslow (1968) called 'the psychopathology of the average'. We have a great gift, the gift of humanity, which when fully realised confers on us as a species nobility and virtue. Any psychology that has in its vision of personhood an expanded sense of awareness, authenticity, an empowered sense of being and a capacity for compassion, for joy and the transcendent in life, subverts all that operates within the social sphere of our lives to suppress human potential.

References

Ahern L, Fisher D 2001 Recovery at your own pace. Journal of Psychosocial Nursing and Mental Health Services 39:4

Ahmed T, Webb-Johnson A 1995 Voluntary groups. In: Fernando S (ed) Mental Health in a Multi Ethnic Society. Routledge, London

Ainsworth M 1991 Attachments and other affectional bonds across the life cycle. In: Parkes C, et al (eds) Attachment Across the Life Cycle. Tavistock/Routledge, London

Argyle M 1994 The Psychology of Interpersonal Behaviour. Penguin, London

Arnold L 1995 Women and Self-Injury – A Survey of 76 Women. Bristol Crisis Service for Women

Barham P, Hayward R 1995 Relocating Madness. From the Mental Patient to the Person. Free Association Books, London

Barker P 1999 The Philosophy and Practice of Psychiatric Nursing. Churchill Livingstone, Edinburgh

Barker P, Buchanan-Barker P 2004 Spirituality and Mental Health. Whurr, London

Barker P, Buchanan-Barker P 2005 The Tidal Model. Brunner-Routledge, Hove

Barker P, Reynolds W, Stevenson C 1997 The human science basis of psychiatric nursing, theory and practice. Journal of Advanced Nursing 25:660–667

Barker P, Manos E, Novak V, Reynolds B 1998 The wounded healer and the myth of mental wellbeing: ethical issues concerning the mental health status of psychiatric nurses. In: Barker P, Davidson B (eds) Ethical Strife. Arnold, London

Barker P, Campbell P, Davidson C (eds) 1999 From the Ashes of Experience. Reflections on Madness, Survival and Growth. Whurr, London

Barrowclough C, Tarrier N 1997 Families of Schizophrenic Patients. Cognitive Behavioural Interventions. Stanley Thorne, Cheltenham

Barry K L, Zeber J E, Blow F C, et al 2003 Effects of strengths model versus assertive community treatment of participant outcomes and utilization: two year follow up. Psychiatric Rehabilitation Journal 26(3):268–277

Bebbington P, Kuipers E 1994 The predictive utility of expressed emotion in schizophrenia: an aggregate analysis. Psychological Medicine 21:707–718

Bentall R 1990 Reconstructing Schizophrenia. Routledge, London

Bentall R 2003 Madness Explained. Psychosis and Human Nature. Allen Lane, London

Berke J 2003 The right to be at risk. Lecture given at the Critical Psychiatry Network Conference. London, June 2003

Birchwood M, Tarrier N 1994 Psychological Management of Schizophrenia. Wiley, Chichester

Birchwood M, MacMillan F, Smith J 1994 Early intervention. In: Birchwood M, Tarrier N (eds) Psychological Management of Schizophrenia. Wiley, Chichester

Birchwood M, Todd P, Jackson C 1998 Early intervention in psychosis: the critical hypothesis. British Journal of Psychiatry 172 (Suppl 33):53–59

Birchwood M, Iqbal Z, Chadwick P 2000 Cognitive approaches to depression and suicidal thinking in psychosis. 1: Ontogeny of post psychotic depression. British Journal of Psychiatry 177:512–516

Bird L 1999 The Fundamental Facts. Mental Health Foundation, London

Bly R 1990 Iron John. Element Books, Longmead, Dorset

Bowlby J 1969 Attachment and Loss: Vol. 1 Attachment (2nd edn 1982). Hogarth, London

Bowlby J 1973 Attachment and Loss: Vol. 2 Separation, Anxiety and Anger. Hogarth, London

Bowlby J 1980 Attachment and Loss: Vol. 3 Loss, Sadness and Depression. Hogarth, London

Bowlby J 1988 A Secure Base. Clinical Applications of Attachment Theory. Routledge, London

Bozarth J, Motomasa N 2005 Searching for the core: the interface of client centred principles with other therapies. In: Joseph S, Worsley R (eds) Person Centred Psychopathology. PCCS Books, Ross-on-Wye

Brandon D 1976 Zen in the Art of Helping. Routledge, London

Brandon D 1997 The Trick of Being Ordinary. Anglia Polytechnic University, Cambridge

Brazier D (ed) 1993 Beyond Carl Rogers. Constable, London

Breggin P 1993 Toxic Psychiatry. Harper Collins, London

Breggin P 1996 Spearheading a transformation. In: Breggin P, Stern M (eds) Psychosocial Approaches to Deeply Disturbed Persons. Haworth Press, New York

Breggin P 1997 The Heart of Being Helpful. Springer, New York

Breggin P, Stern M (eds) Psychosocial Approaches to Deeply Disturbed Persons. Haworth Press, New York

Brown D, Pedder J 1991 Introduction to Psychotherapy. An Outline of Psychodynamic Principles in Practice. Routledge, London

Brown G 1996 Life Events, Loss and Depressive Disorders. In: Heller T, et al (eds) Mental Health Matters. Macmillan, Basingstoke

Butterworth T, Faugier J 1992 Clinical Supervision and Mentorship in Nursing. Chapman & Hall, London

Butzlaff R L, Hooey J M 1999 Expressed emotion and psychiatric relapse: a meta analysis. Archives of General Psychiatry 55:547–552

Byng-Hall J 1995 Rewriting Family Scripts. Guilford Press, New York

Campbell P 1996 Working with service users. In: Sandford T, Gourney K (eds) Perspectives in Mental Health Nursing. Baillière Tindall, London

Campbell P 2000 Challenging the loss of power. In: Read J, Reynolds J (eds) Speaking Our Minds: An Anthology. Palgrave Macmillan, Basingstoke

Campbell P, Lindow V 1997 Changing Practice. Mental Health Nursing and User Empowerment. Royal College of Nursing, London

Camus A 1955 The Myth of Sisyphus. Penguin, London

Casement P 1985 On Learning from the Patient. Tavistock Publications, London

Chadwick P K 1997 Schizophrenia: The Positive Perspective. In Search of Dignity for Schizophrenic People. Routledge, London

Chadwick P 2006 Person-based Cognitive Therapy for Distressing Psychosis. Wiley, Chichester

Chadwick P, Birchwood M, Trower P 1996 Cognitive Therapy for Delusions, Voices and Paranoia. Wiley, Chichester

Chamberlin J 1999a Confessions of a non-compliant patient. Newsletter Articles: National Empowerment Centre. Online. Available: http://power2u.org./articals/recovery/confessions.html

Chamberlin J 1999b The medical model and harm. In: Barker P, et al (eds) From the Ashes of Experience. Whurr, London

Charles R 2004 Intuition in Psychotherapy and Counselling. Whurr, London

Chisholm A, Ford R 2004 Transforming Mental Health Care: Assertive Outreach and Crisis Resolution in Practice. Sainsbury Centre for Mental Health, London

Clarkson P 1989 Gestalt Counselling in Action. Sage, London

Clarkson P 1993 On Psychotherapy. Whurr, London

Clarkson P 1995 The Therapeutic Relationship. Whurr, London

Clarkson P 2004 Gestalt Counselling in Action. Sage, London

Clay S 1999 Madness and reality. In: Barker P, et al (eds) From the Ashes of Experience. Whurr, London

Coleman R 1998 Politics of the Madhouse. Handsell Publishing, Runcorn

Coleman R 1999 Recovery an Alien Concept. Handsell Publishing, Gloucester

Copsey N 1997 Keeping Faith. The Provision of Community Mental Health Services Within A Multi Faith Context. Sainsbury Centre for Mental Health, London

Cormack D 1976 Psychiatric Nursing Observed. Royal College of Nursing, London

Dass R, Gorman P 1989 How Can I Help? Rider, London

Davidson B 1998 The role of the psychiatric nurse. In: Barker P, Davidson B (eds) Psychiatric Nursing. Ethical Strife. Arnold, London

Davis A, Wainwright J 1996 Poverty, work and the mental health services. Breakthrough 1(1):47–55

Davis H, Fallowfield L (eds) 1991 Counselling and Communication in Health Care. Wiley, Chichester

Deegan P 1988 Recovery: The lived experience of rehabilitation. Psychosocial Rehabilitation Journal 11:12–19

Deegan P 1992 The independent living movement and people with psychiatric disabilities: taking back control over our own lives. Psychosocial Rehabilitation Journal 15(3):4–19

Deegan P 1996 Recovery as a journey of the heart. Psychiatric Rehabilitation Journal 19:91–97

Deegan P 1997 Recovery and empowerment for people with psychiatric disabilities. Social Work in Health Care 25(3):11–24

De Girolamo G 1996 WHO studies of schizophrenia: an overview of results and their implications for an understanding of the disorder. In: Breggin P, Stern E M (eds) Psychosocial Approaches to Deeply Disturbed Persons. Haworth Press, New York

Department of Health 1994 Working in Partnership. Collaborative Approach to Care. HMSO, London

Department of Health 1999a National Service Framework for Mental Health. Modern Standards and Service Models. HMSO, London

Department of Health 1999b Modernising Mental Health Services – Safe, Sound and Supportive. Department of Health Publications, London

Department of Health 1999c Safer Services: National Confidential Inquiry into Suicide and Homicide by People Who Are Mentally Ill. Department of Health Publications, London

Department of Health 1999d ECT: A Survey Covering the Period from January 1999 in England. Statistical Bulletin. Government Statistical Service, London

Department of Health 2000 Looking Beyond Labels. Widening Employment Opportunities for Disabled People in the NHS. Department of Health Publications, London

Department of Health 2001a The Journey of Recovery: The Government's Vision for Mental Health Care. Department of Health, London

Department of Health 2001b Mental Health Policy Implementation Guide. Department of Health, London

Department of Health 2002a Women's Mental Health. Strategic Development of Mental Health Care for Women. Department of Health Publications, London

Department of Health 2002b Women's Mental Health: Into the Mainstream. Department of Health Publications, London

Department of Health 2002c Developing Services for Carers and Families of People with Mental Illness. Department of Health, London

Department of Health 2005a Delivering Race Equality in Mental Health Care. Department of Health Publications, London

Department of Health 2005b Women's Mental Health: Into the Mainstream. Strategic Development of Mental Health Care for Women. Department of Health Publications, London

Dossey L 2001 Healing Beyond the Body. Medicine and the Infinite Reach of the Mind. Time Warner, London

Dyson J, Cobb M, Forman D 1997 The meaning of spirituality: a literature review. Journal of Advanced Nursing 26:1183–1188

Egan G 1994 The Skilled Helper. A Problem Management Approach to Helping, 5th edn. Brooks Cole, Pacific Grove

Egan G 2006 The Skilled Helper. A Problem Management and Opportunity Development Approach to Helping. Brooks Cole, Pacific Grove

Fadden G, Kuipers L, Bebbington P 1987 The burden of care: the impact of functional psychiatric illness on the patient's family. British Journal of Psychiatry 150:285–292

Falloon I 1992 Early intervention for first episode schizophrenia. British Journal of Psychiatry 31:257–278

Falloon I, Coverdale J, Tannis M, et al 1998 Early intervention for schizophrenic disorders: implementing optimal treatment strategies in routine clinical services. British Journal of Psychiatry (Supplement) 172(33):33–38

Faugier J 1992 The supervisory relationship. In: Butterworth C, Faugier J (eds) Clinical Supervision and Mentorship in Nursing. Chapman & Hall, London

Fernando S 2002 Mental Health, Race and Culture, 2nd edn. Palgrave, Basingstoke

Fisher D 1999 Hope, humanity and voice in recovery from mental illness. In Barker P, et al (eds) From the Ashes of Experience. Whurr, London

Fisher D, Deegan P 1999 Final Report of Research on Recovery from Mental Illness. National Empowerment Centre, Lawrence, MA

Frame L, Morrison A P 2001 Causes of PTSD in psychosis. Archives of General Psychiatry 58:305–307

259

Frankl V 2004 Man's Search for Meaning. Rider, London

Fromm E 1979 To Have or To Be. Sphere Books, London

Fromm E 1993 The Art of Being. Constable, London

Gallop R 1998 Abuse of power in the nurse client relationship. Nursing Standard 12(37):43–47

Gendlin E 1981 Focusing. Bantam Books, London

Gergen K 1990 Therapeutic professionals and the diffusion of deficit. Journal of Mind and Behaviour 11:353–368

Gersie A 1991 Storymaking in Bereavement. Jessica Kingsley, London

Gilbert P 2005 Compassion: Conceptualisation, Research and Use in Psychotherapy. Routledge, London

Gleeson L, Larson T, Mcgorry P 2003 Psychological treatment in pre and early psychosis. Journal of the American Academy of Psychoanalysis 31:229–245

Goodman L, Rosenberg S, Meuser K, Drake R 1997 Physical and sexual assault history in women with serious mental illness: prevalence, correlates, treatment, and future research directions. Schizophrenia Bulletin 23:685–696

Grayley-Wetherell R, Morgan S 2001 Active Outreach: An Independent User Evaluation of a Model of Assertive Outreach. Sainsbury Centre for Mental Health, London

Griffiths P, Leach G 1998 Psychosocial nursing: a model learnt from experience. In: Barnes E, et al (eds) Face to Face with Distress. Butterworth-Heinemann, Oxford

Groves P 1998 Doing and being: a Buddhist perspective on craving and addiction. In: Barker P, Davidson B (eds) Ethical Strife. Arnold, London

Harding S 2006 Animate Earth – Science, Intuition and Gaia. Green Books, Dartington

Hardy A 1979 The Spiritual Nature of Man. Oxford University Press, Oxford

Hargie O, Saunders C, Dickson D 1994 Social Skills in Interpersonal Communication. Routledge, London

Harrison G, Hopper K, Craig J, et al 2001 Recovery from psychotic illness. Journal of Psychiatry 178:506–517

Hawkins P, Shohet R 2000 Supervision in the Helping Professions. Open University Press, Buckingham

Hay D 1990 Religious Experience Today: Studying The Facts. Mowbray, London

Heron J 2001 Helping the Client. A Creative and Practical Guide, 5th edn. Sage, London

Heron J, Reason P 2000 The practice of cooperative enquiry: research 'with' rather than 'on' people. In: Reason P, Bradbury H (eds) Handbook of Action Research. Sage, London

Hill R, Hardy P, Sheppard G 1996 Perspectives on Manic Depression. Sainsbury Centre for Mental Health, London

Hillman J 1995 A psyche the size of the earth: a psychological forward. In: Roszak T, Gomes M E, Kanner A D (eds) Ecopsychology. Sierra Club Books, San Francisco

Hopton J 1997 Towards anti-oppressive practice in mental health nursing. British Journal of Nursing 6(15):874–878

Horsfall J 1997 Psychiatric nursing. Epistemological contradictions. Advances in Nursing Science 20:56–65

Illich I 1977 Limits to Medicine. Penguin, London

Inglesby E 1998 Creating from chaos. In: Barker P, Davidson B (eds) Ethical strife. Arnold, London

Johannesson O 2004 The development of early intervention services. In: Read J, et al (eds) Models of Madness. Brunner-Routledge, Hove

Johns C 1993 Professional supervision. Journal of Nursing Management 1:9–18

Joseph S, Worsley R (eds) 2005 Person Centred Psychopathology. PCCS Books, Ross-on-Wye

Josselson R 1987 Finding Herself: Pathways to Identity Development in Women. Jossey-Bass, London

Kanter J 1985 Case management of the young adult chronic patient: a clinical perspective. New Directions for Mental Health Services 27:77–92

Kavanagh D 1992 Recent developments in expressed emotion and schizophrenia. British Journal of Psychiatry 160:601–620

Kirkpatrick M 2004 The feminization of psychiatry? Some ruminations. Journal of the American Academy of Psychoanalysis 32(1):201–212

Kirschenbaum H, Henderson V (eds) 1990 The Carl Rogers Reader. Constable, London

Knowles M 1991 The Adult Learner: A Neglected Species. Gulf Publishing, London

Kuipers L, Leff J, Lam D 2002 Family Work for Schizophrenia. A Practical Guide, 2nd edn. Gaskell/Royal College of Psychiatrists, London

Lane J 2006 The Spirit of Silence: Making Space for Creativity. Green Books, Dartington

Levitt B E (ed) 2005 Embracing Non-Directivity. Re-assessing Person Centred Theory and Practice in the 21st Century. PCCS Books, Ross-on-Wye

Lidmila A 1992 The way of supervision. Counselling May: 97–100

Link B, Phelan J 2001 Conceptualising stigma. Annual Review of Sociology 27:363–385

Littlewood R, Lipsedge M 1997 Aliens and Alienists. Ethnic Minorities and Psychiatry, 3rd edn. Brunner-Routledge, Hove

Lynch G 1997 Words and silence: counselling and psychotherapy after Wittgenstein. Counselling May: 126–128

McDermott G 1998 Relapse: helping clients to recognise early signs. Mental Health Nursing 18:22–23

MacGabhann L 2000 Are nurses responding to the needs of patents in acute mental health care? Mental Health and Learning Disabilities Care 4(3):85–88

McGowry P, Yung A, Francey S, et al 2002 Randomized controlled trial of interventions designed to reduce the risk of progression to first episode psychosis in a clinical sample with sub-threshold symptoms. Archives of General Psychiatry 59:921–928

McLeod J 1998 The politics of counselling. In: An Introduction to Counselling. Open University Press, Buckingham

Macmin L, Foskett J 2004 'Don't be afraid to tell.' The spiritual and religious experience of mental health service users in Somerset. Mental Health Religion and Culture 7(1):23–40

McNiff J, Whitehead J 2006 All You Need To Know About Action Research. Sage, London

Marks I, Connelly J, Muijen M 1994 Home based versus hospital based care for people with severe mental illness. British Journal of Psychiatry 165:179–194

Maslow A 1968 Towards a Psychology of Being. Van Nostrand, New York

Maslow A 1970 Religions, Values and Peak Experiences. Viking Press, New York

Maslow A 1973 The Farther Reaches of Human Nature. Penguin, New York

Maslow A 1987 Motivation and Personality, 3rd edn. Harper & Row, New York

Masson J 1988 Against Therapy. Fontana, London

May R 2001 Taking a stand. Online. Available: http://www.brad.ac.uk/health/research/cccmh/files/RefusMayonRadio4-TakingaStand.doc

May R 2006 Understanding psychotic experiences and working towards recovery. Online. Available: spiritualrecoveries.bogspot.com

Mearns D, Thorne B 1999 Person Centred Counselling in Action. Sage, London

Mearns D, Thorne B 2000 Person Centred Therapy Today. Sage, London

Mental Health Act Commission 1997 The National Visit: A One Day Visit to 309 Acute Psychiatric Wards. HMSO, London

Mental Health Act Commission 2005 Count Me In Report. Mental Health Act Commission, London

Mental Health Foundation 1997 Knowing Our Own Minds. A Survey of How People in Emotional Distress Take Control of their Lives. Mental Health Foundation, London

Mental Health Foundation 2000 Strategies for Living: A Report of User Led Research into People's Strategies for Living with Mental Distress. Mental Health Foundation, London

Mental Health Foundation 2002 Taken Seriously: The Somerset Spirituality Project. Mental Health Foundation, London

Miller J 2000 Personal consciousness integration: the next phase of recovery. Psychiatric Rehabilitation Journal 23(4):342–352

Minghella E, Ford R, Freeman T, et al 1998 Open All Hours :24 Hour Response to People with Mental Health Emergencies. Sainsbury Centre for Mental Health, London

Moore C 1996 The Re-enchantment of Everyday Life. Hodder & Stoughton, London

Morgan S 1998 Assessing and Managing Risk. Pavilion Publishing, Brighton

Morgan S 2004a Strengths based practice. Open Mind 126 (March/April)

Morgan S 2004b Risk taking. In: Ryan P, Morgan S Assertive Outreach. A Strengths Approach to Policy and Practice. Churchill Livingstone, Edinburgh

Morgan S, Hemming M 1999 Balancing care and control: risk management and compulsory community treatment. Mental Health Care 3:19–21

Morrison A, Frame L, Larkin W 2003 Relationship between trauma and psychosis: A review and integration. British Journal of Clinical Psychology 42:331–353

Mortenson P, Juel K 1993 Mortality and the causes of death in first admitted schizophrenic patients. British Journal of Psychiatry 163:183–189

261

Mosher B, Burti L 1994 Community Mental Health. A Practical Guide. W W Norton, London

Mullen A, Murray L, Happell B 2002 Multiple family group interventions in first episode psychosis: enhancing knowledge and understanding. International Journal of Mental Health Nursing 11:225–232

Museer K, Goodman L, Trubetta S, et al 1998 Trauma and post traumatic stress disorder in severe mental illness. Journal of Consulting and Clinical Psychology 66:493–499

National Institute for Health and Clinical Excellence 2002 Schizophrenia: core interventions in the treatment and management of schizophrenia in primary and secondary care. Online. Available: www.nice.org.uk

National Institute for Mental Health in England 2003 Cases for change: hospital services. Online. Available: www.nimhe.org.uk

National Institute for Mental Health in England 2005 NIMHE Guiding Statement on Recovery. Online. Available: http://www.nimhe.csip.or.uk/home

National Suicide Prevention Strategy for England 2002 Department of Health Publications, London

Nolan P, Crawford P 1997 Towards a rhetoric of spirituality in mental health care. Journal of Advanced Nursing 26:289–294

Norman C 2006 The Fountain House Movement: an alternative rehabilitation model for people with mental health problems: members' description of what works. Scandinavian Journal of Caring Sciences 20:184–192

Office for National Statistics 2000 Labour Force Survey 1998–1999. Office for National Statistics, London

Onyett S 1998 Case Management in Mental Health. Stanley Thorne, Cheltenham

O'Rourke M, Bird L 2001 Risk Management in Mental Health. Mental Health Foundation, London

Payne S 1998 Hit and miss: success and failure of psychiatric services for women. In: Doyle L (ed) Women and Health Services. Open University Press, Buckingham

O'Toole M S, Ohlsen R I, Taylor T M, et al 2004 Treating first episode psychosis – the service user's perspective: focus group evaluation. Journal of Psychiatric and Mental Health Nursing 11:319–326

Peplau H 1988 Interpersonal Relations in Nursing. Macmillan, Basingstoke

Perkins R E 1999 My three psychiatric careers. In: Barker P, Campbell P, Davidson B (eds) From the Ashes of Experience. Whurr, London

Perkins R, Repper J 1996 Working Alongside People With Long Term Mental Health Problems. Chapman & Hall, London

Perry C 1991 Listen To The Voice Within. SPCK, London

Phillips A 1988 Winnicott. Fontana, London

Podvoll E 2003 Recovering Sanity: A Compassionate Approach to Understanding and Treating Psychosis. Shambhala, Boston

Power N, Elkins K, Adlard S, et al 1998 Analysis of the initial treatment phase in first episode psychosis. British Journal of Psychiatry 172(Suppl):71–76

Rapp C A 1998 The Strengths Model: Case Management with People Suffering from Severe and Persistent Mental Illness. Oxford University Press, New York

Read J 2004 Poverty, ethnicity and gender. In: Read J, Mosher L, Bentall R (eds) Models of Madness. Brunner-Routledge, Hove

Read J, Reynolds J 2000 Speaking Our Minds: An Anthology. Palgrave Macmillan, Basingstoke

Redfield Jamison K 1995 The Unquiet Mind: A Memoir of Moods and Madness. Picador, London

Repper J, Perkins R 2003 Social Inclusion and Recovery. A Model for Mental Health Practice. Baillière Tindall, Edinburgh

Roberts G, Wolfson P 2004 The rediscovery of recovery: open to all. Advances in Psychiatric Treatment 10:37–49

Rogers A, Pilgrim D 1994 Service users' views on psychiatric nurses. British Journal of Nursing 3(1):16–18

Rogers C 1967 On Becoming a Person. Constable, London

Rogers C 1970 Encounter Groups. Penguin Books, London

Rogers C 1977 The politics of the helping professions. In: Kirschenbaum H, Henderson V (eds) (1990) The Carl Rogers Reader. Constable, London

Rogers C 1978a Do we need a reality. In: Kirschenbaum H, Henderson V (eds) (1990) The Carl Rogers Reader. Constable, London

Rogers C 1978b On Personal Power. Inner Strength and its Revolutionary Impact. Constable, London

Rogers C 1980 A Way of Being. Houghton Mifflin, Boston

Rogers C 1986a A client centred/person centred approach to therapy. In: Kirschenbaum H, Henderson V (eds) (1990) The Carl Rogers Reader. Constable, London

Rogers C 1986b Reflections on feelings and transference. In: Kirschenbaum H, Henderson V (eds) (1990) The Carl Rogers Reader. Constable, London

Rogers C, Freiberg H J 1994 Freedom to learn, 3rd edn. Merrill, New York

Romme M 1998 Understanding Voices. Coping with Auditory Hallucinations and Confusing Realities. Handsell Publications, Runcorn

Romme M, Escher S 1993 Accepting Voices. MIND Publications, London

Romme M, Escher S 2000 Making Sense of Voices. MIND Publications, London

Roszak T, Gomes M, Kanner Allen D 1995 Ecopsychology. Restoring the Earth, Healing the Mind. Sierra Club Books, San Francisco

Rowan J 2001 Ordinary Ecstasy. The Dialectics of Humanistic Psychology, 3rd edn. Brunner-Routledge, Hove

Ryan P, Morgan S 2004 Assertive Outreach: A Strengths Approach to Policy and Practice. Churchill Livingstone, Edinburgh

Ryan P, Ford R, Clifford P 1991 Case Management and Community Care. Research and Development for Psychiatry, London

Sainsbury Centre 1997 Pulling Together. The Role and Training of Mental Health Staff. Sainsbury Centre for Mental Health, London

Sainsbury Centre 1998a Keys To Engagement. Review of Care for People with Severe Mental Illness Who Are Hard To Engage with Services. Sainsbury Centre for Mental Health, London

Sainsbury Centre 1998b Acute Problems: A Survey of the Quality of Care in Acute Psychiatric Wards. Sainsbury Centre for Mental Health, London

Santa-Maria C 1998 Professional burnout. Breakthrough 2(2):21–31

Sayce L 2000 From Psychiatric Patient to Citizen. Overcoming Discrimination and Social Exclusion. Macmillan, London

Sayce L 2001 Not just service users but contributors to society: the opportunities of the disability rights agenda. Mental Health Review 6:25–28

Schon D 1991 The Reflective Practitioner. Basic Books, London

Schultz W 1973 Elements of Encounter. Joy Press, Big Sur

Schultz W 1989 Joy: 20 Years Later. 10 Speed Press, Berkeley

Schultz W 1993 Elements of Encounter. Joy Press, Big Sur

Seligman M 1975 Helplessness: On Depression, Development and Health. Freeman, San Francisco

Seligman M 2002 Authentic Happiness. Free Press, New York

Senior P, Croal J 1993 Helping to Heal. The Arts in Health Care. Calouste Gulbenkian Foundation, London

Shaw J 2006 Down and Out in London. Amnesty International, London

Shaw K, McFarlane A, Bookless C, Air T 2002 The aetiology of post-psychotic post-traumatic stress disorder following a psychotic episode. Journal of Traumatic Stress 15:39–47

Sheehy G 1997 New Passages. Predictable Crises of Adult Life. Harper Collins, London

Sheppard M 1993 Client satisfaction, extended intervention and interpersonal skills in community mental health. Journal of Advanced Nursing 18:246–259

Smail D 1998 Taking Care. An Alternative to Therapy. Constable, London

Smail D 1999 Origins of Unhappiness: A New Understanding of Personal Distress. Constable, London

Smith P 1992 The Emotional Labour of Nursing. Macmillan Education, Basingstoke

Sommerbeck L 2005 An evaluation of research, concepts and experiences pertaining to the universality of CCT and its applications in psychiatric settings. In: Joseph S, Worsley R (eds) Person Centred Psychopathology. PCCS Books, Ross-on-Wye

Storr A 1988 Solitude. Flamingo/Harper Collins, London

Strathdee G, Thompson K, Carr S 1997 What service users want from mental health services. In: Thompson K, et al (eds) Mental Health Service Development Skills Workbook. Sainsbury Centre for Mental Health, London

Sullivan H S 1953 The Interpersonal Theory of Psychiatry. W W Norton, New York

Tait L, Birchwood M, Trower P 2003 Predicting engagement with services for psychosis: insight, symptoms and recovery style. British Journal of Psychiatry 182:123–128

Tarrier N, Beckett R, Harwood S, et al 1993 A trial of two cognitive behavioural methods of treatment of drug resistant psychotic symptoms in schizophrenic patients: outcomes. British Journal of Psychiatry 162:524–532

263

Tatton T, Tarrier N 2000 The expressed emotion of case managers of the seriously mentally ill. Psychological Medicine 30:195–204

Teall W 2003 The Start model: a profile of using art as a tool in recovery. Online. Available: http://www.startmc.org.uk

Teall W, Tortora A, Cunningham J 2005 Getting to know Alfred Wallis part 2. Online: Available: artsednews.squarespace.com/storage/Getting-to-know-wallis-pt-22.pdf

Thich Nhat Hanh 1975 The Miracle of Mindfulness. Rider, London

Thomas B 1997 Management strategies to tackle stress in mental health nursing. Mental Health Care 1:15–17

Thomas P, Bracken P 2004 Critical psychiatry in practice. Advances in Psychiatric Treatment 10:361–370

Thorne B 1992 Carl Rogers. Sage, London

UKCC 1998 Guidelines for Mental Health and Learning Disability Nursing. United Kingdom Central Council for Nursing Midwifery and Health Visiting, London

UKCC 1999 Practitioner–Client Relationships and the Prevention of Abuse. United Kingdom Central Council for Nursing Midwifery and Health Visiting, London

Watkins C 1989 Transference phenomena in counselling situations. In: Dryden W (ed) Key Issues for Counselling in Action. Sage, London

Watkins P N 1995 Dramatherapy in the Education of Mental Health Professionals. Dissertation, University of Nottingham

Watkins P N 2007 Recovery in Mental Health. Elsevier Science, Oxford

White M 1987 Family Therapy and Schizophrenia. Addressing the 'in the Corner' Lifestyle. Dulwich Centre Newsletter (Dulwich Centre Publications), Spring

White M 1997 Narratives of Therapists' Lives. Dulwich Centre Publications, Adelaide

White M, Epston D 1990 Narrative Means to Therapeutic Ends. W W Norton, London

Whitmore D 2004 Psychosynthesis Counselling in Action. Sage, London

Wilkins P 2005 Assessment and diagnosis in person centred therapy. In: Joseph S, Worsley R (eds) Person Centred Psychopathology. PCCS Books, Ross-on-Wye

Williams J, Watson G 1996 Mental health that empowers women. In: Heller T, et al (eds) Mental Health Matters. Macmillan, Basingstoke

Williams M, Teasdale J, Segal Z, Kabat-Zinn J 2007 The Mindful Way through Depression: Freeing Yourself from Chronic Unhappiness. Guilford Press, New York

Winship G 1995 The unconscious impact of caring for acutely disturbed patients: a perspective for supervision. Journal of Psychiatric and Mental Health Nursing 2:227–231

Worsley R 2005 The concept of evil as a key to the therapist use of self. In: Person Centred Psychopathology: A Positive Psychology of Mental Health. PCCS Books, Ross-on-Wye

Zubin J, Spring B 1977 Vulnerability – a new view of schizophrenia. Journal of Abnormal Psychology 86:103–126

Index

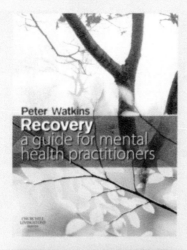
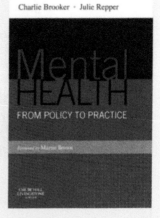
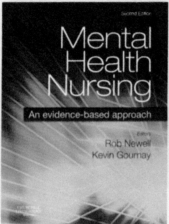
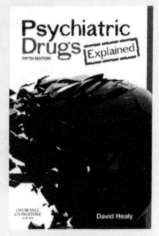

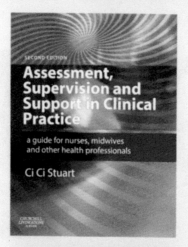

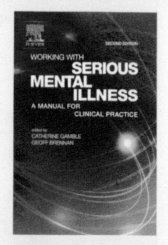

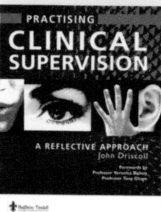

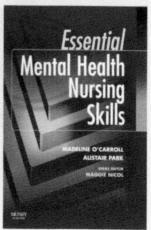

You can order these, or any other Elsevier title (Churchill Livingstone, Saunders, Mosby, Baillière Tindall, Butterworth-Heinemann), from your local bookshop, or, in case of difficulty, direct from us on:

EUROPE, MIDDLE EAST & AFRICA
Tel: +44 (0) 1865 474000
www.elsevierhealth.com

CANADA
Tel: +1 866 276 5533
www.elsevier.ca

AUSTRALIA
Tel: +61 (0) 2 9517 8999
www.elsevierhealth.com

USA
Tel: +1 800 545 2522
www.us.elsevierhealth.com

ELSEVIER

Printed and bound by CPI Group (UK) Ltd, Croydon, CR0 4YY

03/10/2024

01040349-0014